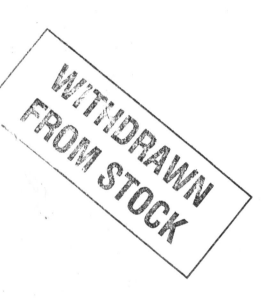

CELLULAR AND MOLECULAR
RENEWAL IN THE MAMMALIAN BODY

CELL BIOLOGY: A Series of Monographs

EDITORS

D. E. BUETOW

*Department of Physiology
and Biophysics
University of Illinois
Urbana, Illinois*

I. L. CAMERON

*Department of Anatomy
University of Texas
Medical School at San Antonio
San Antonio, Texas*

G. M. PADILLA

*Department of Physiology and Pharmacology
Duke University Medical Center
Durham, North Carolina*

G. M. Padilla, G. L. Whitson, and I. L. Cameron (editors). THE CELL CYCLE:
Gene-Enzyme Interactions, 1969

A. M. Zimmerman (editor). HIGH PRESSURE EFFECTS ON CELLULAR
PROCESSES, 1970

I. L. Cameron and J. D. Thrasher (editors). CELLULAR AND MOLECULAR
RENEWAL IN THE MAMMALIAN BODY, 1971

I. L. Cameron, G. M. Padilla, and A. M. Zimmerman (editors). DEVELOPMENTAL
ASPECTS OF THE CELL CYCLE, 1971

P. F. Smith. THE BIOLOGY OF MYCOPLASMAS, in preparation

Cellular and Molecular Renewal in the Mammalian Body

EDITED BY

IVAN L. CAMERON

DEPARTMENT OF ANATOMY
THE UNIVERSITY OF TEXAS
MEDICAL SCHOOL AT SAN ANTONIO
SAN ANTONIO, TEXAS

AND

JACK D. THRASHER

DEPARTMENT OF ANATOMY
SCHOOL OF MEDICINE
UNIVERSITY OF CALIFORNIA AT LOS ANGELES
LOS ANGELES, CALIFORNIA

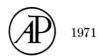 1971

ACADEMIC PRESS   New York and London

ACADEMIC PRESS, INC.
111 Fifth Avenue, New York, New York 10003

United Kingdom Edition published by
ACADEMIC PRESS, INC. (LONDON) LTD.
Berkeley Square House, London W1X 6BA

LIBRARY OF CONGRESS CATALOG CARD NUMBER: 76-137622

PRINTED IN THE UNITED STATES OF AMERICA

CONTENTS

List of Contributors   xi
Preface   xiii

1. Approaches to the Study of Molecular and Cellular Renewal

David J. Lehmiller

I. Introduction   1
II. Cell Populations and Renewal   2
III. Subcellular Renewal   16
References   21

2. The Metabolic Stability of Nuclear DNA

Erle K. Adrian, Jr.

I. Introduction   25
II. DNA Constancy   26
III. DNA Stability   35
IV. Conclusions   37
References   38

3. Cell Proliferation and Renewal in the Mammalian Body

Ivan L. Cameron

I. Introduction   45
II. Cell Proliferation and Growth during the Embryonic and Postnatal
Periods   46

  III. Methods Used to Visualize and to Measure Cell Proliferation and
        Cell Renewal 48
  IV. Classification of Cell Populations Based on Their Proliferative
        Behavior 64
    V. Regulation of Cell Proliferation 74
      References 79

4. Cellular Content and Cellular Proliferation Changes in the Tissues and Organs of the Aging Mammal

D. E. Buetow

     I. Introduction 87
    II. Changes in Numbers of Cells and Nerve Fibers 88
  III. Changes in Mitotic Rates 97
  IV. Changes in Mucosal Cells of the Intestine 97
    V. Discussion 101
      References 104

5. RNA Molecules in Cells and Tissues, *in Vivo* and *in Vitro*

Jack D. Thrasher

     I. Introduction 108
    II. Intracellular Sites of RNA Synthesis 108
  III. Nuclear Sites of RNA Synthesis 112
  IV. The Biosynthesis of RNA Molecules 113
    V. Nucleic Acids of Mitochondria 124
  VI. RNA Synthesis in Special Cell Systems 129
  VII. RNA Synthesis over the Cell Cycle 139
      References 142

6. Turnover of Intracellular Proteins

Jack D. Thrasher

     I. Introduction 153
    II. Proteins of the Nucleus 155
  III. Turnover of Proteins in Cytoplasmic Systems 169
  IV. Proteins and the Cell Cycle 178
    V. Protein Metabolism in Special Cell Systems 184
      References 205

7. The Dynamics of Extracellular and Cell Surface Protein Interactions

Harold C. Slavkin

I.	Introduction	221
II.	Epigenetic Controls Regulating Differentiation: The Problem	223
III.	Outer Cell Surface Properties and Their Role in the Formation of Metazoan Systems	228
IV.	Epithelial–Mesenchymal Interactions	239
V.	The Extracellular Matrix Influences upon Cellular Differentiation	248
	References	267

8. Synthesis, Localization, and Renewal of Lipids in Mammalian Tissues

Sandra Sabatini-Smith

I.	Introduction	277
II.	Fatty Acids and Triglycerides	279
III.	Cholesterol	293
IV.	Sphingolipids	302
V.	Phospholipids	305
VI.	Brown Adipose Tissue	317
VII.	Summary	321
	References	321

9. Localization, Identification, and Renewal of Carbohydrates in Tissues and Cells

T. John Leppi

I.	Introduction	331
II.	Histochemistry of Mucins	334
III.	Histochemistry of Polysaccharides	353
	References	366

10. Calcification

George W. Bernard

Text	373
References	378

AUTHOR INDEX	381
SUBJECT INDEX	401

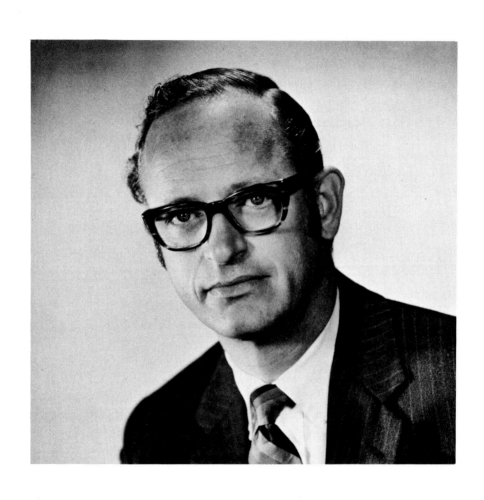

This book is dedicated to

Professor Richard Curtis Greulich

who has taught us and continues to teach others
the excitement of visualizing
the dynamic nature of body constituents.

LIST OF CONTRIBUTORS

Numbers in parentheses indicate the pages on which the authors' contributions begin.

ERLE K. ADRIAN, JR. (25), Department of Anatomy, The University of Texas Medical School at San Antonio, San Antonio, Texas

GEORGE W. BERNARD (373), Department of Oral Biology, School of Dentistry, and Department of Anatomy, School of Medicine, University of California at Los Angeles, Los Angeles, California

D. E. BUETOW (87), Department of Physiology and Biophysics, University of Illinois, Urbana, Illinois

IVAN L. CAMERON (45), Department of Anatomy, The University of Texas Medical School at San Antonio, San Antonio, Texas

DAVID J. LEHMILLER (1), Department of Anatomy, The University of Texas Medical School at San Antonio, San Antonio, Texas

T. JOHN LEPPI (331), Department of Anatomy, The University of New Mexico School of Medicine, Albuquerque, New Mexico

SANDRA SABATINI-SMITH (277), Department of Pharmacology, University of Texas Medical School at San Antonio, San Antonio, Texas

HAROLD C. SLAVKIN (221), Department of Biochemistry, School of Dentistry, and The Graduate Program in Cellular and Molecular Biology, University of Southern California, Los Angeles, California

JACK D. THRASHER (107, 153), Department of Anatomy, School of Medicine, University of California at Los Angeles, Los Angeles, California

PREFACE

This book concerns the dynamic nature of body constituents at the molecular, the organelle, and cellular level of structural organization. Information dealing with cellular and molecular renewal is scattered throughout the literature in a fragmentary manner. It is the intent of this book to bring together much of this information into concise, individual chapters, each of which deals with one of the body's major macromolecular classes, i.e., DNA, RNA, proteins, lipids, and carbohydrates, or with calcification, cell proliferation, cell renewal, and cell loss. The contributors have attempted to concentrate the mass of information into what they consider the essential elements. The use of figures, diagrams, and tables as a means of presenting the information in as concise a manner as possible has been encouraged. Visualization of the renewal process by means of radioautography has been a key part of several of the chapters. However, other methods and approaches have not been ignored, and are included to give as complete a picture of the subject as possible.

Not since the publication of "The Dynamic State of Body Constituents" in 1942 by Rudolph Schoenheimer has an attempt been made to cover this subject in a single volume. The work and concepts reported in Schoenheimer's book arose from the introduction of biological precursor molecules which were labeled with stable isotopes such as deuterium and heavy hydrogen. Since that time, biological precursor molecules labeled with radioactive isotopes have been introduced along with numerous other technological advances which now enable us to fractionate the constituents of the body and to measure the radioactivity incorporated into the fractions. The ability to visualize and localize radioactive molecules at the molecular and ultrastructural level has advanced tremendously. Thus the new techniques and findings now lead us to an ever expanding and refined concept of the dynamic nature of cells and molecules in the mammalian body.

We hope that this volume will provide a stimulus for students and investigators to become aware of the dynamic nature of body constituents and that it will influence their analysis and experimentation of normal, disease, and repair processes within the body. This book should, therefore, not only appeal to those interested in the basic biological processes which operate in the body but to those concerned with the application of this new and dynamic information as it relates to the applied sciences as well.

IVAN L. CAMERON
JACK D. THRASHER

CHAPTER 1

Approaches to the Study of Molecular and Cellular Renewal

David J. Lehmiller

I.	Introduction	1
II.	Cell Populations and Renewal	2
	A. The Cell Cycle	2
	B. Factors Affecting the Cell Cycle	3
	C. Cell Populations	7
	D. Methods for Studying Cell Renewal	9
III.	Subcellular Renewal	16
	A. General Considerations	16
	B. Organelles	18
	C. Macromolecules	19
	D. Minerals, Electrolytes, and Water	21
	References	21

I. Introduction

The purpose of this chapter is to outline the available techniques for studying cellular and molecular renewal. Depending upon individual application, the concept of renewing can be interpreted with a variety of meanings such as replacing, repeating, restoring, or regenerating. Whatever its intended use may be, renewal always indicates a dynamic quality. In a broad sense renewal implies proliferative activity when discussing cell populations and the concept of turnover when applied to the molecular level.

Factors such as accessibility, function, and stability have made the investigation of certain cell types and molecules more feasible and practical than others. A number of different methods have evolved for approaching the dynamic nature of renewal, although each has inherent restrictions

1

which often limit application to special cell and molecule situations. It may well be that by concentrating in certain areas of renewal, the existing techniques have clouded out other possible approaches to uncovering additional knowledge. The reader should bear in mind that some assumptions are always made in a given scientific experiment, and for every successful endeavor expounded, there are criticisms and suggestions that a better method could be devised.

II. Cell Populations and Renewal

A. THE CELL CYCLE

As a practical consideration, cell proliferation is best identified with the phenomenon of mitosis. However, mitosis is actually a discrete event in which one cell divides into two daughter cells. Cell proliferation encompasses the overall dynamics of a cell in passing from its initial resting state through the entire division procedure, including its interaction with the remaining cell population. It is therefore better equated with the mitotic activity at a given time within a tissue. A cell must pass through a series of synthetic steps before it can replicate, and it is equally proper to relate proliferation to activity levels in stages other than mitosis. The chain of events which a cell passes through while proceeding toward division has been termed the cell cycle. Measurements on the time duration of the cell cycle in germinal cells yield objective values of proliferation and renewal.

Howard and Pelc (1953) have partitioned the cell cycle into four separate time periods: the pre-DNA synthetic stage (G_1), the period of DNA replication (S), the post-DNA synthetic and premitotic phase (G_2), and actual mitosis (M). This scheme is very practical since it is structured around two very specific markers in the cell cycle; these are mitosis, which is readily detected visually, and the finite replication time of DNA, which can easily be monitored by administering radioactive DNA percursors. The assumption is made that cells retaining germinal properties reenter the G_1 phase following mitosis. In normal mammalian cell populations, the duration of the S, G_2, and M periods is relatively constant, while it is in the G_1 period that most of the time variations in the overall cell cycle between different tissues occurs (Baserga, 1965; and see Chapter 3). There is some question as to whether or not all cell populations with germinating capacity are normally undergoing proliferation at all times. In the case of the liver, it appears that mitotic activity is virtually nonexistent in the adult unless specific perturbations are introduced. This has resulted in a modification of the Howard and Pelc model in which a resting stage (G_0) is incorporated (Patt and Quastler, 1963). This period, during which potential germinal cells may lie dormant for extended time intervals, is defined as being distinct from G_1. It is mentioned that several investigators have recently postulated the existence of a resting period which cells may temporarily enter from the G_2 period (Epifanova and Terskikh, 1969). Bullough (1965) defines the cell cycle in a different fashion from Howard and Pelc (1953), but there are many similar overtones.

The analysis of dissecting out the phases of the cell cycle is referred to as cell kinetics, and it has become an elaborate subspecialty within the realm of cell proliferation. Current investigators have begun to dwell on the sequence and timing of the actual biosynthetic events which occur within the dividing cell (Baserga, 1968; Petersen et al., 1969). It is only a question of time before more markers are discovered and the cell cycle defined in more precise biochemical events. Of course it is anticipated that eventually the cycle will be describable in terms of gene–RNA–enzyme interactions. In general, such specialization becomes quite cumbersome to apply to multicellular mammalian tissues in which one is desirous of knowing the cell proliferation patterns. This chapter will therefore attempt to relate those associations which have direct application in an experimental approach to measure cell proliferation within an *in vivo* mammalian tissue.

B. Factors Affecting the Cell Cycle

In analyzing cell renewal within a selected tissue, the scientist is desirous of making determinations on either a normal state or an abnormal situation. An inherent difficulty arises in controlling a multitude of factors which can potentially alter the dynamics of the cell cycle. Not having an awareness of all variables and their respective influence could obviously have detrimental effects on the final conclusions. It may not be a simple procedure to identify or establish normal conditions on a meaningful basis, and the maintenance of normalcy during the experiment may be a monumental undertaking. The proper design of the experiment is not only necessary from the investigator's viewpoint, but it is equally important that the readers among the scientific community also recognize important experimental variables so that their acceptance is through critical scrutiny and not blind faith. Listed below are some of the major factors that should be considered in selecting experimental approaches to cell proliferation *in vivo* (Fig. 1 summarizes several of the factors which control cell proliferation).

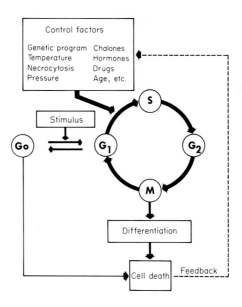

FIG. 1. Factors which control the cell cycle and the regulation of cell proliferation (see text for details).

1. *Anesthetics*

When animals are transferred from the cage to the experiment or are placed in restrainers by personnel, it is a common procedure to use local and/or systemic anesthetics and tranquilizers. The application of these pharmacological agents has been found to have an inhibitory effect upon mitotic activity. The duration and degree of inhibition is dependent upon the choice of drug, the dosage, and the method of administration. The corneal epithelium has been extensively studied in this respect (Buschke *et al.*, 1943; Buschke, 1949).

2. *Temperature*

Watanabe and Okada (1967) found that lowering the ambient temperature from 37° to 31°C prolonged the overall generation time in tissue-cultured mammalian cells by 2.4 times, with the G_1 and S stages of the cell cycle exhibiting the greatest changes. In investigating *in vivo* proliferation, it should be expected that temperature would be an influential parameter in studies where body metabolism is lowered, in epidermal tissues, and when internal organs are exposed. Comparisons between renewal activity in remote tissues like the eye or ear to other regions of higher body temperature are not in order.

3. Age

Intuition tells us that it would not be proper to correlate cell renewal in a newborn mammal to a mature and aging adult. Strehler (1962) has studied aging and demonstrated that many reasons (see Chapters 3 and 4) may exist to explain the decreasing ability of cells to divide and differentiate as age increases. Some hypotheses that are noteworthy are (1) the inability of germinal cells to repair internal damage from effects such as radiation, and (2) the accumulation of harmful metabolic side products in germinal cells over a long period of time.

4. Nutrition

Blumenthal (1950) found that there was a general suppression of mitotic activity during periods of starvation. Unfortunately, many experimental animals, particularly those which receive anesthetics, have their food trays removed many hours prior to the experiment. This is done to eliminate regurgitation problems and potential aspiration. Consequential effects on the cell cycle are intimately related to time duration, depletion of liver glycogen, and endocrine interplay.

5. Stress

When conducting an experiment, test animals are frequently exposed to stressful situations such as handling, isolation, restraints, injections, and physical trauma. Such conditions must at least temporarily alter the normal functioning of the animals' autonomic and endocrine systems. Cameron (1968) showed that just confining mice to small cylindrical holes lowered mitotic activity.

6. Diurnal Variation

This phenomenon has been widely recorded by many investigators. Most observations conclude that cell proliferation is lowest during the waking hours and maximal during rest (Bullough and Laurence, 1961; Vasama and Vasama, 1958). The cause is difficult to determine owing to the multiple interplay of body metabolism and endocrine function. Bullough and Laurence (1961) feel that body activity effects on circulating epinephrine levels is the major factor. The variations in mitotic activity are significant, and repetitive time tables to standardize such effects are a necessity when daily experimentation is performed.

7. Hormones

The relationships of circulating hormones to cell proliferation are complex and not well understood. It is probably a reasonable assumption to state that hormones do not initiate new reactions within cells but only influence existing ones. The presence or absence of a given hormone can stimulate long-lasting, sizable responses on mitotic activity or may only induce a short-acting minor change. Antagonistic or counterbalancing effects on mitotic rate also exist between hormones; an example of this was demonstrated in the case of testosterone and thyroxin (Eartly *et al.*, 1951). The actions of hormones on cell proliferation are indirectly implied to some degree in each of the above-listed conditional factors. However, it additionally becomes necessary in the experimental plan to consider the sex of the test animals, the state of reproductive cycles, the maturity and functioning of all endocrine systems, and the possible upsetting of hormonal control and balance by impingement of the experimental procedure.

8. Tissue Autoregulators

Several ideas have been proposed to explain the partial autoregulation by the individual body tissues. A degree of tissue independence from external factors is apparent in the attainment of the final thickness and size of given cellular layers. One prominent hypothesis is the chalone theory postulated by Bullough (1965). Chalones are tissue-specific mitotic inhibitors elaborated by the tissue cells which are said to control growth. Whenever the concentration of the chalone locally falls below a certain level, the germinal cells are enticed to proliferate to bring the cell population back to normal. If too many cells are present, the chalone concentration is higher than normal and mitotic activity is depressed. Teir *et al.* (1967) state that the breakdown products of cellular necrobiosis may influence the equilibrium between cell production and elimination. Indeed, abnormal proliferation responses are seen in damaged tissues. However, both of these concepts may be explained solely on the basis of the physiology established by a given cell population density in relation to its environment (Lehmiller, 1970). It should be apparent that any experiment which alters the number of viable cells or isolates a small tissue section for observation will create alterations in the normal proliferation patterns (see Chapter 3 for additional discussion of this subject).

9. Toxic Effects

Any foreign chemical compound administered to test animals should be viewed with caution. Metabolic poisons, enzyme inhibitors, and other physiological manifestation are all too commonly used without regard to their proliferative effects.

What happens after mitosis? A single daughter cell may retain germinal properties, undergo differentiation while still retaining germinal potential, or undergo irreversible differentiation and relinquish any proliferation function. The importance of this question is exceedingly dependent upon the type of cell population under investigation. The future of the two daughter cells arising from a parent mitosis has an entirely different significance in embryonic tissue than in steady-state renewing tissue in the adult. Inherent in this consideration is genetic programing, but other factors must be present to regulate the organization, growth, and maintenance of each tissue within the entire body at the cellular level. Leblond (1964) studied the stratified squamous epithelium of the esophagus and concluded that the fate of each daughter cell was largely determined by local environment; he particularly cited intercellular pressure. Extracellular environmental influences are undoubtedly important controllers and regulators, but certainly intracellular changes must also occur.

C. CELL POPULATIONS

Mammalian cells are normally classified into groups or tissues through a combination of knowledge on embryonic origin, physiological function, and morphological identification. In most cases an organ contains both a characteristic cell type, such as the parenchymal cell of the liver, as well as supporting cell populations, such as blood vessels, connective tissue, and nerve cells. The liver cannot therefore be considered a homogeneous cell population. Even the organization of the liver is described in different ways by people from different disciplines. For example, liver parenchymal cells are obviously scrutinized through different eyes: by the anatomist who describe the organization of the liver in terms of lobules, by the pathologist who is concerned with the functional unit (the acinus) (see Chapters 6 and 7), and by the biochemist or physiologist who may not be concerned with the detailed structural organization of the liver. The cell populations comprising a group may then be further subdivided on a basis of cytological differences or enzymatic activity. Thus, even when one is careful to define the exact cell population he is concerned with, he is usually defining the average cell and should be aware that the real cells in the population demonstrate variability around this average cell.

The assessment of cell proliferation as applied to mammalian tissues also has relevance with respect to a "mean." There is no evidence to indicate that germinating cells within a selected tissue proliferate in an identical temporal manner. Each cell in a sense established its own cell cycle consistent with its genetic components and the local physiological conditions. The questionable fate of daughter cells following mitosis was previously mentioned. Final conclusions are necessarily average measurements, and the homogeneity existing within the respective tissue should be assessed to indicate the true value of the results.

A wide variation in proliferative behavior exists among the numerous tissues within the mammalian body (see Chapter 3 for specific examples). The differences are such that separate technical approaches must be employed to secure adequate measurements on all of the populations. Thus, no single approach can give the information needed to classify all of the cell populations on the basis of their proliferative behavior. The following general classification scheme is presented to illustrate the different types of cell proliferative patterns that are encountered within the bodies many tissues.

1. *Steady-State Tissues*

The total cell population in this case is assumed to remain constant, and the rate of cell loss is offset by a corresponding rate of cell production. Steady-state populations are very convenient to examine for proliferation characteristics and this tends to foster hypothetical and idealized situations that are often not warranted. Classic examples of this tissue category are the epidermis and the epithelial lining of the alimentary tract. Structurally these tissues can be described with a germinal layer, a transitional or differentiation region, and a layer of cell death and sloughing from the surface.

2. *Tissues during Embryonic and Hyperplastic Growth*

These states are characterized by an absolute increase in the total cell population. Cell production exceeds cell death, although demonstration of cell death can be difficult to evaluate or detect in many tissues during this time. Rat embryos have been shown to have an exponential increase in total body cells almost up to the time of birth before a gradual decrease occurred in the proliferation rate (Enesco and Leblond, 1962).

3. *Very Slow and Nonrenewing Tissues*

Tissues in this category are relatively stagnant or inert with respect to cell proliferation. The level of mitotic activity that is present in some adult tissues like the adrenal medulla is slight, and it is a vague matter to assign this proliferation to steady-state or growth systems. Other tissues like adult skeletal muscle evidently do not display mitotic activity except under very unusual circumstances. Neurons are devoid of proliferative capacity.

4. Decaying Tissues

The total number of cells in these tissues is decreasing with time. This may be a gradual phenomenon seen in old age where cell death exceeds cell production, or it may occur when there is a decline in a fixed cell population owing to a diseased state. The thymus during development and the ovary during reproductive years are other examples.

5. Tissues with Transient Response Characteristics

Certain circumstances may transform tissues with steady-state or very slow renewing rates into transient supralevels of proliferation. There are several types.

a. Replenishment of Depletion. Bone marrow stimulation by the humoral factor erythropoietin can trigger the release of many stem cells to undergo proliferation and differentiation (Lajtha, 1967). Acute blood losses of great magnitude can be rapidly replaced through the effects of this control factor.

b. Immunological System. Peripheral circulating lymphocytes are actively stimulated in response to processed antigen to undergo proliferation and produce antibody-forming cells (Craddock et al., 1967).

c. Wound Repair. Connective tissue elements and epithelial cells exhibit very marked and exaggerated proliferative activity in response to penetrating wounds (Lehmiller, 1970; McMinn, 1969). Mitotic indices can be observed which are many times higher than normal levels.

6. Neoplastic Tissues

The abnormal cells comprising a tumor generally display proliferative activity that is quite independent and self-determined. Spectra of growth rates are present for both benign and malignant neoplasms, and outside factors such as hormones and the immunological responses can be implicated as contributing to growth potential in some instances.

D. METHODS FOR STUDYING CELL RENEWAL

The gross morphology of an organ or tissue can supply some indication of proliferative activity. Simple measurements on size, weight, and rate of growth can yield clues as well as subjective observations on damage repair or disease response. Techniques providing more precise information on a given cell population necessitate an analysis at the cellular level. Usually a single technique can only extract one element of data about the cell cycle, and the final determination of cell proliferation in a tissue requires the knowledge obtained from several methods before the cell cycle can be adequately described. It should be readily appreciated that most tissues are comprised of vast numbers of cells, and the application of any technique must make extensive use of extrapolation.

1. *Cell Counting*

If the total cell population can be counted, then cell proliferation can be evaluated by monitoring variations in the total count with time. This approach is quite limited since few mammalian cell populations can be practically subjected to a total count. Red blood cells can be directly counted with a hemocytometer or electronically with a Coulter cell counter (Mattern *et al.*, 1957). Frequently the Coulter cell counter is used to count suspensions of tissue culture cells, and additionally it may provide information on cell size (Harris, 1959). The rate of entry of new cells into the total cell population or the rate of removal of existing ones can also indicate levels of cell proliferation. The life span of red blood cells can be determined by tagging them with radioactive markers and then following the rate of disappearance of radioactivity from the circulation after injection (Shemen and Rittenberg, 1946).

2. *Counting Mitotic Figures*

The ratio of cells in a tissue that are undergoing mitosis to the total number of cells capable of dividing is called the mitotic index. This is a useful parameter for comparing proliferative activity, and it can be a direct measure of cell renewal if the time duration of the mitotic phase of the cell cycle can be learned. The mitotic rate can be calculated by dividing the mitotic index by the time interval required for mitosis. Usually the time for passage through the mitotic phase is estimated, but there are significant tissue differences in this regard.

This method finds its widest application in those tissues where cell turnover is relatively quick and a high level of mitotic activity is present, such as the alimentary epithelium and the hemopoietic system. The presence of mitotic figures in even a moderately active proliferative tissue like the corneal epithelium is so sparse that the tedious task of visually counting thousands of cells under the microscope must be done each time to attain reliable statistics (Buschke *et al.*, 1943). As tissue mitotic activity decreases, the collection of a greater number of cell counts is required, and this may magnify the significance of a potential source of error in this procedure. It is often difficult to recognize the early prophase stage of mitosis from artifact of tissue preparation, and this makes the final results dependent to some degree upon the subjectiveness of the individual observer.

3. x-Rays

A spectrum of changes can be associated with x-irradiation of living cells. There may be destruction of enzymatic systems and membranes or disruption of DNA–RNA functioning leading to cell death. On the other hand, some portion of the mitotic process may be slightly altered, resulting in a longer cell cycle or possibly abnormal progeny. These results are very much dose related, but there is also a cell population dependence. In man, bone marrow supression can occur at doses well below 300 rads, while CNS effects may not be evident until levels exceeding 6000 rads are used.

x-Ray doses greater than 300 rads interfere with the synthesis of DNA in human bone marrow cultures. This effect on the S period is not seen between 200 and 300 rads, but there are substantial alterations in the G_1 period and approximately 50% of these cells are not seen to enter the S phase (Lajtha *et al.*, 1958). Sublethal doses of x-irradiation have been found which cause a temporary block late in the G_2 period in HeLa cells, but have no observable effects on either the DNA synthetic period or the postmitotic period (Yamada and Puck, 1961). At the lowest dose studied of 9 rads on HeLa cells, Puck and Steffen (1963) observed that x-irradiation produced a definite delay in the entrance of G_2 cells into mitosis.

If proliferating cells can be selectively blocked in the G_2 period by x-rays, then those cells which had just entered the mitotic phase would continue to divide and a time-cell gap would temporarily appear in the cycle. By measuring the rate of disappearance of mitotic figures after x-irradiation, the acutal time for mitosis can be derived. Knowlton and Widner (1950) did this for seven different *in vivo* mouse tissues, and since they jointly recorded mitotic index data from control mice, they could determine actual proliferation data about the tissues (mitotic rate = mitotic index ÷ mitotic time).

This technique is subjected to quite a bit of criticism. The question immediately arises as to whether or not the mitotic procedure is immune from low dose x-ray effects. The selection of the actual dose, the penetration aspect of *in vivo* tissues, the method of irradiating, and the influence of damaged neighbor cells are all other considerations with which to contend. However, this method is one of the few ways in which to measure the mitotic time, and the final results of its application to cell proliferation rates is comparable to other known approaches.

4. *Microcinematography*

Time-lapse photography can be filmed through a microscope to record the intermitotic times of mammalian cells in tissue cultures (Sisken and Kinosita, 1961). Precise measurements can be achieved on individual cells, but it is not uncommon to find wide variations present among cells of the same strain and culture. This spread cannot be explained on the bases of external physiological environment, and proper evaluation of collected data can be very perplexing. The time of the actual mitotic process is an important by-product that can be extrapolated for use with techniques which determine the mitotic index. Microcinematography can be combined with biochemical markers to elicit the duration of various stages of the cell cycle (Sisken, 1963).

5. *DNA Content of the Nucleus*

The total nuclear DNA of a proliferating cell is doubled during the S stage and is retained throughout the G_2 phase, prophase, and metaphase. There are two related methods that can be directly employed with a fixed tissue section to analyze individual cell DNA and thereby make an assessment on cell proliferation. Both techniques incorporate photographic principles.

Nuclear DNA can be specifically stained with the Feulgen reaction, and the intensity of the stain is directly related to the concentration of DNA present. In this approach, a tissue section is Feulgen stained, photographed under an ordinary light microscope, and then the negative is scanned with a microdensitometer to record density tracings of cell nuclei. Cell nuclei with higher DNA contents will have absorbed more light and consequently will be less dense in the negative. The statistical compilation of the nuclear densities will show a percentage of nuclei with a baseline DNA content or the unreplicated genome (G_1), a transitional spectrum of increasing densities corresponding to cells in the S stage, and an upper level of DNA representing the replicated genome (Walker and Yates, 1952). Combinations with other techniques may provide precise timing information on the cell cycle stages.

There is another method that can be used to obtain a similar type of photographic negative for densitometry analysis. Nucleic acids strongly absorb ultraviolet light in the spectral band around 260 mμ. Since this ultraviolet absorption is also directly related to the nuclear concentrations, a photograph of an unstained tissue section taken through an ultraviolet microscope using illumination at 260 mμ will produce an equivalent film negative (Walker and Yates, 1952).

Difficulties arise with these approaches primarily in the densitometry assay. This is a meticulous process, and the calibration procedure involving film selection, illumination, exposure time, optical parameters, negative developing, and response characteristics of the density recording apparatus makes this portion of the experiment a science unto itself. Proper analysis of light absorption phenomena through photography is appreciated by very few persons.

6. *Colchicine*

In vivo administration of colchicine causes proliferating cells which enter the mitotic phase to be arrested in metaphase. These metaphase cells are blocked from progressing farther along in the division sequence for a period of time on the order of 6 to 8 hours, and the net result is an accumulation of mitotic figures with time. Correspondingly anaphases and telophases diminish with increasing duration of the drug's influence. The exact mechanism of this phenomenum appears related to colchicine binding to subunit proteins of microtubules, creating interference with the spindle apparatus formation that is necessary for continuance of the mitotic process (Borisym and Taylor, 1967). The dosage of colchicine required to produce this effect varies according to species and weight, and the optimum range should be separately investigated and identified. Too much colchicine precipitates tissue necrosis and toxicity in test animals, but circulating concentrations that are too low permit cells to escape early from the arrested metaphase state and complete mitosis. After colchicine is administered, there is a lag period before onset of its action which is dependent upon the selected delivery mode and the physiology of the specific cell population.

Colchicine has been frequently employed in the evaluation of cell proliferation. Metaphase accumulation is induced for a specified time period (allowances made for the lag period) at which point the animal is quickly sacrificed, the selected tissue fixed and processed, and then the colchicine mitotic index is determined. When the numerical difference between the colchicine mitotic index and the normal control mitotic index is divided by the effective time duration of drug action, the resultant yield is the rate of accumulation of mitotic figures or simply the mitotic rate. The reciprocal of the mitotic rate is the intermitotic time or the cell turnover time.

The assumption is made that colchicine does not interfere with the remainder of the cell cycle, and particularly does not disturb cell progression through the S, G_2, and prophase stages. Stimulation or retardation of these cells during the experiment would substantially alter the colchicine mitotic index. Hell and Cox (1963) demonstrated an average 14% reduction in DNA synthesis in incubated slices of guinea pig epidermis which had been treated with colchicine. They could not differentiate whether this was owing to arrested cells in the S period or failure of G_1 cells to enter the S period. Other investigators have shown in normal and regenerating rat livers that colchicine causes a drop in ATP concentration and an increase in the concentrations of AMP and NAD (Wang *et al.*, 1963). Henry *et al.* (1952) conducted an extensive study on the mitotic activity in the rabbit oral epithelium with colchicine and found a decreased incidence of prophases over a 6-hour interval. They recorded this depression and made corresponding allowances in their colchicine mitotic index. However, Stevens-Hooper (1961) found no change in the rate of entry of cells into prophase in her colchicine investigations on rat intestinal epithelium. Bertalanffy (1964) also shares the viewpoint that colchicine does not affect the dynamics of cell entry into mitosis. Thus there appears to be some question as to whether or not colchicine-arrested metaphases represent an unbiased accumulation of proliferating cells proceeding through the cell cycle. It would be a wise decision to include provisions for monitoring the prophase population and perhaps the S phase kinetics in a planned procedure utilizing colchicine.

7. *Tritiated Thymidine*

Currently, the most popular method for investigating cell proliferation involves the use of radioactive isotopes of thymidine, especially tritiated thymidine. Since thymidine is a specific precursor for DNA, the basic concept is to make tritiated thymidine available extracellularly where cells synthesizing DNA can directly incorporate the tagged molecule into the nucleus. Cells containing tritiated thymidine can be identified through the process of autoradiography and are referred to as labeled cells. The presence of labeled cells infers certain kinetic parameters about quantities and rates of cells progressing through the cell cycle, and thus leads to information about cell proliferation.

There are a number of basic assumptions made when utilizing tritiated thymidine *in vivo*, and the reader is referred to several texts which dwell in depth upon the proper use and interpretation of tritiated thymidine (Cleaver, 1967; Feinendegen, 1967). Briefly stated, several of the more important considerations are that cells other than those synthesizing DNA may take up the thymidine isotope, chromosome damage can result after incorporation, high concentrations promote radioactive lethality, breakdown products of dead cells may be reused, and uneven distribution of tritiated thymidine may occur to the given cell population. These possible problem areas are usually minimal perturbations but they may be significant sources of error in certain experimental situations. Most tritiated thymidine studies depend upon the "pulse" concept. After administration to the test animal, it is assumed that any tritiated thymidine that was not immediately taken up by DNA-synthesizing cells would be quickly cleared from the tissues and metabolized by the liver. No pooling of the tagged molecule would occur extracellularly, and therefore the time it was available to the cell population would be very short compared to the total duration of the S period; i.e., a pulse effect.

In tissues such as the epidermis where mature cells remain in the cell population for periods of time greater than the duration of the cell cycle, a specialized employment of tritiated thymidine can be made to analyze proliferation. A single pulse is given to test animals, and then the ratio of labeled basal (germinal) cells to the total number of labeled cells is followed with respect to time. This ratio would initially be 1.0, and it would gradually fall off to 0.5 as each labeled basal cell divided and formed two cells. However, at a later time, corresponding to the duration of the cell cycle, the ratio would become less than 0.5 as the original labeled basal cells began to divide again (Wimber, 1963; Brown and Oliver, 1968).

In those tissues which have a rapid turnover of mature cells, cell proliferation can be assessed by examining only the germinal cells. The technique is to pulse label a group of S period cells and then to follow them as they repeatedly evolve through the cell cycle. After administration of the precursor, the ratio of the number of labeled mitoses to the total number of mitoses is plotted with respect to time. Soon after pulsing, the ratio advances from zero to 1.0 and remains plateaued at this level for a period of time before it begins to decrease. Later, the ratio begins to increase once more as the origin cells divide again, and a second plateau period is recorded. The time between the midpoints of the two plateaus is the cell cycle time (Wimber, 1963; Brown and Oliver, 1968).

Double labeling is another method for determining the duration of the S period. A single pulse of tritiated thymidine is administered, and after a controlled time interval, a second pulse is given with ¹⁴C-labeled thymidine. The two isotopes can be separately identified with autoradiography owing to the difference in β-particle emission energies. Owing to the different times of availability of the thymidine compounds to the cell population, a differential analysis can be applied to cells which completed synthesis of DNA and were only labeled with tritiated thymidine compared to those which were labeled with ¹⁴C-thymidine or both isotopes.

The duration of the S period can be derived from the following equality:

No. of cells labeled only with ³H-thymidine
―――――――――――――――――――――――――――――
No. of cells labeled with ¹⁴C-thymidine

$$= \frac{\text{control time between isotope application}}{\text{duration of the S period}}$$

The reader is directed to a complete illustrated discussion of this technique by Wimber (1963). Shortly after a cell population has been pulse labeled with tritiated thymidine, the ratio of the number of labeled cells to the total number of germinal cells can be determined. This calculation yields the S stage index, and when this value is divided by the known time duration of the S period, the result is the cell turnover time. This is analogous to the scheme involving mitotic index and mitotic duration.

There are other methods for employing tritiated thymidine in cell kinetics. Tissue cultures can be labeled and the cell cycle statistically derived by monitoring the dilution of the isotope subsequent to cell division. The complete time for a tissue to renew its entire population can be estimated by continuously administering tritiated thymidine until all cells are labeled. It is common to use tritiated thymidine in combination with either colchicine, Feulgen staining, or x-irradiation to obtain time measurements on various phases of the cell cycle.

III. Subcellular Renewal

A. GENERAL CONSIDERATIONS

The study of cell proliferation harbors a fundamental property that readily lends the analysis to direct observation. The fixed tissue section is examined with respect to the chosen marker, and the differential counting between marked and unmarked cells is a simple task since the uniformity of tissue structure is preserved. At the molecular level, any direct attempt to assess turnover is confronted with the dilemma that any marker chosen to establish identity will be on the same order of physical magnitude as the selected molecule for study. Consequently, there is little freedom of choice in the available methods, and nearly all approaches are built around the use of isotopes.

What we do essentially when we use isotopes to study molecular renewal is to make a direct substitution of one atom for a slightly different one, and then we assume that we have not disturbed the systemic equilibrium. Tracer elements can be applied in three molecular formations: (a) elemental states which are primarily employed for mineral and electrolyte turnover studies; (b) labeled amino acids or other precursors which would be incorporated into a synthesized macromolecule; and (c) labeled biomolecules which can be used for comparison in extracellular fluid spaces. Either radioactive isotopes or stable isotopes can be utilized as the label marker. The radioactive compounds are used more frequently because they can be easily detected by scintillation counters or autoradiography. Common radioactive tracers are ^3H, ^{14}C, ^{32}P, ^{35}S, ^{51}Cr, ^{131}I, and ^{45}Ca. The stable isotopes must be measured with a mass spectrometer, and this is definitely not a convenient apparatus. However, some elements are not available in radioactive forms for either atomic or economic reasons, and nonradioactive isotopes do have applications. The more common stable isotopes are ^2H, ^{13}C, ^{15}N, and ^{18}O.

There are several aspects that should be considered depending upon the choice of isotope, how it is used, and where it is located on the labeled molecule (Feinendegen, 1967).

1. Kinetic Effects

Owing to differences introduced by the tracer element, the rates of chemical reactions may be altered. This has been particularly noticed in several experiments where tritium bonds were important reactant parameters. Heavier masses tend to retard reaction rates, and some effects may also be expected when ^{15}N or ^{18}O is used.

2. Enzyme Specificity

The isotope may change conformational and chemical makeup of a precursor such that interactions with synthetic enzymes will result in different utilization rates compared to a nonlabeled precursor. Such discrimination of the tracer compound could cause selective intracellular retention or pooling.

3. Homeostasis

We could hardly expect to flood extracellular compartments with unusual precursors and not induce changes in the internal equilibrium conditions of the cell. The presence of just an external source of some of the synthetic substrates may be enough to alter the intracellular pools of precursors by upsetting feedback control networks.

4. Transmutation Effects

When the unstable radioisotope decays, it can significantly disrupt the local atomic environment. Involvement encompasses the emitted β- and x-rays, the spontaneous changes in charge distribution and nuclear chemistry, and the recoil energy of the transmuted nucleus. Damage may not necessarily be confined to the molecule where the transmutation occurred, and this phenomenon has been particularly implicated for producing alterations in nucleic acids (genes).

There are two special situations where molecular renewal can be investigated without utilizing isotopes, but they are both areas involving a transient effect. The concept of molecular turnover in each instance is quite restrictive, and both conditions are outside the realm of normal physiology.

1. The synthesis of certain biomolecules may not occur unless a specific stimulus such as a hormone or foreign protein is present. Such a molecule can be examined with respect to its rate of appearance after an exogenous stimulating pulse is administered, and the subsequent rate of disappearance can also be followed. If the molecule was strictly confined to an intracellular lifetime, then its activity levels could be monitored indirectly through special stains and fluorescent antibody methods, or directly by spectrophotometry and chemical assay. Extracellular circulating molecules can easily be evaluated with direct concentration determinations. Practical examples falling into this overall category are the pregnancy and immunological competency tests.

2. The lifetimes of some molecules, especially the circulating plasma proteins, can be derived by abruptly interfering with their production and then measuring the rate of disappearance. This can be accomplished by poisoning synthetic enzyme systems, by resecting the organ responsible for production, or by eliminating a source of synthetic stimulus. Endocrine systems are particularly suited to this type of analysis.

B. ORGANELLES

Investigations of cell organelle turnover represent complex undertakings Since we have only partial knowledge of the structural composition and physiology of these subcellular units, it is practically impossible to differentiate turnover of isolated compounds within the organelle versus the synthesis and anabolism of the entire organelle. Also, labeling methods are confounded by the inability to distinguish if reuse of labeled materials occurs and whether or not intracellular pools of subunits exist.

A classic example of how one might approach renewal of organelles is illustrated in the double labeling method employed by Fletcher and Sanadi (1961) (also see Chapter 8). They labeled mitochondria in rat livers with both ^{35}S-methionine and ^{14}C-acetate to establish a broad base of marked precursors within structural elements. After incorporation, they followed the rate of loss of each label in four separate mitochondrial components: the soluble protein, the insoluble protein, the lipid, and the cytochrome. The observed rates of loss of each tracer from the four components fell within experimental error, and this led them to conclude that the mitochondria were turning over as a whole unit with a half-life of 10.3 days for rat liver.

C. MACROMOLECULES

Metabolic renewal of proteins (Chapters 6 and 7), lipids (Chapter 8), and carbohydrates (Chapter 9) may be assayed in extracellular spaces, in entire cells, and in intracellular compartments. There is an endless number of different macromolecules that can be evaluated with respect to turnover, and each is subject to its own physiological and homeostatic controlling mechanisms. Since the synthesis of the body's macromolecules is an intracellular event, the basic scheme of introducing labeled synthetic precursors into the extracellular fluids readily follows. The more commonly used isotope-tagged compounds are the amino acids, glucose, nucleic acid precursors, cholesterol, and intermediary metabolites. A given precursor may have selective specificity for certain synthetic pathways such as thymidine for DNA, and this would obviously be a desirable characteristic whenever possible. On the other hand, some precursors can be utilized in a number of separate structural patterns and would definitely not be specific indicators. Further complications arise if the precursor is biologically unstable or prone to undergo interconversion or catabolism. To preclude the possibility of falsely interpreting the tracer results, it is a wise practice to cross-check the experiment with a different labeled precursor (double-labeling method). There should be no difference in the rate of disappearance of either isotope in the final product.

Isotopically labeled precursors provide information on the synthetic steps that transpire in the catabolism of macromolecules. By varying the position of the marker within the same precursor, it is possible to extract data on molecular position, stepwise progression, and contributions of precursor fragments. Several experiments have been performed using radioautography to show the intracellular progression of labeled precursors from entry into the cell through synthesis of carbohydrate and protein complexes in secretory granules (Caro and Palade, 1964; Peterson and Leblond, 1964; also see Chapters 5, 8, and 9). These time sequential studies provided vivid demonstrations of the roles of the rough endoplasmic reticulum and the Golgi complex in the synthesis pathway of cell secretions.

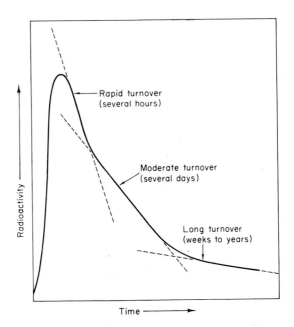

FIG. 2. Time curves of radioactivity in macromolecules (such as protein) following a single injection of radioactive amino acid. The curve suggests the existence of three species of protein with different turnover times.

Aside from variations in normal physiology owing to stimulating factors or phases of the cell cycle, the turnover of intracellular macromolecules can be categorized into three groups: rapid, slow, and very slow or non-renewing molecules. Often three separate decay curves illustrating these components can be extracted by monitoring the rate of tracer disappearance from an entire cell which had been labeled with a nonspecific amino acid (see Fig. 2). Cell secretory products generally have short intracellular life-times and therefore would have rapid turnover rates. Miller *et al.* (1951) demonstrated that ^{14}C-lysine was rapidly removed from the circulation by liver parenchyma, and it subsequently appeared in the plasma albumin and globulin fractions within several hours. Intracellular structural components and enzymes usually have longer survival times. ^{14}C-labeled glycine incorporated into muscle aldolase has been found to disappear exponentially with a half-life of approximately 20 days (Schapira *et al.*, 1960). Hemoglobin in the intact red blood cell does not exhibit renewal (Grinstein *et al.*, 1949).

The stability-renewal status of DNA is apparently controversial, and this facet will receive ample coverage in another chapter of this book (see Chapter 2). An investigator should be aware that a nonrenewing macromolecule will not incorporate radioactive precursors and he should understand that the way to get such a macromolecule labeled is to apply the precursor during a period of synthesis, i.e., during embryogenesis or growth.

D. Minerals, Electrolytes, and Water

Determinations on turnover of the minerals and electrolytes can only be accomplished by using parent-related isotopes (see Comar and Bronner, 1962). Compartmentization of the intracellular and extracellular spaces is the major obstacle confronting investigators in these areas. A single mineral may be found in the mammalian body in the free state, in an inorganic molecule, chelated to a protein carrier, or bound in a protein molecule (see Chapter 10). It should therefore be appreciated that turnover of a specific element would be related to how it was handled within the body. Turnover of electrolytes is directly related to bodily intake and excretion. The exchangeable electrolytes are greatly influenced by the presence of cellular membranes, and are also influenced by the great variation in the diffusible equilibrium rates among the various tissues.

Tritium-labeled water rapidly diffuses throughout the body and has been extensively utilized to monitor water turnover (see review by Feinendegen, 1967). A small fraction is observed to be directly incorporated into tissue constituents, and some of the tritium exchanges with hydrogen bounds. Otherwise, the half-life of tritiated water in man is approximately 8–10 days.

REFERENCES

Baserga, R. (1965). The relationship of the cell cycle to tumor growth and control of cell division: a review. *Cancer Res.* **25,** 581–595.

Baserga, R. (1968). Biochemistry of the cell cycle: a review. *Cell Tissue Kinet.* **1,** 167–191.

Bertalanffy, F. D. (1964). Tritiated thymidine versus colchicine technique in the study of cell population cytodynamics. *Lab. Invest.* **13,** 871–886.

Blumenthal, H. T. (1950). The nature of cycle variations in mitotic activity: the relation of alimentation and nutrition to this phenomena. *Growth* **14,** 231–249.

Borisy, G. G., and Taylor, E. W. (1967). The mechanism of action of colchicine. *J. Cell Biol.* **34,** 525–533.

Brown, J. M., and Oliver, R. (1968). A new method of estimating the cell cycle time in epithelial tissues of long generation time. *Cell Tissue Kinet.* **1,** 11–21.

Bullough, W. S. (1965). Mitotic and functional homeostasis: a speculative review. *Cancer Res.* **25,** 1683–1727.

Bullough, W. S., and Laurence, E. B. (1961). Stress and adrenaline in relation to the diurnal cycle of epidermal mitotic activity in adult male mice. *Proc. Roy. Soc. Ser.* **B154**, 540–556.

Buschke, W. (1949). Experimentelle studien zur Patho-physiologie des Hornautepithels: zell-bewegungen bei der Wundheilung, zell-teilung, Mitospemmung und andere Kernphenomene. *Ophthalmologica* **118**, 407–439.

Buschke, W., Friedenwald, J. S., and Fleischmann, W. (1943). Studies on the mitotic activity of the corneal epithelium. *Bull. Johns Hopkins Hosp.* **73**, 143–168.

Cameron, I. L. (1968). A method for the study of cell proliferation and renewal in the tissues of mammals. *In* "Methods in Cell Physiology" (David M. Prescott, ed.), Vol. III, pp. 261–276. Academic Press, New York.

Caro, L. G., and Palade, G. E. (1964). Protein synthesis, storage, and discharge in the pancreatic exocrine cell. An autoradiographic study. *J. Cell Biol.* **20**, 473–495.

Cleaver, J. E. (1967) "Thymidine Metabolism and Cell Kinetics." North-Holland, Amsterdam.

Comar, C. L., and Bronner, F. (1962). "Mineral Metabolism," Vol. II, Part B. Academic Press, New York.

Craddock, C. G., Winkelstein, A., Matsuyuki, Y, and Lawrence, J. S. (1967). Observations on the relationship of thymus to hemapoiesis and lymphopoiesis. *In* "Control of Cellular Growth in Adult Organisms" (H. Teir and T. Rytömaa, eds.), pp. 153–170. Academic Press, New York.

Eartly, H., Grad, B., and Leblond, C. P. (1951). The antagonistic relationship between testosterone and thyroxine in maintaining the epidermis of the male rat. *Endocrinology* **49**, 677–686.

Enesco, M., and Leblond, C. P. (1962). Increase in cell number as a factor in the growth of the organs and tissues of the young male rat. *J. Embryol. Exp. Morphol.* **10**, 530–562.

Epifanova, O. I., and Tershikh, V. V. (1969). On the resting periods in the cell life cycle. *Cell Tissue Kinet.* **2**, 75–93.

Feinendegen, L. E. (1967). "Tritium-labeled Molecules in Biology and Medicine." Academic Press, New York.

Feinendegen, L. E. (1968). Problems associated with the use of labeled molecules in biology and medicine: general review. *In* "Biological Effects of Transmutation and Decay of Incorporated Radioisosopes, Panel Proceedings Series." International Atomic Energy Agency, Vienna.

Fletcher, M. J., and Sanadi, D. R. (1961). Turnover of rat-liver mitochondria. *Biochem. Biophys. Acta* **21**, 356–360.

Grinstein, M., Kamen, M. D., and Moore, C. V. (1949). The utilization of glycine in the bioshythesis of hemoglobin. *J. Biol. Chem.* **179**, 359–364.

Harris, M. (1959). Growth measurements on monolayer cultures with an electronic cell counter. *Cancer Res.* **19**, 1020–1024.

Hell, E., and Cox, D. G. (1963). Effects of colchicine and colchemid on synthesis of deoxyribonucleic acid in the skin of guinea pig's ear *in vitro*. *Nature (London)* **197**, 287–288.

Henry, J. L., Meyer, J., Weinmann, J. P., and Schour, I. (1952). Pattern of mitotic activity in oral epithelium of rabbits. *Arch. Pathol.* **54**, 281–297.

Howard, A., and Pelc, S. R. (1953). Synthesis of desoxyribonucleic acid in normal and irradiated cells and its relation to chromosome breakage. *Heredity Suppl.* **6**, 261–273.

Knowlton, N. P., and Widner, W. R. (1950). The use of x-rays to determine the mitotic and intermitotic time of various mouse tissues. *Cancer Res.* **10**, 59–63.

Lajtha, L. G. (1967). Proliferation kinetics of steady state cell populations. *In* "Cellular Growth in Adult Organisms" (H. Teir and T. Rytömaa, eds.), pp. 97–105, Academic Press, New York.

Lajtha, L. G., Oliver, R., Kumatori, T., and Ellis, F. (1958). On the mechanism of radiation effect on DNA synthesis. *Radiat. Res.* **8,** 1–16.

Leblond, C. P. (1964). Classification of cell populations on the basis of their proliferative behavior. *Nat. Cancer Inst. Monogr.* **14,** 119–150.

Lehmiller, D. J. (1970). Cell migration and proliferation during repair of superficial corneal wounds produced by a carbon dioxide laser. *Tech. Rept.* 70–29. School of Aerospace Medicine, Brooks Air Force Base.

Mattern, C. F. T., Brackett, F. S., and Olson, B. J. (1957). Determination of number and size of particles by electronic gating: blood cells. *J. Appl. Physiol.* **10,** 56–70.

McMinn, R. M. H. (1969). "Tissue Repair." Academic Press, New York.

Miller, L. L., Bly, C. G., Watson, M. L., and Bale, W. F. (1951). The dominant role of the liver in plasma protein synthesis. *J. Exp. Med.* **94,** 431–453.

Patt, H. M., and Quastler, H. (1963). Radiation effects on cell renewal and related systems. *Physiol. Rev.* **43,** 357–396.

Petersen, D. F., Tobey, R. A., and Anderson, E. C. (1969). Essential biosynthetic activity in synchronized mammalian cells. *In* "The Cell Cycle" (G. M. Padilla, G. L. Whitson, and I. L. Cameron, eds.), pp. 341–359. Academic Press, New York.

Peterson, M., and Leblond, C. P. (1964). Synthesis of complex carbohydrates in the golgi region, as shown by radioautography after injection of labeled glucose. *J. Cell Biol.* **21,** 143–148.

Puck, T. T., and Steffen, J. (1963). Life cycle analysis of mammalian cells. I. A method for localizing metabolic events within the life cycle, and its application to the action of colcemide and sublethal doses of x-irradiation. *Biophys. J.* **3,** 379–397.

Schapira, G., Kruh, J., Dreyfus, J. C., and Schapira, F. (1960). The molecular turnover of muscle aldolase. *J. Biol. Chem.* **235,** 1738–1741.

Shemen, D., and Rittenberg, D. (1946). The life span of the human red blood cell. *J. Biol. Chem.* **166,** 627–636.

Sisken, J. E. (1963). Analysis of variations in intermitotic time. *In* "Cinemicrography in Cell Biology" (George G. Rose, ed.), pp. 143–168. Academic Press, New York.

Sisken, J. E., and Kinosita, R. (1961). Timing of DNA synthesis in the mitotic cycle *in vitro. J. Biophys. Biochem. Cytol.* **9,** 509–518.

Stevens-Hooper, C. E. (1961). Use of colchicine for the measurement of mitotic rate in the intestinal epithelium. *Amer. J. Anat.* **108,** 231–244.

Strehler, B. L. (1962). "Time, Cells, and Aging." Academic Press, New York.

Teir, H., Lahtiharju, A., Alho, A., and Forsell, K.-J. (1967). Autoregulation of growth by tissue breakdown products. *In* "Control of Cellular Growth in Adult Organisms" (H. Teir and T. Rytömaa, eds.), pp. 67–82. Academic Press, New York.

Vasama, Raimo, and Vasama, Ritva (1958). On the diurnal cycle of mitotic activity in the corneal epithelium of mice. *Acta Anat.* **33,** 230–237.

Walker, P. M. B., and Yates, H. B. (1952). Nuclear components of dividing cells. *Proc. Royal Soc. Ser.* **B140,** 274–299.

Wang, D. Y., Greenbaum, A. L., and Harkness, R. D. (1963). The effect of colchicine on the acid-soluble ribonucleotides of normal and regenerating rat liver. *Biochem. J.* **86,** 62–64.

Watanabe, I., and Okada, S. (1967). Effects of temperature on growth rate of cultured mammalian cells (L 5178 Y). *J. Cell Biol.* **32,** 309–323.

Wimber, D. E. (1963). Methods for studying cell proliferation with emphasis on DNA
    labels. *In* "Cell Proliferation" (L. F. Lamerton and R. J. M. Fry, eds.), pp. 1–36.
    Blackwell, Oxford.
Yamada, M., and Puck, T. T. (1961). Action of radiation on mammalian cells. IV.
    Reversible mitotic lag in the S_3 Hela cell produced by low doses of x-ray. *Proc. Nat.
    Acad. Sci. U.S.* **47,** 1181–1191.

CHAPTER 2

The Metabolic Stability of Nuclear DNA*

Erle K. Adrian, Jr.

I. Introduction.. 25
II. DNA Constancy... 26
    A. The Constancy Hypothesis................................ 26
    B. Deviations from DNA Constancy.......................... 27
III. DNA Stability.. 35
IV. Conclusions.. 37
    References.. 38

I. Introduction

For more than 20 years, in spite of numerous claims to the contrary, the ideas of DNA constancy and DNA stability have been generally accepted, almost to the point of their being declared fundamental principles of biology. Although DNA constancy and DNA stability are closely related, they are not synonymous. DNA constancy refers to the quantity of DNA possessed by a chromosome set, which according to the constancy hypothesis should be the same for every cell within a given species. Obviously, the amount of a material may be quite constant, while at the same time undergoing a rapid turnover. The concept of DNA stability, which refers to its lack of turnover, is therefore much more restrictive than that of DNA constancy.

The early biochemical and cytophotometric experiments which established the relative constancy of nuclear DNA were not sufficiently exact to rule out small variations in the absolute DNA content of the nucleus. Many of the experiments claiming to demonstrate DNA turn-

*Supported by Public Health Service Grant #NS08949.

over or variations in the absolute amount of DNA per nucleus, however, either have been directly contradicted or have not been confirmed. The purpose of this chapter is to examine the evidence both for and against the metabolic stability of the DNA of the nucleus. Other general review articles which cover various aspects of this topic are those by Swift (1953), Vendrely and Vendrely (1956), Lima-de-Faria (1962a) Roels (1966), and Cleaver (1967).

II. DNA Constancy

A. THE CONSTANCY HYPOTHESIS

The early work on DNA constancy was largely directed toward the establishment of DNA as the primary genetic material. Thus, it was desirable to demonstrate a proportionality between the number of chromosomes and the DNA content of the nucleus. In 1947, Mirsky and Ris showed that most of the chromosomal nucleic acid is DNA, and Boivin and Vendrely (1947) theorized that genes are macromolecules of DNA. By measuring the total amount of DNA in nuclear suspensions from which estimates of the total number of nuclei had been made, it was possible to calculate the amount of DNA per nucleus. A remarkable uniformity in DNA content was found in nuclei from somatic cells of the same species, and this value was shown to be twice that found in sperm nuclei from the same species (Boivin et al., 1948; Vendrely and Vendrely, 1948, 1949a, 1949b; Mirsky and Ris, 1949). Subsequently, numerous biochemical investigations confirmed these observations (reviewed by Davidson and Leslie, 1950). When single nuclei were examined cytophotometrically, the results were in agreement with the theory of DNA constancy, and a direct proportionality was evident between DNA content and the number of chromosomes (Ris and Mirsky, 1949; Swift, 1950; Leuchtenberger et al., 1951; Pollister et al., 1951; Frazer and Davidson, 1953). Although some published results were inconsistent with the constancy hypothesis (Pasteels and Lison, 1950), examination of the same tissues by other investigators (Alfert and Swift, 1953) did not confirm these deviations from constancy, but instead added further support for the constancy hypothesis. The majority of the early cytophotometric studies on the amount of DNA per nucleus were in agreement with the general conclusion that DNA is ". . . a quantitatively constant element of the nucleus" (Vendrely and Vendrely, 1956).

B. Deviations from DNA Constancy

1. *Insects*

a. Polytene Chromosomes of Dipteran Larvae. Exceptions to the constancy hypothesis soon became apparent, however. The giant chromosomes of dipteran larvae, long considered polytene (T. S. Painter, 1941), were shown to possess approximately 1000 times more DNA than the chromosomes from diploid nuclei from the same larvae (Kurnick and Herskovitz, 1952). The puffs or bulbs that are characteristic of these giant chromosomes were shown by Breuer and Pavan (1955) to be associated with an accumulation of DNA (Feulgen) several times greater than the amount present in the same bands of the chromosome before puff formation. These localized increases in the amount of DNA, which at first seemed to be independent of the endomitotic process, did not occur in the same bands in polytene chromosomes from different tissues. Although Pelc and Howard (1956), using ¹⁴C-labeled adenine, were unable to demonstrate DNA synthesis in these chromosomal bands, Ficq and Pavan (1957) were able to do so with tritiated thymidine. Since the greatest incorporation of the isotope was found in areas of active puff formation, these authors interpreted their data as being consistent with ". . . an increase in the number of specific genes" directly related to gene activity. Using ultraviolet microspectrophotometry, Rudkin and Corlette (1957) found a doubling of the DNA content of the puffed regions relative to adjacent nonpuffed areas on the chromosome. However, they determined that the localized increases in DNA represented such a small proportion of the total nuclear DNA that they would not be detectable in methods where the total nuclear DNA was measured. Again the idea was brought forth that extra DNA was synthesized in areas of increased gene activity.

It was then shown that the formation of these DNA-rich puffs on giant chromosomes could be prevented by placing the larvae in the cold (Stich and Naylor, 1958). Within 2 days after returning the larvae to a warmer environment, however, the puffs appeared with some regions having as much as an eightfold increase in DNA. When the larvae were again placed in the cold, there was a gradual disappearance of the accumulated DNA. This apparent synthesis and subsequent disappearance of the excess DNA gave rise to the concept of "metabolic DNA" (Pavan, 1959), which has been defined as ". . . any DNA which is produced by the multiplication of chromosome loci, either in excess or independent of the process of genome multiplication" (Pavan, 1965).

Although the data thus far presented seemed to indicate that the puffs were sites of DNA synthesis which occurred independent of the replicative process, additional work raised doubts as to the validity of this idea. Using tritiated thymidine, Steffensen (1963) showed that DNA synthesis in the polytene chromosomes occurred almost entirely in the chromosomal bands and that regions with few bands and puffs showed little radioactivity. In some puffs, however, there seemed to be a total absence of thymidine uptake. Keyl (1963) failed to detect any increase in the DNA content of the puffs of *Glyptotendipes*, the organism which had been used in the temperature studies of Stich and Naylor (1958). Plaut (1963), using pulse labeling with tritiated thymidine, noted the appearance of a number of discrete labeling sites, indicating several independent points of DNA synthesis that were not obviously related to the development of puffs. Evidence was then presented that although there was a disproportionate synthesis of DNA in the regions of the puffs, it was probably part of an asynchronous replication process with both initial and terminal labeling appearing in the puff sites (Gabrusewycz-Garcia, 1964). Further evidence that the increased amounts of DNA found in the chromosomal puffs were associated with additional rounds of replication was presented by Keyl (1965). In hybrids of two subspecies of *Chironomus*, certain crossbands of the giant chromosomes were found to have either 2, 4, 8, or 16 times as much DNA as were found in homologous crossbands. The bands containing the increased amounts of DNA required more time in replication than their homologs. Crouse and Keyl (1968) then studied the development of a single puff and found a similar stepwise geometric increase in the amount of DNA in one of the bands forming a subunit of the puff, while no such increase was found in closely adjacent bands. No evidence was found for subsequent loss of the additional DNA, which seemed to be integrated into the chromosome (Crouse, 1968). The newly synthesized DNA in the puffs appeared therefore to be derived from additional isolated rounds of the replication process rather than being entirely independent of it as suggested by Pavan (1959, 1965). The results of Nash and Bell (1968) were consistent with this idea. In a study of DNA synthesis throughout the replicative cycle of the polytene chromosomes, they found spatially continuous DNA synthesis in the early phases of the cycle with discontinuous labeling in the terminal phases. Rodman (1968) also found continuous DNA synthesis at the beginning of the cycle, but Howard and Plaut (1968) were unable to find any single region that was completely early or late replicating.

b. *DNA Bodies in Oocytes.* In the oocytes of at least three insect genera, *Tipula, Dytiscus,* and *Acheta*, extrachromosomal DNA-containing bodies have been identified (Lima-de-Faria, 1962b, Lima-de-Faria *et al.*, 1968; Cave and Allen, 1969). In nuclei of premeiotic interphase cells, these structures first appear as intranucleolar masses of dense chromatin. In early meiotic prophase, they are the sites of intense DNA synthesis. Reaching a maximum size by midpachytene, the shape of these bodies in *Acheta* changes to resemble that of a chromosome puff. During late pachytene and early diplotene the body becomes less compact, and by the end of diplotene, disintegration begins with subsequent release of the DNA. These DNA-containing bodies have been interpreted as representing hundreds of copies of the operons of the nucleolar organizing region or neighboring regions (Lima-de-Faria and Moses, 1966).

2. Amphibians

a. Nucleolar DNA. For many years structures similar to the DNA-containing bodies of insect oocytes have been known to be present in the very large oocytes of amphibians. They were shown to be extrachromosomal DNA associated with the multiple nucleoli characteristic of these cells (T. S. Painter and Taylor, 1942). Miller (1964, 1966) suggested that the multiplicity of DNA-containing nucleoli were the result of an "amplification" of the cistrons for ribosomal RNA in the absence of replication of the rest of the genome. The result of this amplification was the accumulation and storage of ribosomes for use during the early developmental stages of the embryo. The extra DNA was thought to be produced either by a repetitive duplication and subsequent detachment of the copies at the nucleolar organizer loci or by the formation of a limited number of copies which then moved to the nuclear envelope and underwent a series of additional duplications.

When the ovaries of *Xenopus laevis* were cultured in the presence of tritiated thymidine, a marked uptake of isotope was detected in the nucleolar granules in the pachytene stage but no label was found in the chromosomes (Gall, 1967, 1968). The labeled DNA appeared to be metabolically stable, and it was present in association with the nucleoli throughout the period of oogenesis. The nucleus of the amphibian oocyte is required to furnish massive amounts of RNA to a quantity of cytoplasm many times greater than that found in somatic cells. Apparently this problem has been surmounted by specific replication of the nucleolar organizer region during meiotic prophase with the formation of additional organizers to serve as templates for RNA precursors (Gall, 1968). Perkowska et al.(1968) determined that these cells contain from 1400 to 1600 nucleoli along with more than 5000 nucleolar cores. The additional DNA associated with these structures results in an increase of the total DNA content from 4C to 14C (Macgregor, 1968). The sites of tritiated thymidine labeling were found to be consistent with the suggestion of

Miller (1966) that there is duplication of one or more copies of the nucleolar organizer with subsequent replication of the detached copies. This additional DNA has been calculated to represent a factor of gene amplification of about 2600 times (Perkowska *et al.*, 1968). D. D. Brown and David (1968) found the ratio of rDNA to 4 S DNA to be at least 5 times higher in amphibian oocytes than in sperm from the same species. The synthesis of RNA occurred only during oogenesis, and there was no further duplication of the nonchromosomal DNA after meiotic prophase.

b. Lampbrush Chromosomes. The lampbrush chromosomes, which have been identified in the oocytes of many vertebrates and a few invertebrates, are particularly evident in amphibians (Callan, 1963; E. H. Davidson, 1968). The DNA content of these chromosomes has been shown to be about 4 times that found in the chromosomes of other cell types in the same animal (Izawa *et al.*, 1963). The high protein to DNA and RNA to DNA ratios which characterize these chromosomes are thought to be related to widespread activity throughout the length of the chromosomes. The extra DNA found in these chromosomes has been suggested to be replicates of single genes, a form of gene amplification necessary because of the great mass of cytoplasm of the amphibian oocyte (Callan and Lloyd, 1960).

3. Mammals

a. Adrenal Medulla. Changes in the DNA content of adrenal medullary nuclei following periods of increased or decreased cellular activity have been reported. Cold stress has been the most frequent means by which adrenal medullary activity has been modified, although other types of stimuli have been used. Leeman (1959a), using the Lison cytophotometric technique, found a decrease in DNA-Feulgen in rat adrenal medullary nuclei following splanchnicectomy and an increase following insulin administration. After rats were exposed to low temperature (4°C) for 2 weeks, an 11.4% increase in mean DNA content over control levels was found in their adrenal medullary nuclei (Leeman, 1959b). In a similar experiment in which rats were subjected to low temperatures for a period of 2 weeks, Roels and Lagasse (1961) reported an increase in nuclear dry weight of the cells in the adrenal medulla as measured by interference microphotometry. In contrast, the results of Viola-Magni (1965, 1966a, 1966b) and Tongiani and Viola-Magni (1969) consistently showed a loss of nuclear DNA from the cells of the adrenal medulla following intermittent exposure to cold (15 hours at 4°C and 9 hours at room temperature, daily). This decrease in nuclear DNA was stated to be equally distributed over all the nuclei, and it reached a maximum mean value of 40.1% after a total of 300 hours exposure to cold (Viola-Magni, 1965). However, in rats that were returned to room temperature for a period of 10 days following the 300 hours of exposure to cold, the DNA values per adrenal medullary nucleus had a mean increase of 17.5% over control values. The amount of DNA per nucleus was measured by Feulgen cytophotometry, by determinations of the nuclear dry mass before and after treatment with DNase, and by biochemical methods. The results obtained by the three methods were essentially in agreement except that no increase in DNA per nucleus following the 10 days of exposure to room temperature was observed with the biochemical method. The DNA content of untreated adrenal medullary nuclei was found by all methods to be greater than that of kidney nuclei. When tritiated thymidine was given to rats brought to room temperature after 300 hours of intermittent cold exposure, labeling was noted in the adrenal medulla during the first 3 days of recovery, but no mitoses were identified (Viola-Magni, 1966a). Since all the injected animals had at least an 8-hour interval between injection and sacrifice and since smears were studied rather than sections, the question of the type of cells which were labeled is raised. When four injections of tritiated thymidine were administered over an 8-hour period, the labeling index increased by a factor of 10, suggesting short periods of synthetic activity.

Injections of tritiated thymidine were given after periods of intermittent exposure to cold which ranged in length from 100 to 750 hours (Viola-Magni, 1966b). At first, labeled cells were found only after injections given at the beginning of the 9-hour period of room temperature. After 350 hours of intermittent exposure to cold, DNA synthesis was detected during the periods of exposure to cold as well as during the periods at room temperature. Again, the length of time between injection of labeled thymidine and sacrifice (either 9 or 15 hours) and the absence of photographs showing labeling in unmistakable adrenal medullary cells raise some question as to the identification of the labeled cells.

A single injection of tritiated thymidine was then given to two groups of rats that had been exposed to the cold intermittently for 300 hours (Pelc and Viola-Magni, 1969). One group was thereafter kept continuously at room temperature and the other group was exposed to the cold as before. The percentage of labeled cells decreased with time in both groups but did so at a more rapid rate in the group subjected to intermittent cold exposure. In the animals left continuously at room temperature, the daily loss of labeled "metabolic" DNA was calculated to be more than 2%. If this loss occurs at a constant rate, the DNA of the adrenal medulla should turn over at least once every 50 days, and this turnover should thus be detectable in long-term labeling experiments. Where tritiated thymidine has been administered for long periods of time in drinking water of mice, labeling has been observed in adrenal medullary cells, but it occurs at such

a slow rate that renewal of the entire population would not occur during
the life span of the animal (Cameron, 1970). Although the labeling index
of the rats exposed to cold decreased with time, the average grain count of
the labeled cells showed no change. This observation has also been interpreted as being indicative of loss of metabolic DNA. However, it can
equally well be explained by the presence in the adrenal medulla of labeled
migratory cells, a factor which has not been considered in any of the fore-
going experiments.

The results of at least two cytophotometric studies (Cohn and Van
Duijn, 1967; Arold and Sandritter, 1967) have failed to confirm the loss
of DNA from adrenal medullary nuclei following intermittent exposure
to cold.

b. *Leukocytes.* The DNA content of leukocytes has been extensively
investigated by Feulgen cytophotometry, and many of the reported exceptions to the constancy hypothesis have been in this diverse group of
cells. Although the earliest cytophotometric studies reported DNA values
for leukocytes which did not differ significantly from the values found in
other somatic cells (Swift, 1950; J. N. Davidson *et al.*, 1950), lower values
were soon reported (Atkins and Richards, 1956). Hale (1963) made a
study of the variables involved in Feulgen cytophotometry of leukocytes
and found approximately 10% less DNA in mature leukocytes than was
found in nuclei of gastric epithelium, liver, and kidney. The decreased
DNA value for leukocytes could not be explained by differences in the
Feulgen technique, mitotic activity, chromosome number, or spectral
absorption curves of the various cell types measured.

Den Tonkelaar and Van Duijn (1964), using photographic colorimetry
and scanning cytophotometry, found no difference in the Feulgen-DNA
content of rat leukocytes and liver and kidney cells. Garcia (1964a,b),
on the other hand, found that while the mean DNA content of peripheral
leukocytes of both the rabbit and the human was within the diploid range,
there were differences in mean DNA content between the granulocytes
and mononuclear cells and between individual cells in these groups which
could not be accounted for by instrumental variation, distributional error,
or differences in Feulgen hydrolysis. Similar results were reported for
rat leukocytes (Garcia and Iorio, 1968). When rabbit leukocytes were
subjected to hypotonic treatment, however, their DNA values were found
to be increased from 7 to 12% over those of controls (Garcia, 1969a).
Evidence was presented that the reactivity of dye-binding sites in the
deoxyribonucleoprotein molecules is related to the physical state of these
molecules in such a way that there appears to be an increased amount of
DNA when these molecules become more diffuse. The relationships be-

tween the degree of coiling of the deoxyribonucleoprotein complex and the Feulgen reaction have recently been reviewed by Garcia (1969b). When the DNA values of large leukocytes and the small condensed nuclei of erythrocytes of birds, amphibians, and fishes were compared, there was again a positive correlation between total dye content and nuclear size (Rasch et al., 1969). Mayall (1969) has also found differences in the apparent DNA content of monocytes, small lymphocytes, and neutrophiles.

c. *Liver*. The DNA content of hepatic cell nuclei has been investigated extensively, and values for these cells were published in most of the early biochemical and cytophotometric studies on the quantity and constancy of nuclear DNA (Vendrely and Vendrely, 1956). The effects of diet, growth, and sex on the composition of hepatic cells were investigated by Campbell and Kosterlitz (1947, 1948, 1950), who could detect no significant alterations in DNA content per nucleus. Ely and Ross (1951), however, reported 50% more DNA per nucleus in livers from rats on a protein-free diet than was found in rats on a high protein diet, but this finding was not confirmed by Campbell and Kosterlitz (1952). Increased amounts of DNA per unit whole liver were also reported following alloxan administration (Diermeier et al., 1951), but no change was found in rats which were diabetic as a result of depancreatization (Diermeier et al., 1952). When growth hormone was given to hypophysectomized rats, no change in the amount of DNA-Feulgen per nucleus could be detected cytophotometrically, although biochemical analysis showed an apparent increase in DNA per unit of whole liver (Di Stefano et al., 1952, 1955). This apparent increase in DNA per unit weight was shown by cytophotometry to be due to a decrease in the RNA and protein content of these cells. Bergerard and Tuchmann-Duplessis (1953) found a decreased amount of DNA per nucleus following hypophysectomy and a return to normal after the administration of growth hormone. Decreases in the amount of hepatic cell DNA have also been reported following cortisone treatment (Lowe and Rand, 1956; Lowe et al., 1959).

When the left lobe of the liver was made ischemic by ligation, the mean Feulgen-DNA content per nucleus was reduced by about 25% (James, 1968). This decrease was shown to result from irreversible damage to the hepatic cells and subsequent loss of DNA as a part of the necrotic process.

d. *Adrenal Cortex and Thyroid*. Changes in the nuclear DNA content of the cells in the adrenal cortex and in the thyroid gland have been frequently reported, and this work has been reviewed extensively by Roels (1966). Apparent increases in DNA content were found in functionally active nuclei, a state in which the nucleus was usually reported to be enlarged. States of decreased activity, such as that following hypophysectomy, resulted in apparent decreases in nuclear DNA content. Alfert *et al.* (1953, 1955) studied thyroid follicular epithelium in hypophysectomized, normal, and propylthiouracil-treated rats. While they found the nuclear volumes of these three groups of animals to be in the ratios 1:2:3, respectively, all the nuclei had identical DNA contents which were typical of diploid cells.

e. *Sperm.* The DNA content of sperm nuclei has been used as the reference standard for the haploid amount of DNA in many of the determinations of nuclear DNA content (Vendrely and Vendrely, 1956). Decreases in the amount of DNA per sperm nucleus have been reported in cases of infertility (Leuchtenberger and Leuchtenberger, 1960) and following refrigeration of semen (Salisbury *et al.*, 1961). When microfluorometry and microspectrophotometry in visible and ultraviolet light were used to measure the DNA content of a large population of bull spermatozoa, a wider distribution of values was found than could be explained by instrumental and technical variation (Bahr and Wied, 1966). An hypothesis was brought forth that there is a distribution of redundant chromosomal DNA in such cells. Gledhill *et al.* (1966) found that although there was a considerable reduction in Feulgen reactivity when spermatids differentiated into testicular spermatozoa, there was no change in the DNA content as measured by absorption at 2650 Å. Therefore, it seemed likely that there were changes in the dye-binding capacity related to physical changes in the deoxyribonucleoprotein molecules and to chemical changes in the histones. Mayall (1966) pointed out that if the hypothesis of DNA constancy is assumed, then the absolute amount of DNA per nucleus should be greater in diploid cells from females than in those from males and X and Y sperm should differ by about 4.6% in DNA content. In a series of measurements of human sperm using an integrating cytophotometer and a two-wavelength microspectrophotometer, he was able to demonstrate a bimodal distribution of two equal populations with mean DNA content differing by about 4%.

f. *Keratinizing Epithelia.* Both Feulgen cytophotometry (Bern *et al.*, 1957) and radioautography with tritiated thymidine (Pelc, 1958a) show loss of DNA from differentiating cells in keratinizing epithelia. The nuclei of such cells first swell and then shrink with both changes being accompanied by loss of DNA. Following tritiated thymidine injection, there is a loss of about 72% of the label between the second and third days. This loss occurs during the period of differentiation, at the same time that keratin is being synthesized by the nuclei of the differentiating cells.

III. DNA Stability

The role of DNA as a carrier of genetic information would seemingly require it to possess a unique metabolic stability. Using radioactive labels a number of investigators were able to show that DNA had a very low rate of turnover which seemed to be correlated only with mitotic activity (Hevesy and Ottesen, 1943; Brues et al., 1944; Hammarsten and Hevesy, 1946; G. B. Brown, 1948; Furst et al., 1950; Barton, 1954; Fresco et al., 1955; Healy et al., 1956; Hecht and Potter, 1956; Révész et al., 1956). By 1959, it was clear that turnover or exchange of DNA, as distinguished from synthesis of new DNA in preparation for division or polyploidy, was an exceptional occurrence, if, indeed, it occurred at all (Hughes, 1959). Since that time, a number of authors have claimed to demonstrate losses of DNA followed by synthetic replacement not associated with subsequent division. In addition, evidence has been presented which would indicate periodic replacement of DNA in some cell types. This section will review the evidence for DNA turnover in mammalian cells.

In a long series of experiments (Lasnitzki and Pelc, 1957; Pelc, 1958b; Pelc and Gahan, 1959; Pelc, 1959, 1963a,b; 1964, 1967), Pelc and his associates have used radioactive DNA precursors to demonstrate DNA synthesis in the seminal vesicle and other organs of the mouse in which mitotic figures are rare. Because of the disparity between the large number of labeled cells and the small number of mitotic figures detected by these workers, they concluded that the observed DNA synthesis did not always lead to mitosis but instead might serve some metabolic function. Gall and Johnson (1960) addressed themselves to this problem by measuring the DNA content of cells in the seminal vesicle that were labeled 6 hours after a single injection of tritiated thymidine. Pelc (1959) had reported that virtually all the nuclei in the seminal vesicle were in the diploid range, but Gall and Johnson (1960) found that only slightly more than a third of the labeled nuclei were in the 2C class with the rest having Feulgen dye contents above the upper limit for the diploid amount. Obviously, then, the labeled nuclei had synthesized varying amounts of DNA in the period between injection and sacrifice which were in addition to the normal diploid complement and which did not represent turnover. A correlation was also observed between the grain counts of the labeled cells and their Feulgen dye content. Out of 101 labeled nuclei studied, 6 were found in division and 37 had a diploid value, suggesting that they had completed division between injection and sacrifice. A ratio of labeled cells to mitoses calculated from this data would be very much lower than that observed in Pelc's experiments and would be more in accord with such ratios observed in other tissues. In contrast to the ratio of labeled cells to mitotic figures calculated by Pelc and Gahan (1959), which was 88, Messier and Leblond (1960) found this ratio to be 6.7 for the seminal vesicle of rats and 6.5 and 3.0 in two mice, figures completely consistent with premitotic DNA synthesis as an explanation for all the observed labeling.

Pelc (1962) also made the observation that following high doses of tritiated thymidine, or low doses with long exposure times, weakly labeled nuclei were found in the seminal vesicle, liver, smooth muscle, and in the interstitial cells of the testis. Instead of a continuous distribution of grain counts, a distinctly bimodal distribution of grain counts was observed, with one group having between 5 and 44 grains per nucleus and the other group having nuclei too heavily labeled for the grains to be counted. The weakly labeled nuclei were estimated to be incorporating the label at about 2% of the rate of the heavily labeled nuclei, which were assumed to be in premitotic DNA synthesis. It has been suggested that this low rate of DNA synthesis represents replacement of DNA in some gene loci (Pelc, 1963b).

Cells incorporating tritiated thymidine at the full rate which subsequently fail to divide have also been described in bone (Owen and MacPherson, 1963), cardiac muscle, smooth muscle, testicular interstitial cells, hepatic cells, mast cells, nerve cells (Pelc, 1963b), and intestinal epithelium (Appleton et al., 1969). The suggestion has been made that incorporation of DNA precursors at a rate equivalent to premitotic synthesis without subsequent division is an indication of metabolic activity of DNA or repair of aged cells (Pelc, 1963b, 1964, 1967).

When DNA was extracted from heart, muscle, and intestine of mice killed at either 12, 23, or 48 hours after a single injection of tritiated thymidine, two molecular weight classes of DNA with different specific activities were found (Stroun et al., 1967). The ratio of the specific activity of the low molecular weight fraction to that of the high molecular weight fraction ranged from 14.6 in muscle to 4.6 in intestine. An assumption was made that the low molecular weight fraction is metabolic DNA or contains metabolic DNA.

Based on the data thus far cited, Pelc (1968) has published an hypothesis that metabolic DNA consists of extra copies of active genes, molecules which are subject to wear and tear and which are lost from the cell and periodically replaced. This metabolic DNA is considered to be present in addition to the stable "genetic" DNA and is thought to be formed after the last division in some cells.

A great deal of evidence has been presented which demonstrates the occurrence of DNA repair processes in bacteria following ultraviolet irradiation (Setlow and Carrier, 1964; Boyce and Howard-Flanders, 1964; Pettijohn and Hanawalt, 1964; Hanawalt et al., 1968; Howard-Flanders *et al.*, 1968; Setlow *et al.*, 1968). Reviews of this subject have been written by Howard-Flanders (1968) and Strauss (1968). These repair processes are characterized by the excision of damaged areas containing thymine dimers followed by a nonconservative replication of DNA.

When mammalian cells in culture were subjected to ultraviolet irradiation and then placed in a medium containing tritiated thymidine, there was a great increase in the number of labeled cells over that found in unirradiated controls (Rasmussen and R. B. Painter, 1964). Even cells in mitosis were found to take up tritiated thymidine. Incorporation of tritiated thymidine was detectable in all cells even after low doses of ultraviolet irradiation. This DNA synthesis was not semiconservative, and it occurred in cells that were not in the normal DNA synthesis phase (Rasmussen and R. B. Painter, 1966). This unscheduled DNA synthesis was found to occur after doses of ultraviolet irradiation where 90% or more of the cells survive and after doses of x-rays where survival approaches 50% (R. B. Painter, 1968).

Cultured leukocytes have also been shown to repair radiation-induced breaks in the DNA molecule (Lett *et al.*, 1967). Ninety percent of human leukocytes that were incubated for 2 hours in a medium containing tritiated thymidine following ultraviolet irradiation incorporated the label into their DNA, whereas only 0.2% of unirradiated cells was labeled (Evans and Norman, 1968). However, the amount of tritiated thymidine taken up per labeled cell was 10 times greater in the normal cells, which were presumably undergoing premitotic DNA synthesis.

DNA synthesis has also been demonstrated in the skin of hairless mice following ultraviolet irradiation (Epstein *et al.*, 1968). Although normal DNA synthetic activity in the basal layer is depressed immediately after radiation, there is a much more generalized appearance of weak labeling in cells in the basal, Malpighian, and granular layers which reaches a peak at 20 minutes after irradiation and which is markedly reduced by 2 hours. This phenomenon may represent DNA repair, which has been described by Cleaver (1968) in normal skin fibroblasts following ultraviolet irradiation. Cleaver (1968) has shown that cells from patients with xeroderma pigmentosum have a reduced or absent repair replication in comparison with normal fibroblasts. Since patients with this disease develop fatal skin cancers when exposed to sunlight, an association has been made between the defective repair mechanism and carcinogenesis.

IV. Conclusions

The experimental data cited in this chapter show that exceptions to DNA constancy and DNA stability do occur. Gene amplification in polytene chromosomes and in the oocytes of insects and amphibia seems to be well established and may represent phenomena that generally occur but are less easily detectable in other types of cells (Cahn et al., 1968). Deviations from DNA constancy may occur in mammals, and the experimental work on the adrenal medulla is of particular interest (Viola-Magni, 1966a,b; Pelc and Viola-Magni, 1969). However, physical changes in the deoxyribonucleoprotein molecule have been shown to influence the Feulgen-DNA content of nuclei (Gledhill et al., 1966; Garcia, 1969a), and such changes have not been ruled out in most of the work where variations in nuclear DNA content have been reported. The effects of physical changes in the nuclear material on other quantitative methods should also be investigated. The claim that DNA synthesis at a rate equivalent to premitotic doubling does not lead to mitosis in some cells (Pelc and Gahan, 1959; Pelc, 1959, 1963a,b) has been the object of considerable doubt (Gall and Johnson, 1960; Messier and Leblond, 1960; Cleaver, 1967). However, the observation of weak tritiated thymidine labeling in some tissues (Pelc, 1962) may possibly be related to DNA repair similar to that observed in cultured mammalian cells (Rasmussen and R. B. Painter, 1964, 1966; R. B. Painter, 1968; Cleaver, 1968) and in vivo (Epstein et al., 1968). In summary, although the tenets of DNA constancy and DNA stability rest on relatively firm ground, exceptions to both doctrines definitely occur and will undoubtedly be shown to have major importance in the understanding of gene action, differentiation, carcinogenesis, and other areas of biological research.

REFERENCES

Alfert, M., and Swift, H. (1953). Nuclear DNA constancy: A critical evaluation of some exceptions reported by Lison and Pasteels. Exp. Cell Res. 5, 455–460.

Alfert, M., Bern, H. A., and Kahn, R. (1953). Karyometric and cytochemical studies on the rat thyroid gland. Anat. Rec. 117, 585–586.

Alfert, M., Bern, H. A., and Kahn, R. (1955). Hormonal influence on nuclear synthesis. IV. Karyometric and microspectrophotometric studies of rat thyroid nuclei in different functional states. Acta Anat. 23, 185–205.

Appleton, T. C., Pelc. S. R., and Tarbit, M. H. (1969). Formation and loss of DNA in intestinal epithelium. J. Cell Sci. 5, 45–55.

Arold, R., and Sandritter, W. (1967). Zytophotometrische Bestimmungen des DNS-Gehaltes von Zellkernen des Nebennierenmarkes, der Nebennierenrinde und der Schilddruse unter verschiendenen experimentellen Bedingungen. Histochemie 10, 88–97.

Atkins, N. G., and Richards, B. M. (1956). Deoxyribonucleic acid in human tumors as measured by microspectrophotometry of Feulgen stain: a comparison of tumors arising at different sites. Brit. J. Cancer 10, 769–786.

Bahr, G. F., and Wied, G. L. (1966). Cytochemical determinations of DNA and basic protein in bull spermatozoa. Ultraviolet spectrophotometry, cytophotometry, and microfluorometry. Acta Cytol. 10, 393–412.

Barton, A. D. (1954). Evidence for the biochemical stability of desoxyribosenucleic acid (DNA). *Fed. Proc. Fed. Amer. Soc. Exp. Biol.* **13**, 422.

Bergerard, J., and Tuchmann-Duplessis, H. (1953). Effet de l'hypophysectomie et action de l'hormon somatotrope sur la teneur en ADN des noyaux hépatiques chez le rat. *Compt. Rend.* **236**, 1080–1082.

Bern, H. A., Alfert, M., and Blair, S. M. (1957). Cytochemical studies of keratin formation and of epithelial metaplasia in the rodent vagina and prostate. *J. Histochem. Cytochem.* **5**, 105–119.

Boivin, A., and Vendrely, R. (1947). Sur le role possible des deux acides nucléiques dans la cellule vivante. *Experientia* **3**, 32–34.

Boivin, A. R., Vendrely, R., and Vendrely, C. (1948). L'acide désoxyribonucléique du noyau cellulaire dépositaire des caractères héréditaires; arguments d'ordre analytique. *Compt. Rend.* **226**, 1061–1063.

Boyce, R. P., and Howard-Flanders, P. (1964). Release of ultraviolet light-induced thymine dimers from DNA in E. coli K-12. *Proc. Nat. Acad. Sci. U. S.* **51**, 293–300.

Breuer, M. E., and Pavan, C. (1955). Behavior of polytene chromosomes of Rynchosciara angelae at different stages of larvae development. *Chromosoma* **7**, 371–386.

Brown, D. D., and David, I. B. (1968). Specific gene amplification in oocytes. *Science* **160**, 272–280.

Brown, G. B. (1948). Studies of purine metabolism. *Cold Spring Harbor Symp. Quant. Biol.* **13**, 43–51.

Brues, A. M., Tracy, M. M., and Cohn, W. E. (1944.) Nucleic acid of rat liver and hepatoma: their metabolic turnover in relation to growth. *J. Biol. Chem.* **155**, 619–633.

Cahn, R. D., Solursh, M., and Lasher, R. (1968). Selective gene amplification as a mechanism for stability of specialized cellular differentiation. *J. Cell Biol.* **39**, 20a.

Callan, H. G. (1963). The nature of lampbrush chromosomes. *Int. Rev. Cytol.* **15**, 1–34.

Callan, H. G., and Lloyd, L. (1960). Lampbrush chromosomes of crested newts *Triturus cristatus* (Laurenti). *Phil. Trans. Roy. Soc. London Ser. B* **243**, 135–219.

Cameron, I. L. (1970). Cell renewal in the organs and tissues of non-growing adult mouse. *Texas Rep. Biol. Med.*, in press.

Campbell, R. M., and Kosterlitz, H. W. (1947). Ribonucleic acid as a constituent of labile liver cytoplasm. *J. Physiol.* **106**, 12–13P.

Campbell, R. M., and Kosterlitz, H. W. (1948). The effect of dietary protein on the turnover of phospholipides, ribonucleic acid, and deoxyribonucleic acid in the liver. *J. Biol. Chem.* **175**, 980–990.

Campbell, R. M., and Kosterlitz, H. W. (1950). The effects of growth and sex on the composition of the liver cells of the rat. *J. Endocrinol.* **6**, 308–318.

Campbell, R. M., and Kosterlitz, H. W. (1952). The absence of dietary effects on the DNA content of liver nuclei of the adult rat. *Science* **115**, 84.

Cave, M. D., and Allen, E. R. (1969). Extra-chromosomal DNA in early stages of oogenesis in *Acheta domesticus*. *J. Cell Sci.* **4**, 593–609.

Cleaver, J. E. (1967). "Thymidine Metabolism and Cell Kinetics." Wiley, New York.

Cleaver, J. E. (1968). Defective repair replication of DNA in xeroderma pigmentosum. *Nature (London)* **218**, 652–656.

Cohn, N. S., and Van Duijn, P. (1967). Constancy of DNA content in adrenal medulla nuclei of cold-treated rats. *J. Cell Biol.* **33**, 349–354.

Crouse, H. V. (1968). The role of ecdysone in DNA-puff formation and DNA synthesis in the polytene chromosomes of *Sciara coprophila*. *Proc. Nat. Acad. Sci. U. S.* **61**, 971–978.

Crouse, H. V., and Keyl, H.-G. (1968). Extra replications in the "DNA-puffs" of Sciara coprophila. *Chromosoma* **25**, 357–364.

Davidson, E. H. (1968). "Gene Activity in Early Development." Academic Press, New York.

Davidson, J. N., and Leslie, I. (1950). Nucleic acids in relation to tissue growth: a review. *Cancer Res.* **10**, 587–594.

Davidson, J. N., Leslie, I., Smellie, R. M. S., and Thomson, R. Y. (1950). Chemical changes in the developing chick embryo related to the deoxyribonucleic acid content of the nucleus. *Biochem. J.* **46**, Proc. XL.

Den Tonkelaar, E. M., and Van Duijn, P. (1964). Photographic colorimetry as quantitative cytochemical method. II. Determination of relative amounts of DNA in cell nuclei. *Histochemie* **4**, 10–15.

Diermeir, H. F., di Stefano, H., Tepperman, J., and Bass, A. D. (1951). Effect of alloxan administration on liver nucleoproteins. *Proc. Soc. Exp. Biol. Med.* **77, 769–771**.

Deirmeier, H. F., di Stefano, H., and Bass, A. D. (1952). Effect of alloxan administration on liver DNA (desoxyribose nucleic acid). *Fed. Proc. Fed. Amer. Soc. Exp. Biol.* **11**, 338–339.

Di Stefano, H. S., Bass, A. D., Diermeier, H. F., and Tepperman, J. (1952). Nucleic acid patterns in rat liver following hypophysectomy and growth hormone administration. *Endocrinology* **51**, 386–393.

Di Stefano, H. S., Deirmeier, H. F., and Tepperman, J. (1955). Effects of growth hormone on nucleic acid and protein content of rat liver cells. *Endocrinology* **57**, 158–167.

Ely, J. O., and Ross, M. H. (1951). Desoxyribonucleic acid content of rat liver nuclei influenced by diet. *Science* **114**, 70–73.

Epstein, J. H., Fukuyama, K., and Epstein, W. L. (1968). UVL induced stimulation of DNA synthesis in hairless mouse epidermis. *J. Invest. Derm.* **51**, 445–453.

Evans, R. G., and Norman, A. (1968). Radiation stimulated incorporation of thymidine into the DNA of human lymphocytes. *Nature (London)* **217**, 455–456.

Ficq, A., and Pavan, C. (1957). Autoradiography of polytene chromosomes of *Rhynchosciara angelae* at different stages of larvae development. *Nature (London)* **180**, 983–984.

Frazer, S. C., and Davidson, J. N. (1953). Photometric estimations of deoxyribonucleic acid in individual cell nuclei. *Exp. Cell Res.* **4**, 316–332.

Fresco, J. R., Bendich, A., and Russell, P. J. (1955). Metabolic stability of deoxyribonucleic acid (DNA) in nongrowing tissue. *Fed. Proc. Fed. Amer. Soc. Exp. Biol.* **14**, 214.

Furst, S. S., Roll, P. N., and Brown, G. B. (1950). On the renewal of the purines of the desoxypentose and pentose nucleic acids. *J. Biol. Chem.* **83**, 251–266.

Gabrusewycz-Garcia, N. (1964). Cytological and autoradiographic studies in *Sciara coprophila* salivary gland chromosomes. *Chromosoma* **15**, 312–344.

Gall, J. G. (1967). Synthesis of nucleolar DNA in amphibian oocytes. *J. Cell Biol.* **35**, 43a–44a.

Gall, J. G. (1968). Differential synthesis of the genes for ribosomal RNA during amphibian oogenesis. *Proc. Nat. Acad. Sci. U. S.* **60**, 553–560.

Gall, J. G., and Johnson, W. W. (1960). Is there "metabolic" DNA in the mouse seminal vesicle? *J. Biophys. Biochem. Cytol.* **7**, 657–666.

Garcia, A. M. (1964a). Studies on DNA in leucocytes and related cells of mammals. III. The Feulgen-DNA content of human leucocytes. *Acta Histochem.* **17**, 230–345.

Garcia, A. M. (1964b). Studies on DNA in leucocytes and related cells of mammals. IV. The Feulgen-DNA content of peripheral leucocytes, megakaryocytes and other bone marrow cell types of the rabbit. *Acta Histochem.* **17**, 246–258.

Garcia, A. M. (1969a). Studies on deoxyribonucleic acid in leukocytes and related cells of mammals. VI. The Feulgen-deoxyribonucleic acid content of rabbit leukocytes after hypotonic treatment. *J. Histochem. Cytochem.* **17,** 47–55.

Garcia, A. M. (1969b). Cytophotometric studies on haploid and diploid cells with different degrees of chromatin coiling. *Ann. N. Y. Acad. Sci.* **157,** 237–249.

Garcia, A. M., and Iorio, R. (1968). Studies on DNA in leukocytes and related cells of mammals. V. The fast-green-histone and the Feulgen-DNA content of rat leukocytes. *Acta Cytol.* **12,** 46–51.

Gledhill, B. L., Gledhill, M. P., Ridgler, R., Jr., and Ringertz, N. R. (1966). Changes in deoxyribonucleoprotein during spermiogenesis in the bull. *Exp. Cell Res.* **41,** 652–665.

Hale, A. J. (1963). The leucocytes as a possible exception to the theory of deoxyribonucleic acid constancy. *J. Pathol. Bacteriol.* **85,** 311–326.

Hammarsten, E., and Hevesy, G. (1946). Rate of renewal of ribo-and desoxyribo-nucleic acids. *Acta Physiol. Scand.* **11,** 335–343.

Hanawalt, P. C., Pettijohn, D. E., Pauling, E. C., Brunk, C. F., Smith, D. W., Kanner, L. C., and Couch, J. L. (1968). Repair replication of DNA *in vivo. Cold Spring Harbor Symp. Quant. Biol.* **33,** 187–194.

Healy, G. M., Siminovitch, L., Parker, R. C., and Graham, A. F. (1956). Conservation of desoxyribonucleic acid phosphorus in animal cells propagated *in vitro. Biochim. Biophys. Acta* **20,** 425–426.

Hecht, L. T., and Potter, V. R. (1956). Nucleic acid metabolism in regenerating rat liver. I. The rate of deoxyribonucleic acid synthesis *in vivo. Cancer Res.* **16,** 988–993.

Hevesy, G., and Ottesen, J. (1943). Rate of formation of nucleic acid in the organs of the rat. *Acta Physiol. Scand.* **5,** 237–247.

Howard, E. F., and Plaut, W. (1968). Chromosomal DNA synthesis in *Drosophila melanogaster. J. Cell Biol.* **39,** 415–429.

Howard-Flanders, P. (1968). DNA repair. *Annu. Rev. Biochem.* **37,** 175–200.

Howard-Flanders, P., Rupp, W. D., Wilkins, B. M., and Cole, R. S. (1968). DNA replication and recombination after UV irradiation. *Cold Spring Harbor Symp. Quant. Biol.* **33,** 195–205.

Hughes, W. L. (1959). The metabolic stability of deoxyribonucleic acid. In "The Kinetics of Cellular Proliferation" (F. Stohlman, ed.), pp. 83–94. Grune & Stratton, New York.

Izawa, M., Allfrey, V. G., and Mirsky, A. E. (1963). Composition of the nucleus and chromosomes in the lampbrush stage of the newt oocyte. *Proc. Nat. Acad. Sci. U. S.* **50,** 811–817.

James, J. (1968). Feulgen-DNA changes in rat liver cell nuclei during the early phase of ischaemic necrosis. *Histochemie* **13,** 312–322.

Keyl, H.-G. (1963). DNS-Konstanz im Heterochromatin von *Glyptotendipes. Exp. Cell Res.* **30,** 245–247.

Keyl, H.-G. (1965). A demonstrable local and geometric increase in the chromosomal DNA of Chironomus. *Experientia* **21,** 191–193.

Kurnick, N. B., and Herskovitz, I. (1952). The estimation of polyteny in Drosophila salivary gland nuclei based on termination of deoxyribonucleic acid content. *J. Cell. Comp. Physiol.* **39,** 281–299.

Lasnitzki, I., and Pelc, S. R. (1957). Effect of 2-methylcholanthrene on DNA synthesis in mouse prostates grown *in vitro. Exp. Cell Res.* **13,** 140–146.

Leeman, L. (1959a). La teneur en DNA de la médullo-surrénale aprés splanchnicectomie bilatérale et aprés injection d'insuline chez le rat blanc. *Exp. Cell Res.* **16,** 686–688.

Leeman, L. (1959b). Deoxyribonucleic acid content of the cell nuclei in the adrenal medulla after exposure to low temperature. *Nature (London)* **183,** 1188.

Lett, J. T., Caldwell, I., Dean, C. J., and Alexander, P. (1967). Rejoining of x-ray induced breaks in the DNA of leukaemia cells. *Nature (London)* **214,** 790–792.

Leuchtenberger, C., and Leuchtenberger, R. (1960). Quantitative cytochemical studies on the relation of deoxyribonucleic acid of cells to various pathological conditions. *Biochem. Pharmacol.* **4,** 128–163.

Leuchtenberger, C., Vendrely, R., and Vendrely, C. (1951). A comparison of the content of desoxyribosenucleic acid (DNA) in isolated animal nuclei by cytochemical and chemical methods. *Proc. Nat. Acad. Sci. U. S.* **37,** 33–38.

Lima-de-Faria, A. (1962a). Progress in tritium autoradiography. *Progr. Biophys. Biophys. Chem.* **12,** 281–317.

Lima-de-Faria, A. (1962b). Metabolic DNA in *Tipula oleracea. Chromosoma* **13,** 47–59.

Lima-de-Faria, A., and Moses, M. J. (1966). Ultrastructure and cytochemistry of metabolic DNA in *Tipula. J. Cell Biol.* **30,** 177–192.

Lima-de-Faria, A., Nilsson, B., Cave, D., Puga, A., and Javorska, H. (1968). Tritium labelling and cytochemistry of extra DNA in *Acheta. Chromosoma* **25,** 1–20.

Lowe, C. U., and Rand, R. N. (1956). Alterations in biochemical composition and ribonucleic acid metabolism induced in rat liver by cortisone. *J. Biophys. Biochem. Cytol.* **2,** 331–350.

Lowe, C. U., Box, H., Venkataraman, P. R., and Sarkaria, D. S. (1959). Cytophotometric study of desoxyribonucleic acid in cortisone treated rat hepatocytes. *J. Biophys. Biochem. Cytol.* **5,** 251–255.

Macgregor, H. C. (1968). Nucleolar DNA in oocytes of *Xenopus laevis. J. Cell Sci.* **3,** 437–444.

Mayall, B. H. (1966). The detection of small differences in DNA content with microspectrophotometric techniques. *J. Cell Biol.* **31,** 74A.

Mayall, B. H. (1969). Deoxyribonucleic acid cytophotometry of stained human leukocytes. I. Differences among cell types. *J. Histochem. Cytochem.* **17,** 249.

Messier, B., and Leblond, C. P. (1960). Cell proliferation and migration as revealed by radioautography after injection of thymidine-H[3] into male rats and mice. *Amer. J. Anat.* **106,** 247–285.

Miller, O. L., Jr. (1964). Extra chromosomal and nucleolar DNA in amphibian oocytes. *J. Cell Biol.* **23,** 60a.

Miller, O. L., Jr. (1966). Structure and composition of peripheral nucleoli of salamander oocytes. *Nat. Cancer Inst. Monogr.* **23,** 53–66.

Mirsky, A. E., and Ris, H. (1947). The chemical compositon of isolated chromosomes. *J. Gen. Physiol.* **31,** 7–18.

Mirsky, A. E., and Ris, H. (1949). Variable and constant components of chromosomes. *Nature (London)* **163,** 666–667.

Nash, D., and Bell, J. (1968). Larval age and the pattern of DNA synthesis of polytene chromosomes. *Can. J. Genet. Cytol.* **10,** 82–90.

Owen, M., and MacPherson, S. (1963). Cell population kinetics of an osteogenic tissue. II. *J. Cell Biol.* **19,** 33–44.

Painter, R. B. (1968). Mechanisms of DNA repair in mammalian cells. *In* "Effects of Radiation on Cellular Proliferation and Differentiation," pp. 91–100. International Atomic Energy Agency, Vienna.

Painter, T. S. (1941). An experimental study of salivary chromosomes. *Cold Spring Harbor Symp. Quant. Biol.* **9,** 47–53.

Painter, T. S., and Taylor, A. N. (1942). Nucleic acid storage in the toad's egg. *Proc. Nat. Acad. Sci. U. S.* **28,** 311–317.

Pasteels, J., and Lison, L. (1950). Teneur des noyaux au repos en acide désoxyribo-nucléique dans different tissus chez le rat. *Compt. Rend.* **230,** 780–782.

Pavan, C. (1959). Morphological and physiological aspects of chromosomal activities. *Proc. Int. Congr. Genet. 10th, Montreal, 1958,* University of Toronto Press pp. 321–336.

Pavan, C. (1965). Nucleic acid metabolism in polytene chromosomes and the problem of differentiation. *Brookhaven Symp. Biol.* **18,** 222–241.

Pelc, S. R. (1958a). The participation of the cell nucleus and its DNA in the formation of keratin. *Exp. Cell Res. Suppl.* **6,** 97–104.

Pelc, S. R. (1958b). Nuclear uptake of labelled adenine in the seminal vesicle of the mouse. *Exp. Cell Res.* **14,** 301–315.

Pelc. S. R. (1959). Metabolic activity of DNA as shown by autoradiographs. *Lab. Invest.* **8,** 225–236.

Pelc, S. R. (1962). Incorporation of tritiated thymidine in various organs of the mouse. *Nature (London)* **193,** 793–795.

Pelc, S. R. (1963a). On the question of renewal of differentiated cells. *Exp. Cell Res.* **29,** 194–198.

Pelc, S. R. (1963b). Incorporation of labelled precursors of DNA in non-dividing cells. *In* "Cell Proliferation" (L. F. Lamerton and R. J. M. Fry, eds.), pp. 94–109. Davis, Philadelphia, Pennsylvania.

Pelc, S. R. (1964). Labelling of DNA and cell division in so called non-dividing tissues. *J. Cell Biol.* **22,** 21–28.

Pelc, S. R. (1967). Renewal of DNA in non-dividing cells and aging. *Exp. Gerontol.* **1,** 215–222.

Pelc, S. R. (1968). Turnover of DNA and function. *Nature (London)* **219,** 162–163.

Pelc, S. R., and Gahan, P. B. (1959). Incorporation of labelled thymidine in the seminal vesicle of the mouse. *Nature (London)* **183,** 335–336.

Pelc, S. R., and Howard, A. (1956). Metabolic activity of salivary gland chromosomes in *Diptera. Exp. Cell Res.* **10,** 549–552.

Pelc, S. R., and Viola-Magni, M. P. (1969). III. Decrease of labeled DNA in cells of the adrenal medulla after intermittent exposure to cold. *J. Cell Biol.* **42,** 460–468.

Perkowska, E., Macgregor, H. C., and Birnstiel, M. L. (1968). Gene amplification in the oocyte nucleus of mutant and wild-type Xenopus laevis. *Nature (London)* **217,** 649–650.

Pettijohn, D., and Hanawalt, P. (1964). Evidence for repair-replication of ultraviolet damaged DNA in bacteria. *J. Mol. Biol.* **9,** 395–410.

Plaut, W. (1963). On the replicative organization of DNA in the polytene chromosome of *Drosophila melanogaster. J. Mol. Biol.* **7,** 632–635.

Pollister, A. W., Swift, H., and Alfert, M. (1951). Studies on the desoxypentose nucleic acid content of animal nuclei. *J. Cell Comp. Physiol.* **38,** [suppl. 1], 101–119.

Rasch, E. M., Pettit, B. J., and Rasch, R. W. (1969). "Constancy versus compaction": a comparative study of DNA-Feulgen staining in blood cell nuclei of birds, amphibians, and fishes. *J. Cell Biol.* **43,** 111–112a.

Rasmussen, R. E., and Painter, R. B. (1964). Evidence for repair of ultra-vilet damaged deoxyribonucleic acid in cultured mammalian cells. *Nature (London)* **203,** 1360–1362.

Rasmussen, R. E., and Painter, R. B. (1966). Radiation-stimulated DNA synthesis in cultured mammalian cells. *J. Cell Biol.* **29,** 11–19.

Révész, L., Forssberg, A., and Klein, G. (1956). Quantitive studies on the multiplication of neoplastic cells *in vivo.* II. Metabolic stability of deoxypentose nucleic acid and the use of labeled tumor cells for the measurement of growth curves. *J. Nat. Cancer Inst.* **17,** 37–47.

Ris, H., and Mirsky, A. E. (1949). Quantitative cytochemical determination of desoxy-ribonucleic acid with the Feulgen nucleal reaction. *J. Gen. Physiol.* **33**, 125–145.

Rodman, T. C. (1968). Relationship of developmental stage to initiation of replication in polytene nuclei. *Chromosoma* **23**, 271–287.

Roels, H. (1966). "Metabolic" DNA: a cytochemical study. *Int. Rev. Cytol.* **19**, 1–34.

Roels, H., and Lagasse, A. (1961). Influence of cold stress on the dry weight of the cells nuclei ofthe adrenal medulla of the white rat. *Exp. Cell Res.* **23**, 408–409.

Rudkin, G. T., and Corlette, S. L. (1957). Disproportionate synthesis of DNA in a polytene chromosome region. *Proc. Nat. Acad. Sci. U. S.* **43**, 964–968.

Salisbury, G. W., Birge, W. J., de la Torre, L., and Lodge, J. R. (1961). Decrease in nuclear Feulgen-positive material (DNA) upon aging and *in vitro* storage of bovine spermatozoa. *J. Biophys. Biochem. Cytol.* **10**, 353–359.

Setlow, R. B., and Carrier, W. L. (1964). The disappearance of thymine dimers from DNA: An error correcting mechanism. *Proc. Nat. Acad. Sci. U. S.* **51**, 226–231.

Setlow, J. K., Randolph, M. L., Boling, M. E., Mattingly, A., Price, G., and Gordon, M. P. (1968). Repair of DNA in *Haemophilus influenzae*. II. Excision repair of single-strand breaks, defects in transformation, and host cell modification in uv-sensitive mutants. *Cold Spring Harbor Symp. Quant. Biol.* **33**, 209, 218.

Steffensen, D. M. (1963). Localization of deoxyribonucleic acid exclusively in the bands of *Drosophila* salivary chromosomes. *Proc. Int. Congr. Genet., 11th, The Hague*, 109.

Stich, H. F., and Naylor, J. M. (1958). Variation of deoxyribonucleic acid content of specific chromosome regions. *Exp. Cell Res.* **14**, 442–445.

Strauss, B. S. (1968). DNA repair mechanisms and their relation to mutation and recombination. *Curr. Topics Microbiol. Immunol.* **44**, 1–85.

Stroun, M., Charles, P., Anker, P., and Pelc, S. R. (1967). Metabolic DNA in heart and skeletal muscle and in intestine of mice. *Nature (London)* **216**, 716–717.

Swift, H. H. (1950). The desoxyribose nucleic acid content of animal nuclei. *Physiol. Zool.* **23**, 169–198.

Swift, H. (1953). Quantitative aspects of nuclear nucleoproteins. *Int. Rev. Cytol.* **2**, 1–76.

Tongiani, R., and Viola-Magni, M. P. (1969). II. Differences in adrenal medulla nuclear DNA content among rats of different strains following intermittent exposure to cold. *J. Cell Biol.* **42**, 452–459.

Vendrely, R., and Vendrely, C. (1948). La Teneur du noyeau cellulaire en acide désoxy-ribonucleique a travers des organes des individus et les espéces animales. *Experientia* **4**, 434–436.

Vendrely, R., and Vendrely, C. (1949a). Nouveaux résultats sur la teneur absolue en acide désoxyribonucleixue du noyau cellulaire. Cas particulier des érythrocytes d'Oiseau. *Compt. Rend.* **228**, 1256–1258.

Vendrely, R., and Vendrely, C. (1949b). The desoxyribonucleic acid content of nuclei of various organs in different species of animals. *Experientia* **5**, 327–329.

Vendrely, R., and Vendrely, C. (1956). The results of cytophotometry in the study of the deoxyribonucleic acid (DNA) content of the nucleus. *Int. Rev. Cytol.* **5**, 171–197.

Viola-Magni, M. P. (1965). Changes in the DNA content of adrenal medulla nuclei of rats intermittently exposed to cold. *J. Cell Biol.* **25**, 415–433.

Viola-Magni, M. P. (1966a). A radioautographic study with H^3-thymidine on adrenal medulla nuclei of rats intermittently exposed to cold. *J. Cell Biol.* **28**, 9–19.

Viola-Magni, M. P. (1966b). An analysis of DNA loss and synthesis in the rat adrenal medulla nuclei upon cold stimulation. *J. Cell Biol.* **30**, 213–225.

CHAPTER 3

Cell Proliferation and Renewal in the Mammalian Body*

Ivan L. Cameron

I. Introduction.. 45
II. Cell Proliferation and Growth during the Embryonic and Postnatal Periods... 46
III. Methods Used to Visualize and to Measure Cell Proliferation and Cell
    Renewal.. 48
    A. Mitosis and the Mitotic Index.................................. 48
    B. Use of Colchicine and Other Drugs Which Arrest Cells in the Process of
       Cell Division... 51
    C. Use of Radioautography in Combination with Tritiated Thymidine as a
       Tool for Studying the Cell Cycle, Cell Proliferation, Cell Migration, and
       Cell Renewal.. 53
IV. Classification of Cell Populations Based on Their Proliferative Behavior...... 64
V. Regulation of Cell Proliferation.................................... 74
    References.. 79

I. Introduction

The present chapter deals in large part with the renewal of cells in the body. The chapter presents information concerning (1) cell proliferation in the growing mammalian body, (2) cell renewal in the adult body, as well as (3) information concerning the stimulation of cell proliferation in non-renewing cell populations.

From the historical point of view the evidence that some cell populations in the body were capable of cell renewal was first reported at the end of the last century. In fact, Bizzozero in 1894 actually proposed that the

* Supported in part by the National Institutes of Health Grant #GM16542 and by the Morrison Trust.

various types of tissues and organs in the body could be classified on the basis of their ability to proliferate. The concept of cell renewal lay relatively dormant until it was revitalized, chiefly by the efforts of Leblond and his associates beginning in the late 1940's.

It is now generally accepted that cells replicate nuclear DNA in preparation for cell division. Thus, with the advent of tritiated thymidine, a radioactive precursor which is specifically incorporated into newly synthesized DNA, it became possible to tag those cells that are preparing for cell division. An injection of tritiated thymidine acts as a pulse of label and that tritiated thymidine which is not incorporated into DNA is rapidly cleared from the circulation. Because tritium has such a soft β-ray the use of tritiated thymidine became a good and useful tool for high resolution radioautographic studies. These facts and techniques now enable us to visualize and trace the fate of those cells which were in the process of nuclear DNA synthesis at the time that tritiated thymidine was injected. The use of this radioautographic technique has led to a rapid accumulation of information concerning the renewal of cells in the various tissues and organs of the mammalian body.

This chapter summarizes evidence that many of the cell populations of the body are in a dynamic state of cell renewal. It includes a temporal analysis of the phases of the cell cycle in numerous cell populations. The chapter contains a discussion of the classification of the cell populations based on their proliferation behavior. It also includes evidence that there are some cell populations that do not normally demonstrate proliferative activity but are capable of initiating cell proliferation upon appropriate stimulation. The chapter ends with the presentation of a model which can be used to explain the control of cell proliferation in the body.

II. Cell Proliferation and Growth during the Embryonic and Postnatal Periods

It is known that the adult mammal is composed of many types of cell populations, all of which have their origin in a single fertilized ovum. Thus, it follows that a great deal of cell proliferation and cell differentiation takes place during development. Starting with the zygote, three basic factors should be considered in order to interpret the growth that takes place in the tissue and organs of the developing animal. These three factors are increase in number of cells, increase in size of individual cells, and increase of extracellular materials. Shortly after the fertilization of a mammalian egg a series of cell divisions occurs (cleavage). This cell cleavage leads to the formation of a solid ball of cells called a morula. The formation of the morula is not accompanied by growth in mass; thus the number of cells increase while size of the individual cells decrease. At about the time that the young embryo reaches the stage of development where it can implant itself into the uterine wall of the mother the relationship between cell growth and cell division changes in such a way that the cells increase in size between cell divisions, and thus a net increase in the mass of the embryos results. These facts are meant to illustrate the importance of understanding growth as measured by such factors as cell number, cell size, and amount of extracellular material.

Once the developing embryo reaches macroscopic size it becomes relatively easy to measure growth on a weight basis, and when the embryo reaches a somewhat larger size the weight gain of individual organs and tissues also becomes measurable. In order to determine the number of cells in the rat embryo, Enesco and Leblond (1962) measured the total amount of DNA of the embryo and then divided by 6.2 pg ($\mu\mu$g) to obtain a calculation of the number of nuclei in the embryo. This calculation is based on the fact that the amount of DNA in the nucleus of a diploid mammalian cell is relatively constant (6.2 pg) in most of the organs and tissues of mammals whatever their age or species (see Vendrely and Vendrely, 1956; Enesco and Leblond, 1962; also Chapter 2). Since there is only one nucleus in most of the cells of the embryo, the number of nuclei approximates the number of cells. Enesco and Leblond (1962) have carried out a number of such measurements and calculations in the developing rat. Their findings indicate that a 12-day rat embryo contains 50 million cells. Calculating backwards to the time of the newly fertilized egg they estimate that about 25 cell generations must have occurred, which suggests that the cell number doubled about twice per day during this period. They indicate that there are 3 billion cells in the rat at the time of birth (after 22 days of gestation); thus they calculate that during the last 10 days of embryonic life only about six cell generations occur. In these calculations one must also assume that there is no cell death and that all cells continue to divide at a regular interval during the period of study. By 90 days after birth there are about 67 billion cells in the rat.

Knowing both the weight of the animal (or the organ or the tissue, as the case may be), as well as the number of cell nuclei in each case, Enesco and Leblond have calculated the weight of material associated with one nucleus at various stages during the development of the rat. The weight per nucleus value varies with the size of cells and with the amount of extracellular materials. Careful analysis of the organs (pancreas, kidney, liver, testis, and adrenal) and of the tissues (striated muscle, epididymal fat pad, and skin) of the young growing rat allowed recognition of three sequential phases or periods of neonatal development: (1) From birth until 17 days of age there was a period of rapid cell proliferation with no change in cell size. (2) From 17 to 48 days of age addition of new cells continues in all organs and tissues while the size of the cells also increases in most of the organs and increases rapidly in the tissues (striated muscle and epididymal fat). (3) From 48 to 90 days the addition of cells to the organs and tissues slows down and in some cases stops completely. Some cell populations such as fat and striated muscle continue to enlarge in cell size but in most of the organs no further increase in cell size was recognized.

Although observations such as those described above give us general information on the growth and cellularity of the organs and tissues of of developing animals, they tell us very little or nothing about the specific types of cells which are involved in cell growth and cell proliferation. Indeed, most of the organs and tissues contain at least two different cell types, including (1) the supporting cells, such as blood vessels and connective tissues elements, and (2) the parenchymal cells which give the organ or tissue its functional specificity (for example, acinar cells of the pancreas, glandular cells of the endocrines, etc.). Neither do these observations by themselves give us any indication if there is a significant loss or renewal of specific cells during the animals' development. The next section of this chapter deals with methods which allow us to visualize and describe the specific cell types involved in cell proliferation as well as to measure the rates of cell proliferation in the various organs and tissues. The resulting information can then be used to classify the specific cell populations based on their proliferative behavior.

III. Methods Used to Visualize and to Measure Cell Proliferation and Cell Renewal

A. Mitosis and the Mitotic Index

The presence of mitotic figures in the histological sections of the organs and tissues of the body indicate that cell proliferation is occurring. Over the years it has come to be generally accepted that new mammalian cells arise exclusively by the process of mitosis. Mitosis occurs not only in the growing organs and tissues but also in a number of organs and tissues of the adult body.

Some of the organs and tissues where mitotic figures are frequently observed are as follows: The hair follicle, which in man assures the continued elongation of the hair shaft; the basal or the deepest cell layer of the epidermis where a basement membrane separates the basal cells from the dermis and does not allow migration of newborn epidermal cells into the dermal area. On the average half of the newborn basal cells move away from the basement membrane and eventually move through the various layers of epidermis toward the surface where they are eventually sloughed off. Another morphological area of intense cell proliferation is found in the small intestine. Mitotic figures are frequent in the crypts of Lieberkühn whereas no epithelial cell mitosis occurs on the slender villi that project away from the crypts toward the lumen of the intestine. Long ago Bizzozero (1892) observed that mitosis in the crypts was very active and he suggested that some of the newborn cells must push up onto the epithelium of the villi; he therefore postulated that the cells were migrating away from the site of their birth. This proposition was extended, refined, and confirmed by the observations of Leblond and Stevens (1948) and others.

Other areas of intense mitotic activity occur in the male and female reproductive system. For example, spermatogonia in the seminiferous tubules of the testis continually display high mitotic activity which leads to the formation of spermatocytes, which then mature into spermatids and eventually become mature spermatozoa. Tissues of the female reproductive system demonstrate a periodic occurrence of numerous mitotic figures at several sites. For example, mitotic activity is periodically high in the developing overian follicles, in the corpus luteum, in the endometrium of the uterus, and the epithelium of the vagina. This mitotic activity is cyclic and correlated with the estrous or menstrual cycle, as the case may be.

Other sites of rapid cell proliferation are found in the bone marrow where stem cells such as the erythroblasts produce a continuous supply of erythrocytes which are released for use in the peripheral circulation. Other cells of the bone marrow also demonstrate considerable mitotic activity including the granulocytes, monocytes, lymphocytes, and the megakaryocytes. Lymphatic tissue, such as thymus, lymph nodes, tonsils, and spleen, show considerable mitotic activity which leads to a constant production of lymphocytes.

Visualization of mitotic activity is always evidence of cell proliferation but in the nongrowing organ or tissue it also suggests that cell renewal is occurring. The next question is: How can one obtain information about the renewal or turnover of the cell population by observations of mitotic frequency in histological sections? Estimates of cell population turnover time can be accomplished by determining the "mitotic index." The mitotic index is the percentage of cells in the population that are in some stage of mitosis at a given time. Cell population turnover time is defined as the time necessary to replace the number of cells present in the entire population. Caution must be exercised in identifying the stages of mitosis that are being counted. Some authors count only the metaphase stage of mitosis, and because metaphase is only one stage of mitosis, it is obvious that those who use metaphases counts will have a lower index of mitosis than those that include all stages of mitosis in the mitotic index estimate.

One necessary and important assumption or parameter needs to be established before turnover time estimates can be made from the mitotic index. This assumption concerns the duration of the mitotic event itself. Unless there is some independent measure of the duration of mitosis, one must assume a value which is generally less than 1 hour and more than 1/2 hour. Obviously the accuracy of the duration of mitosis is of great importance to the final estimates of the cell population turnover time. Indeed, it should be pointed out that not all cell populations spend the same duration of time in mitosis (Leblond, 1959).

If one is dealing with mixed populations of cells, identification of specific cell types at the time of mitosis is difficult. This difficulty arises from the loss of cytological detail which occurs at the time of mitosis. Another problem arises if a dividing nucleus is smaller or larger than the rest of the cells in the population. The size of the dividing cell will influence the frequency of appearance in histological sections. For example, if the cell swells at the time of mitosis one may expect to encounter a higher mitotic frequency in histological section than if the cell did not change in size at the time of mitosis. This size factor can be corrected for by simple procedure (see Abercrombie, 1946). Other factors that are sometimes overlooked concern variations in the duration of mitosis due to the experimental conditions itself, or upon the time of day that the animal is killed. Indeed, many tissues of the body demonstrate a daily variation in the mitotic rate (diurnal rhythm). One can see from the above discussion that if the duration of mitosis is known, and if the mitotic index has been properly, determined, one can estimate the turnover time of any given cell population. It should be pointed out the turnover time in such cases refers to a condition of dynamic equilibrium where cell birth and cell death and loss are balanced in the cell population and where every cell in the population is involved in the renewal process. Thus the turnover time of the whole cell population will approximately equal the mean life span of any given cell in the population. In such an ideal situation if the mitotic index of a cell population is 5% and the duration of mitosis is 1 hour, the turnover time is caluclated to be 20 hours. Thus the use of the mitotic index to determine turnover time in cell populations which are not increasing in cell number (i.e., nongrowing populations) is relatively simple and straightforward, if all of the assumptions are valid.

B. USE OF COLCHICINE AND OTHER DRUGS WHICH ARREST CELLS IN THE PROCESS OF CELL DIVISION

The poleward separation of mitotic chromosomes which starts at the end of metaphase and comprises the anaphase stage of mitosis is dependent on a functional mitotic spindle apparatus. The group of chemicals called spindle poisons causes the dissolution of the spindle apparatus and arrests cells at the metaphase stage of mitosis. Spindle poisons are relatively specific in their action and allow the collection of increased numbers of arrested metaphase figures with time after injection. In general, a spindle poison is allowed to act for 3 to 6 hours after injection. The number of cells in metaphase then increases considerably above normal. For example, if one considers that mitosis lasts approximately 1/2 hour, a collection of 4 hours metaphase figures would be expected to increase the mitotic index about seven- to eightfold.

One of the assumptions that must be made or determined when using mitotic spindle poison is that the posion itself does not disrupt the normal entry of cells into mitosis. This assumption is tested by determining the percentage of cells in prophase throughout the period of drug administration. If the number of prophases stays constant while the percentage of metaphases increases linearly, one may reasonably assume that no detrimental effect has occurred prior to the spindle disruption phase. Figure 1 shows the results of an experiment to determine the duration of mitosis and the turnover time in the ileum of white rats. In this experiment 260-gm male rats were killed at various intervals after colchicine injection (Stevens-Hooper, 1961). The percentages of cells in prophase, metaphse, anaphase, and telophase at increasing intervals of time are shown on this figure. The figure demonstrates that metaphases collect in a roughly linear fashion with time up to 3 hours, whereas the percentage of cells in prophase stays relatively constant throughout the period of study. One also notices that the percentage of anaphase and telophase of cells decreases to zero value by 3 hours, which is to be expected if all cells are inhibited at the metaphase stage. Two problems often encountered in the use of colchicine are that not all tissues will respond in the same manner to the use of the spindle poison, and that some tissues demonstrate a lag between the administration of the drug and its mitotic inhibitory ability. Another factor is that cells stalled in metaphase for 4 or more hours may begin degeneration so that they are no longer recognized and scored as mitotic cells. Indeed, with increased time one might expect normal mitotic feedback mechanisms to sense the lack of cell proliferation and to influence the normal cell renewal process.

The epidermis, corneal epithelium, esophageal epithelium, and other

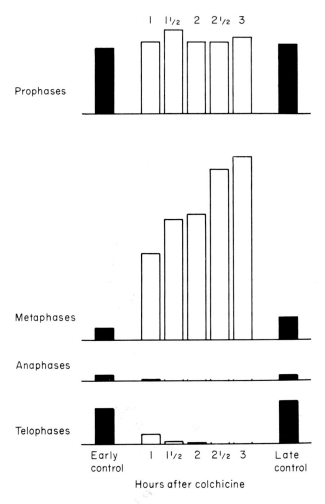

Fig. 1. Data of Stevens-Hooper (1961) on the frequency of mitotic division in the ileum of the white rat, controls (black columns) and at various time intervals after colchicine injection (white columns). The data show no significant change in the frequency of prophases, a progressive increase in the number of metaphases, and a decrease in the number of anaphases and telophases with time. The figure was first published by Leblond (1959) and is reproduced here with permission of the authors and Grune and Stratton N. Y. (see text for details).

cell populations of the body have been shown to demonstrate a striking diurnal rhythm in their mitotic activity, it is therefore important to average the mitotic rate over a 24-hour period in order to obtain an accurate estimate of turnover time in the cell population. One way to do this is to take six groups of animals and kill them at 4-hour intervals over a 24-hour period. Each group of animals is injected with colchicine, or one of the other mitotic spindle poisons, 4 hours prior to the time of killing. In Fig. 1 the duration of individual mitotic stages was calculated as follows: P equals the percent of normal frequency of that stage while the percentage of blocked metaphases has a frequency of Q, and T is the duration of minutes after injection. The formula PT/Q can then be used to calculate the mitotic duration. Using the formula for the data of Fig. 1, one can calculate that the duration of prophase equals 1–1.5 hours, metaphase about 20 minutes, telophase about 47 minutes, and the entire duration of mitosis is estimated at about 2 hours.

Other methods have been used to determine cell turnover and renewal; for example, von Volksman (1950) injected india ink into the basal layer of epidermis; with time the india ink carbon particles reached the epidermal surface. Presumably the particles were carried up with the cells which were displaced from the basal layers. Greulich and Leblond (1953) were perhaps the first to use radioautography techniques to illustrate turnover of the epidermis. Their studies showed that radioactive bicarbonate was rapidly incorporated into macromolecular material in the basal layer of epidermal cells; and with time the radioactivity was found in successively higher layers. The epidermis was, therefore, considered a renewal cell population where the cells are born in the basal cell layer; then some of the newborn cells stay behind to give rise to new stem or progenitor cells while other cells pass up through the successive layers to differentiate and to eventually die and be lost at the surface. As reported below, later studies using more specific isotope precursors have confirmed these early reports.

Another technique that has been used to study cell turnover is to destroy a cell population such as the seminiferous epithelium of the testis by x-ray irradiation and then measure the time necessary to restore the epithelium. This gives a good estimate of the epithelial turnover time (Oakberg, 1956). Similar radiation recovery studies have also been used on blood cells and intestinal epithelium (Patt and Quastler, 1963).

C. Use of Radioautography in Combination with Tritiated Thymidine as a Tool for Studying the Cell Cycle, Cell Proliferation, Cell Migration, and Cell Renewal

Various isotope precursors have been used to label the nuclear DNA of proliferating cells. The earlier precursors include ^{32}P-phosphate and ^{14}C-adenine, but none of these earlier precursors have the advantages that can be obtained by use of ^{14}C- or ^{3}H-labeled thymidine. Tritiated thymidine is especially useful for radioautographic studies because it gives such high radioautographic resolution. Tritiated thymidine is specifically incorporated into the DNA of those cells which are replicating their nuclear DNA in preparation for cell division. When an animal such as rat, mouse, or man is injected interperitoneally, subcutaneously, or intravenously with tritiated thymidine, the isotope is rapidly distributed about the body. Every cell that is in the process of nuclear DNA replication will incorporate the tritiated thymidine into the newly synthesized DNA. The remainder of tritiated thymidine which is not immediately used in the synthesis of DNA is rapidly catabolized from the body pool. Thus, a single injection of tritiated thymidine acts as a pulse of radioisotope, labeling all of those cells in the process of DNA synthesis and no others. It is generally conceded that the nuclear DNA of cells is a stable molecule which is conserved in that cell until the cell dies or is killed. Thus, the use of tritiated thymidine for studying the cell cycle, cell proliferation, and cell renewal in the tissues of most mammals is a powerful tool.

A number of assumptions have to be made concerning the specificity of tritiated thymidine as well as the stability of nuclear DNA; however, these assumptions have already been stated and tested in a number of cases. These assumptions can be summarized as follows: Cells which replicate DNA proceed through the cell cycle to divide. The amount of tritiated thymidine used as a tracer does not alter the normal proliferation kinetics of the animal and is not toxic to the experimental animal. Every cell which is synthesizing DNA during the time the animal is given the tritiated thymidine is labeled. The method of precursor administration does not of itself alter the cell proliferation and renewal characteristics of the animal. These and other assumptions have been dealt with in great detail by Cleaver (1967), and one may say that although the assumptions are not completely true for every tissue and organ population of the body, the exceptions are small and pitfalls can be avoided by a good understanding and proper experimental design. There are enough studies to indicate that high dosages of tritiated thymidine can cause radiation damage and that there is a mechanism by which the breakdown products of labeled DNA are reused in other cells. However, in general it can be stated that the assumptions are sufficiently well founded and tested so that tritiated thymidine in combination with radioautography can be used as an exceptionally reliable and excellent tool for studying cell proliferation.

Figure 2A diagrammatically represents a cell population. The shaded area in this figure represents the percentage of cells in the process of DNA synthesis at the time of pulse exposure to tritiated thymidine. Figures 2B, C, and D indicate what happens to the labeled cohort of cells with time after the pulse labeling. Realize first that the only cytologically observable

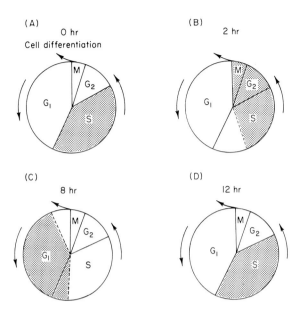

Fɪɢ. 2. Dissection of the phases of a 12-hour cell cycle based on instantaneous pulse labeling of cells in nuclear DNA synthesis with tritiated thymidine. M = mitosis phase, G_1—pre-DNA synthetic phase, S = phase of DNA synthesis, G_2 = post DNA synthetic phase. For simplicity it is assumed that all cells in the population behave exactly alike (that is, there is no variability between individual cells). Time increases between A and D. The cohort of labeled cells in the cell population is indicated by the shaded area. Notice that the cohort of labeled cells moves around the cycle with time. To determine the duration of the phases of the cell cycle, radioautographs of frequently taken samples are prepared and analyzed. One complete cell cycle occurs between A and D. The arrow leading away from the cell cycle shows that in steady-state renewal cell populations half of the cells actually leave the generative cell compartment and differentiate.

event of the cell cycle is that of mitosis and then imagine the cohort of labeled cells must pass through the various stages of the cell cycle. In practice, samples are frequently taken from the entire cell population and then radioautographs of the samples are prepared. In the early samples all of the dividing cells are unlabeled. With time, however, the cohort of labeled cells reaches division and the radioautographic samples now show labeled dividing cells. One can therefore obtain an estimate of the duration of time between injection of the isotope and the appearance of labeled dividing cells. After a longer duration of time all the cells that were originally labeled have passed through mitosis and the percentage of labeled dividing cells drops. At this same time those cells which were in a stage prior to the synthesis of DNA at the time of tritiated thymidine injection (the G_1 stage)

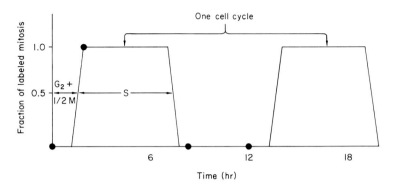

FIG. 3. Fraction of labeled mitosis as a function of time after an instantaneous pulse label of tritiated thymidine. This graph shows an idealized cell population with no variability between individual cells. For comparison the four time values from Fig. 2 are plotted on this figure.

are now coming through cell division. One can easily imagine that the cycle goes on for several cell cycles and if one continues to sample and to plot a graph indicating the percent of labeled cells in mitosis, data of the type shown in Fig. 3 will be obtained. A second peak in percent of labeled mitotic cells indicates that the cohort of labeled cells have come around the cycle a second time. Figure 3 indicates that the cohort of labeled cells has gone through more than one division. One can obtain an estimate of the total duration of the cell cycle by determining the distance between the first peak of labeled dividing cells and the second peak of labeled dividing cells. In Fig. 3 the cell cycle as estimated by the peak-to-peak technique is approximately 12 hours or 720 minutes. A dissection of the cell cycle into individual phases can be obtained from this type of data. For example, the duration of time between the labeling and the appearance of 50% of labeled dividing cells is an estimate of the G_2 plus one-half of the mitosis time. In a nongrowing cell renewal population, that is, a cell population under steady-state renewal conditions such as occurs in the duodenal crypts, one may estimate the duration of mitosis by knowing the mitotic index and the cell cycle duration. For example, if the mitotic index is 6% the fraction of the cell population in mitosis is 0.06. Thus one can multiply the fraction of cells in mitosis times the duration of the cell cycle (720 minutes in this case) to get the duration of mitosis (43.2 minutes).This calculation assumes that all of the cells in the population are actually members of the progenitor cell population pool. This assumption is not always warranted and care should be taken to define the actual progenitor cell population as precisely as possible (for a detailed discussion see Leblond *et al.*, 1964). To get an approximate estimate of the G_2 time one need only subtract half the duration of mitosis (for example, in this case half of 43.2 minutes equals 21.6 minutes) from the G_2 plus one-half of mitosis time value. The time between 50% on the ascending slope of the first curve and the 50% on the descending slope is an estimate of the mean duration of DNA synthesis of the population of cells, which is 5 hours in this example. By subtracting the duration of the G_2 phase, the S phase, and mitosis phase from the total cell cycle time one gets an estimate of the duration of the G_1 portion of the cell cycle.

Numerous other methods for estimating the cell cycle duration and the phases of the cell cycle in populations of mammalian cells have been devised. The reader is referred to Nachtwey and Cameron (1968) for a tabular summary of these methods or Cleaver (1967) for a discussion of the use of the various methods.

It is not the aim of this chapter to describe and make comparisons of the various methods of determining the duration of the phases of the cell cycle. It is important, however, that each investigator be aware of the criticisms and problems that can be encountered by the use of the various techniques. For those readers who are interested in pursuing the use of the various methods and in making comparisons, the following references may be helpful: Thrasher (1966), Cleaver (1967), Feinendegen (1967), Nachtwey and Cameron (1968).

The duration of the phases of the cell cycle has been determined in a large number of cell populations both *in vivo* and *in vitro*. Before continuing our discussion of cell renewal, it seems important to analyze the cell cycle data obtained on the various cell populations in living mammals. Table I lists the duration of the phases of the cell cycle in a number of cell populations in several species of mammals. Analysis of the data from Table I allows one to draw a number of general conclusions regarding the constancy and variation in the duration of the cell cycle phases. Obviously, the total cell cycle time is extremely variable; the shortest duration is approximately 7 hours, the longer durations are 100 hours or more. A most interesting generalization can be made about the duration of the S phase. Here the range of values is concentrated between 5 and 8 hours. The only notable exceptions are the ear epidermis in the mouse, certain types of spermatogonia, and certain cancer and tumor cell populations. The duration of the S phase seems to be somewhat shorter in embryonic and young growing animals than it is in mature animals; however, the difference is not striking. It seems possible that the exceptionally long duration of S phase as found in the ear epidermis and spermatogonia is related to the lower body temperatures found in these regions of the mammalian body. It is apparent in the case of the Ehrlich's ascites tumor cells that the dura-

TABLE I

DURATIONS OF THE PHASES OF THE CELL CYCLE *in Vivo*

Animal and cell population	G_1 (hr)	S (hr)	G_2 (hr)	M (hr)	T (hr)	Ref.[a]
From studies on adult mice						
Duodenum crypt	4.5–5.5	5	~2.0	—	11.5	26
Duodenum crypt	3.6	7.4	1.5	0.7	13	43
Jejunum crypt	1–2	8	1.5	—	11.2	15
Small intestinal crypt	9.0	7.5	1.5	1.0	19	29
Forestomach epithelium	30	9–10	1–2	1–2	43	46
Uterine epithelium (castrated)	31.5	8.5	1.0	1.0	42	10
Uterine epithelium (castrated and estrogen treated)	18.5	5.5	1.0	1.0	26	10
Vaginal epithelium (estrus)	15.4	7.6	~1	~1	25	42
(diestrus)	62.5	7.5	~1	~1	72	42
Hair follicle	2.8	6.0	2.0	—	10.8	19
Ear epidermis	~22 days	30	6.5	3.8	24 days	39
Ear epidermis	7–80	18	3.5	2.0	30–100	33
Antibody forming	1	6.8	0.7	0.5	9	36
Tongue epithelium	17	7	2	1.0	27	5
Esophagus epithelium	171.5	6.9	1.5	1	181	6
Esophagus epithelium	75	7.2	4.1	0.7	87	30
Abdominal epidermis	139	6.2	5.3	0.5	151	30
Forestomach	156	6.9	4.1	1.0	168	30
Adrenal cortex	1863	7.5	—	—	1875	30
From studies on young mice (20 gm)						
Duodenum crypt	5	5.9–6.7	1.0	1.3	10–13.3	17
Jejunum crypt	2.8–3.8	5.8–6.1	0.9	0.6	10.1–13.8	17
Ileum crypt	—	6.2–6.3	0.6	0.8	10.5–11.4	17
Colon crypt	13.5	6.3–6.4	1.1	0.7	21.7	17
Pharynx epithelium	75	5.0–6.0	1.2	1.8	84	17
From studies on mice embryos						
Embryonic tail	1.2	6.3	1.5	—	9	45
Embryo neural tube	2.3	4.0	0.8	1.3	8.4	21
Trophoblasts of 8-day placenta	—	7.0	—	—	9.4	4
Trophoblasts of 12-day placenta	—	6.5	—	—	15	4
From studies on mouse gonadal cells						
Spermatogonia type AII	7.5	7.5	14.0	—	28–30	32
Spermatogonia type AIII	8.0	8.0	11.0	—	26–28	32
Spermatogonia type AIV	9.5	13.0	8.0	—	30–31	32
Spermatogonia type (intermediate)	8.5	14.0	6.0	—	26–28	32
Spermatogonia B	10.5	18.0	4.5	—	29–30	32

TABLE I
DURATIONS OF THE PHASES OF THE CELL CYCLE *in Vivo*—*continued*

Animal and cell population	G_1 (hr)	S (hr)	G_2 (hr)	M (hr)	T (hr)	Ref.[a]
From studies on mouse cancer cells						
Ehrlich ascites	3	8.5	1.5	5.1	18	9
Ehrlich ascites	—	9	—	1	24	25
Ehrlich ascites (5-day diploid)	4–4.5	6.5–7	4	—	15	8
Ehrlich ascites (5-day tetraploid)	~0.17	13–14	6	~1	~38	8
Ehrlich ascites	11	19	5.5	0.5	36	1
Ehrlich ascites (1-day)	0	6.0	1.2	0.8	8	23
Ehrlich ascites (4-day)	—	13	3	—	17	23
Ehrlich ascites (2-day)	2.5	9	—	—	13	14
Ehrlich ascites (4-day)	6	9	—	—	17	14
Ehrlich ascites (12-days	15	21	—	—	40	14
Yoshida sarcoma	2	6.5	3–7	1	11–18	7
Transplantable fibrosarcoma	3.5	5.5	1.0	1	11	13
Epithelial tumor	7.0	6.5	2.0	—	15.5	18
Spindle tumor	3.0	12.0	1.0	—	16	18
Mammary tumor	7 hr–3 days	9–13	1–4	—	1–3.5 days	31
Leukemia L5178Y	1.5	6.9–7.4	2	—	11.5	8
DBAG tumor	3	12	1	—	16	18
DBAH tumor	7.5	6	2.5	—	16	18
From studies on adult rats						
Duodenum crypt	1	8.2	1	—	9.4	28
Jejunum crypt	1	7.7	1	—	9.0	28
Jejunum (crypt bottom, 1–6)	3.5	8.5	1	1	14	3
Jejunum (crypt center, 13–15)	2.0	6.5	1	1	10.5	3
Jejunum (crypt top, 22+)	1.5	6.5	1	1	10	3
Ileum cryptl	1	7.8	1	—	8.9	28
Incisor ameloblasts	16	8	2.5	0.8	27.3	37
Spleen germinal center	—	4.5	1	—	13.4	12
From studies on newborn rats and regenerating rat liver						
Small intestinal crypt	5.6	5.6	1.7	0.6	13.5	30
Salivary gland	8.1	5.7	1.2	0.8	15.8	30
Epidermis	11.0	5.5	1.7	0.7	18.9	30
Tongue epithelium	15.6	5.6	1.6	0.5	23.3	30
Tongue muscle	23.5	6.8	1.9	0.3	32.5	30
Interscapular brown fat	27.2	5.6	1.5	0.4	34.7	30
Cartilage	30.7	7.3	1.8	0.7	40.5	30
Pancreas acinar	31.6	6.2	1.4	1.2	40.4	30
Cardiac muscle	29.9	8	3.3	8	42	30
Growing bone, metaphysis	22	8	2	~1	32	20

TABLE I

DURATIONS OF THE PHASES OF THE CELL CYCLE *in Vivo*—*continued*

Animal and cell population	G_1 (hr)	S (hr)	G_2 (hr)	M (hr)	T (hr)	Ref.[a]
From studies on newborn rats and regenerating rat liver (continued)						
Endosteum	45	8	3	~1	57	20
Periosteum	188	8	3	~1	200	20
Liver (1-day-old rat)	5.0	7.0	1.5	0.3	18.8	34
Liver (3-weeks-old rat)	9.0	9.0	1.8	1.7	21.5	34
Liver (8-week-old rat)	28.0	16.0	1.8	1.7	47.5	34
Liver (regenerating)	—	7.0	4.0	—	—	38
Liver (regenerating)	—	7.2	2–4	1–1.5	—	41
Liver (regenerating)	3.5	8	2.5	1	15	11
From studies on rat cancer cells						
BICR/M1 tumor	8	8	3	—	19	40
BICR/M2 tumor	50	10	3	—	63	40
Yoshida ascites hepatoma	19	24	1	2	45	16
From studies on other mammals						
Hamster pouch epithelium	128	10.2	1.6	2.6	142	35
Hamster pouch epithelium	8.7–11.9	6.1	2.2	0.5	17.5	35
Hamster jejunum crypt	1–1.75	6.7	4.9	—	13.0	2
Hamster jejunum crypt (tumor)	1–1.5	6.1	4.6	—	12.0	2
Hamster fibrosarcoma	~4	8	4	~1	17	8
Canine erythroid precursors	2	6	1	1	10	24
Canine myeloid precursors	2.5	5.5	1	1	10	22
Human colon crypt	~10	11–14	1	—	24	27
Bovine lymphocytes	~0.8	5	~0.5	~0.7	~7	44

[a] Key to references:

1. Baserga (1965)
2. Betts *et al.* (1966)
3. Cairnie *et al.* (1965)
4. Cameron (1964)
5. Cameron (1966)
6. Cameron and Greulich (1963)
7. Chigasaki (1963)
8. Defendi and Manson (1963)
9. Edwards *et al.* (1960)
10. Epifanova (1966)
11. Fabrikant (1968)
12. Fliendner *et al.* (1964)
13. Frindel *et al.* (1967)
14. Frindel *et al.* (1969)
15. Fry *et al.* (1961)
16. Gaetani *et al.* (1964)
17. Galand (1967)
18. Goldfeder (1965a, b)
19. Griem (1966)
20. Young (1962)
21. Kauffman (1966)
22. Lala (unpublished), see Cleaver (1967)
23. Lala and Patt (1966)
24. Lala *et al.* (1966)
25. Lennartz and Maurer (1964)

tion of the cell cycle increases during the growth period of the tumor. It also becomes apparent that the S phase is related to the duration of culture growth period in this tumor cell population. Indeed, the most recent studies by Frindel *et al.* (1969) indicate that the S phase increases as the population density of the Ehrlich's ascites tumor cells increases. This observation helps explain the large variability of S phase values as reported in earlier studies on Ehrlich's ascites tumors. The cells in the growing rat liver also appears to increase the duration of S phase as the liver reaches a growth plateau in the adult state. The majority of reports indicate that mitosis lasts between 0.5 to 1.0 hour. The variability in the G_2 phase is noticeable. In general, it appears that the shorter the cell cycle duration the shorter the G_2 phase; however, the greatest variability in the cell cycle obviously occurs during the G_1 phase. Here the duration of the G_1 value goes from essentially zero in some very rapidly dividing cell populations to many hours and even days in other cell populations.

It therefore seems safe to generalize that the combined durations of the S and G_2 and the mitosis phases are relatively constant and that the G_1 phase is the portion of the cell cycle which contains the greatest amount of temporal variability. Not only is the duration of the G_1 phase variable between different cell types but it is also the most variable within one particular cell population when grown under variations in environmental conditions such as nutrition, pH, and cell population density.

Even though there are exceptions to the general rule that the combined duration of S and G_2 is constant, one is reasonably safe in saying that most somatic cells of the living mammal show a relative constancy of the S and G_2 phase. It appears, therefore, that initiation of DNA synthesis is a controlling point in the growth of cell populations. One may anticipate that the factors which control cell proliferation operate at some point prior to the

---

Footnotes to Table I continued

26. Lesher *et al.* (1961)
27. Lipkin *et al.* (1962)
28. Loran and Crocker (1963)
29. Matsuzawa and Wilson (1964)
30. Maurer *et al.* (1965)
31. Mendelsohn *et al.* (1960)
32. Monesi (1962)
33. Pilgrim *et al.* (1966)
34. Post and Hoffman (1964)
35. Reiskin and Mendelsohn (1964)
36. Sado and Makinodan (1964)

37. Sasaki (1965)
38. Shea (1964)
39. Sherman *et al.* (1961)
40. Steel *et al.* (1966)
41. Stocker and Pfeifer (1967)
42. Thrasher *et al.* (1967)
43. Thrasher and Greulich (1965)
44. Vincent *et al.* (1969)
45. Wimber (1963)
46. Wolfsberg (1964)

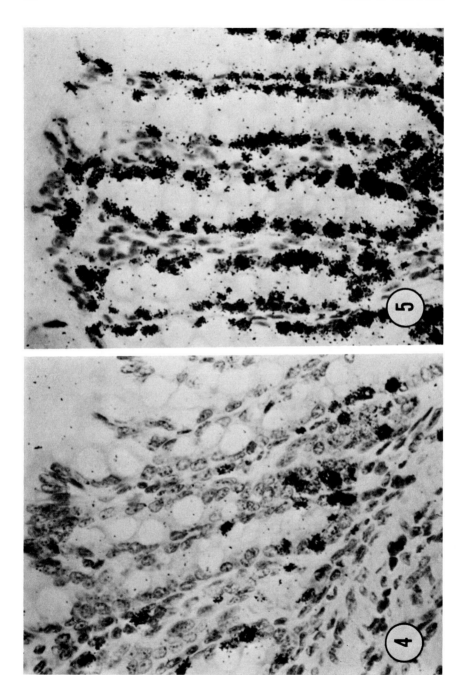

onset of the DNA synthetic phase. It also appears that initiation of DNA synthesis leads almost inevitably to cell mitosis and cell proliferation.

Because the duration of mitosis usually lasts between 0.5 to 1 hour, the task of finding mitotic cells in slowly renewing cell populations of the body is oftentimes difficult or impossible. Since the average duration of nuclear DNA synthesis requires between 5 and 8 hours in almost every mammalian cell population where it has been studied (see Table I), one may inject an organism with tritiated thymidine, kill the animal shortly thereafter, prepare radioautographs of the tissues, and then expect to find about 10 times more labeled cells than dividing cells. It therefore becomes clear that the "DNA synthetic index" as compared to the "mitotic index" is a more sensitive indicator of cell proliferation.

Even by use of the DNA synthetic index one still cannot adequately study cell renewal and growth in very slowly renewing tissues. It would therefore be extermely advantageous to have a technique that would allow labeling of every cell coming into the S phase during long periods of time. A requirement of this technique would be that it does not disturb normal cell proliferation in the animal. In the design of such an experiment, one must take into account that the shortest duration of DNA synthesis would be expected to be more than 4 hours. Thus, an isotope such as tritiated thymidine would have to be administered about once every 4 to 6 hours in order to label every cell coming into DNA synthesis and, therefore cell division. Some of the possible schedules and route of isotope administration are (1) intraperitoneal injection of the isotope at least once every 4 to 6 hours, (2) an indwelling catheter and pump which would chronically administer the isotope, or (3) administration of the isotope in the animal's drinking water. In the latter case one must assume that the animal actually drinks enough water during each 4- to 6-hour period of the day to give an adequate labeling to all of the cells in the animal's body. An experiment was designed to test each of these three possible routes of isotope administration on cell proliferation activity (Cameron, 1968). The results of this experiment show that injection of the isotope every 4 hours over a 1-day period, as well as administration via an indwelling catheter, caused a significant decrease in the number of colchicine-collected metaphases in

---

FIG. 4. Radioautograph from the mucosa of the colon of an animal given tritiated thymidine for 1 hour, then killed. Labeled nuclei are confined to the area toward the bottom of the crypts. 600 ×.

FIG. 5. Radioautograph of the mucosa of the colon of an animal given tritiated thymidine in its drinking water for 48 hours, then killed. All but the most superficial mucosal cell nuclei are labeled. 600 ×.

the progenitor cells of the esophageal epithelium compared to the number of collected metaphases in animals that were given free access to drinking water. Thus, one may conclude from these results that giving isotope by repeated injections or by an indwelling catheter has a significant inhibitory effect on the number of proliferating cells. It is evident from these experimental data that administration of tritiated thymidine in the animal's drinking water is a method of choice.

Knowing that precursor administered via the drinking water is a method of choice, it is also necessary to establish the drinking habits of the animals during one full day. Cameron (1968) has measured the drinking habits of his mice and indicates that under his experimental conditions the animals drink at least once every 4 hours, consuming on the average 1 ml of water every 4 hours. The range of water consumed in any 4-hour period was from 0.60 to 1.72 ml. Thus, it was concluded that administration of tritiated thymidine in the drinking water is frequent enough and in adequate and regular amounts to be a practical means of iostope administration. Thus, by this method one can label every cell coming into DNA synthesis and cell division during long periods of time.

Not only can tritiated thymidine radioautography be used as a method to detect the site of those cells undergoing nuclear DNA synthesis at the time of isotope administration, but it can also be used to follow the migratory fate of these labeled cells with time. For example, Fig.4 illustrates the labeling pattern in the descending colon 1 hour after administration of tritiated thymidine. At this early time the zone of maximum proliferation is shown to be toward the bottom of the intestinal crypts. After 2 days of isotope administration, as illustrated in Fig. 5, essentially all of the mucosal cell nuclei are labeled with the exception of those at the extreme surface. After 3 days all of the columnar absorptive and mucous goblet cells of the colon mucosa had a labeled nucleus. Clearly the mucosal cells are born deep in the crypts of the colon and migrate to the surface and are extruded in less than 3 days.

IV. Classification of Cell Populations Based on Their Proliferative Behavior

It has been established that a number of cell populations in the body continue to demonstrate cell renewal in the adult nongrowing mammal. As was pointed out early in the chapter, such *renewal cell populations* include the epidermis; the epithelial cells lining the alimentary tract; the hemopoietic cells of bone marrow and lymphatic cells of thymus, spleen, lymph node; as well as various reproductive system cell populations, such as the spermatogonia in the seminiferous tubules of the testis and the uterine and vaginal epithelial cell populations in the female. In opposition to these renewal cell popualtions it is also clear that various neurons in the central and peripheral nervous system, as well as cardiac muscle cells of adult mammals, demonstrate no cell proliferation whatsoever in the adult state; these cell populations have therefore, been classified as nonrenewal or *static cell populations*. As reported in Section II of this chapter, Leblond (1964) and Enesco and Leblond (1962) have devised a third classification category for cell populations taken from growing animals. These cell populations include the parenchymal cells of the pancreas, kidney, liver, salivary gland, heart, skeletal muscle, etc. Such cell populations as these are termed *expanding cell populations*.

Tables II and III give a summary of turnover times of cell populations in the mammalian body as taken from the literature. Analysis of Tables II and III permits one to make several generalizations concerning cell renewal in the adult body. The most rapidly renewing cell populations include those of the bone marrow, the hemopoietic and lymphopoietic cells in the bone marrow, and those epithelial cell populations along the gastrointestinal tract. The rate of cell turnover in these populations varies from about 1.4 days to about 5 days. The esophagus and the mucosa of the oral cavity demonstrates cell turnover times of about 3 to 10 days. The epidermis and cornea show turnover times varying from 7 days in the case of the corneal epithelium to as much as 100 days in epidermal populations. In general, however, cell renewal in the Malpighian layer of the skin (with one exception) varies from 10 to 45 days. Comparison of the turnover time values of the epidermis, oral cavity, and alimentary tract, where the reported turnover time values are perhaps most reliable, suggests that there is a variability in turnover times depending on the technique used. The colchicine-collected metaphase technique yields values which are generally a little longer than the tritiated thymidine DNA synthetic index method. The reason for such discrepancies is not readily apparent. Comparison of the values between mouse, man, rat, cat, and dog suggests that there is little species difference in the turnover times of those cell populations that can be compared. However, in the male genital system there appears to be an increase in the duration of spermatogenesis when one compares mice, rat, and man, respectively. Comparison of the values in the respiratory tract and urinary tract on Tables II and III suggests a considerable amount of variability between the various methods and reports. The author has analyzed the original reports and suggests that one possible difference in the values reported by Bertalanffy and Lau (1962a) and others (Leblond *et al.*, 1955) as opposed to those reported by Blenkinsopp (1967, 1969) is

TABLE II

TURNOVER TIMES OF CELL POPULATIONS IN THE MAMMALIAN BODY

Cell population	Species	Technique	Turnover time (days)	Ref.[a]
Epidermis (Malpighian layer) and cornea				
Ear	Rat	Colchicine	34	1
	Mouse	Mitotic index	28	16
Abdomen	Rat	Colchicine	19	1
	Man	Mitotic index	100	15
Thorax	Man	^{3}HT[b]	45	30
Plantar	Rat	Colchicine	19.1	26
Forearm	Man	Mitotic index	13	15
Cheek	Rat	^{3}HT	10	11
Sebaceous gland	Rat	Colchicine	7.8	1
Corneal epithelium	Man	^{3}HT	7	31
	Rat	Colchicine	6.9	5
Oral cavity				
Buccal mucosa	Rat	Colchicine	4.3	2
	Rabbit	Colchicine	8.6	14
	Rat	Colchicine	13.8	27
	Rat	^{3}HT	4.1	11
Tongue				
Superior surface	Rat	^{3}HT	3.2–3.5	11
	Rat	Colchicine	4.9	2
Inferior surface	Rat	^{3}HT	5.1	11
	Rat	Colchicine	5.7	2
Gingiva, free	Rat	^{3}HT	5.6	11
Attached gingiva	Rat	^{3}HT	5.8	11
	Rat	Colchicine	44	27
Epithelial cuff	Rat	^{3}HT	11	27
Crevicular gingiva	Rat	Colchicine	16	27
Crestal gingiva	Rat	Colchicine	22	27
Hard palate	Rat	Colchicine	14.8	27
	Rat	^{3}HT	4.3	11
Soft palate	Rat	^{3}HT	5.2	11
Alimentary tract				
Esophagus	Rat	Colchicine	8.8–11.6	2
Stomach				
Fundus	Rat	Colchicine	3–6.4	25
Surface epithelium	Rat	Colchicine	2.9	25
Mucous neck cells	Rat	Colchicine	6.4	25
Pylorus				
Surface epithelium	Rat	Colchicine	1.9	19
glands	Rat	Colchicine	1.8	19
Cardia	Rat	Colchicine	9.1	2
Duodenum	Rat	Colchicine	1.6	17
	Man	Colchicine	2	7
	Cat	Colchicine	2.2	22

TABLE II

TURNOVER TIMES OF CELL POPULATIONS IN THE MAMMALIAN BODY—*Continued*

Cell population	Species	Technique	Turnover time (days)	Ref.[a]
Jejunum	Rat	Colchicine	1.3	2
	Cat	Colchicine	2.7	22
	Dog	³HT	2.8	32
Ileum	Rat	Colchicine	1.4	17
	Cat	Colchicine	2.7	22
	Dog	³HT	2.6	32
Colon	Rat	Colchicine	10	2
	Rat	³HT	3	33
	Man	³HT	4–6	35
Rectum	Man	³HT	6–8	34
	Rat	Colchicine	6.2	2
Liver				
Hepatocytes	Rat	³HT	400–450	21
Respiratory tract				
Trachea	Rat	Colchicine	47.6	19
	Rat	³HT	111	8
Bronchus	Rat	Colchicine	27	19
Main bronchus	Rat	³HT	126	8
Intermediate bronchus	Rat	³HT	167	8
Bronchioles	Rat	³HT	200	8
Lung				
Nonvacuolated	Rat	Colchicine	8	4
Vacuolated alveolar cells	Mouse	³HT	21	36
	Rat	Colchicine	29	4
Urogenital tract				
Urinary system				
Bladder				
Superficial cells	Rat	Colchicine	33	18
Deep cells	Rat	Colchicine	64	18
Superficial cells	Rat	³HT	~112	9
Deep cells	Rat	³HT	~333	9
Ureter	Rat	Colchicine	49	3
Female genital system				
Vagina	Rat	Colchicine	3.9	6
	Mouse	³HT	4	28
Cervix	Rat	Colchicine	5.5	6
Cervix	Man	³HT	5.7	24
endometrium				
Surface epithelium	Rat	Colchicine	5.9	6
Glands	Rat	Colchicine	10.4	6
Uterine tube	Rat	Colchicine	40.6	6
Ovarian germinal				
Epithelium	Rat	Colchicine	32.8	6

TABLE II

TURNOVER TIMES OF CELL POPULATIONS IN THE MAMMALIAN BODY—*Continued*

Cell population	Species	Technique	Turnover time (days)	Ref.[a]
Urogenital tract continued				
Male genital system				
Duration of spermatogenesis	Mouse	Radiation recovery	34	23
	Rat	³HT	48	10
	Man	³HT	74	13
Lymphopoietic and hemopoietic tissues				
Small lymphocytes				
Bone marrow	Rat	³HT	~4	12
Thymus	Rat	³HT	~7	12
Spleen	Rat	3HT	~15	12
Mesenteric lymph node	Rat	³HT	20	12
Bone marrow	Rat (erythrocyte series)	Mitotic index	2.5	29
	Rat (erythrocyte series)	³HT	2.3	20
	Rat (myclocyte series)	Mitotic index	1.4	29

[a] Key to references:

1. Bertalanffy (1957)
2. Bertalanffy (1960)
3. Bertalanffy and Lau (1962)
4. Bertalanffy and Leblond (1953)
5. Bertalanffy and Lau (1962)
6. Bertalanffy and Lau (1963)
7. Bertalanffy and Nagy (1961)
8. Blenkinsopp (1967)
9. Blenkinsopp (1969)
10. Clermont *et al.* (1959)
11. Cutright and Bauer (1967)
12. Everett and Tyler (Caffrey) (1967)
13. Heller and Clermont (1963)
14. Henry *et al.* (1952)
15. Katzberg (1952)
16. Knowlton and Widner (1950)
17. Leblond and Stevens (1948)
18. Leblond *et al.* (1955)
19. Leblond and Walker (1956)
20. Lord (1968)
21. MacDonald (1961)
22. McMinn (1964)
23. Oakberg (1956)
24. Richart (1963)
25. Stevens and Leblond (1953)
26. Storey and Leblond (1951)
27. Trott and Gorenstein (1963)
28. Walker (1960)
29. Widner *et al.* (1951)
30. Johnson *et al.* (1960)
31. Hanna *et al.* (1961)
32. Knudtson *et al.* (1962)
33. Messier (1960)
34. Cole and McKalen (1961)
35. Cole and McKalen (1963)
36. Spencer and Shorter (1962)

[b] ³HT = tritiated thymidine.

TABLE III

TURNOVER TIMES OF MOUSE CELL POPULATIONS FROM TRITIATED THYMIDINE
RADIOAUTOGRAPHY STUDIES[a]

Cell population	Turnover time in days		
	Cameron	Reported in literature	Ref.[b]
Epidermis (Malpighian layer)			
Dorsal	7–14	6	7
Ear	14–21	22	13
Abdomen	7–14	—	
Plantar	10	—	
Dermal connective tissue	60	—	
Cornea	5–7	6–7	6
Buccal epithelium	5–7	4.4	9
		6	8
Tongue epithelium			
Superior surface	4	4	12
		4	16
		5	3
Pocket of filiform			
Papillae	7–9	—	
Inferior surface	4–5	8	8
Gingiva of molar tooth			
Oral surface	7	10–12	1
Down growing	5–7	10–12	1
Epithelial attachment	4	1–5	1
Soft palate	5	—	
Esophagus, epithelium	5	5	3
Lamina propria cells	125	—	
Stomach			
Forestomach epithelium	4	4	12
Fundus or body			
Surface epithelium	4	4	12
		5	3
Parietal cells	60	—	
Zymogenic (chief) cells	>600	—	
Duodenum, epithelium	3	2–3	3
		2	12
		2	5
Colon, epithelium	2–3	3	12
Respiratory epithelium			
Nasal	100	—	
Olfactory	100	—	
Trachea	90	>58	2
		20	8
Bronchus	130	18	8
		21	15
Bronchioles	100	59	8
Alveolar wall cells of lung	125	71–460	14
		>21	15

69

TABLE III

TURNOVER TIMES OF MOUSE CELL POPULATIONS FROM TRITIATED THYMIDINE
RADIOAUTOGRAPHY STUDIES[a]—*Continued*

Cell population	Turnover time in days		
	Cameron	Reported in literature	Ref.[b]
Kidney			
Proximal and distal tubules	190	—	
Collecting tubules	170	—	
Glomerular tuft	170	—	
Parietal layer of Bowman's capsule	140	—	
Interstitial cells	165	—	
Transitional epithelium of urinary system	>700	Very long	18 or 19
Liver			
hepatocytes	480–620	—	
Littoral cells	160	—	
Pancreas			
Acinar cells	520	—	
Islet cells	150	—	
Submandibular gland			
Alveolar cells	185	—	
Glandular tubular cells	210	—	
Adrenal cortex			
Zona glomerulosa	90–125	30–90	17
Zona fasciculata	380	373	17
zona reticularis	560–1040	>386	17
Interstitial cells	90	—	
Thymus			
Cortex cells	7	3–4	20
Medulla cells	14	—	
Spleen			
White pulp, spenic nodule without pale germinal center	14–21	—	
Pale germinal center	1–2	—	
Red pulp, areas along trabeculae and just beneath capsule	3	—	
Megakaryocytes maturation time	2–3	2–3	11
Erythrocyte maturation time (from proliferative stage to orthochromatic stage)	1–2	—	
Sperm maturation time (from resting primary spermatocyte to mature spermatozoa)	21–30	25 (radiation recovery study)	10
Epididymal epithelium (head part)	380	—	

because Bertalanffy used younger animals still in a state of growth, whereas Blenkinsopp used older animals where growth was minimal. Thus, one suspects that the values obtained by Bertalanffy and others in general yield values that are somewhat shorter owing to growth factors. Table III lists comparative turnover times of mouse cell populations from tritiated thymidine radioautographic studies. Here the turnover time values of a recent report by Cameron (1970) and a number of other reports from the literature on mice cell populations are compared. Once again, a comparison of the turnover time values in the epidermis, the oral cavity, and the alimentary tract shows similar values. Many of the values for cell populations with turnover times of less than 30 days as reported by Cameron (1970) are actually determinations of the time required for 100% of the cell population to become labeled. These turnover time values are, therefore, not estimates but direct determinations from the data. On the other hand, the values of turnover times of more than 30 days are usually estimates determined from such data as are shown in Fig. 6. Figure 6 is actually a plot showing the percentage increase in the number of cells with labeled nuclei as a function of time. Because the percentage of labeled cells appears to increase almost linearly with time, it was assumed that this linear increase would continue. Thus, to get the turnover time values which are listed in Table III under the column marked Cameron, the increase in percent of cells with labeled nuclei was extrapolated to the point where it reached 100%. As can be seen in Table III, the turnover time values for many of the slowly renewing cell populations have not been estimated previously, for example, cell populations in the kidney, liver, pancreas, submandibular gland, as well as cell populations such as the dermal connective tissue and the lamina propria cells in the alimentary tract.

Footnotes to Table III.

  [a] Taken from Cameron (1970).
  [b] Key to references:

1. Beagrie and Skougaard (1962)	11. Odell *et al.* (1969)
2. Blenkinsopp (1967)	12. Oehlert and Buchner (1961)
3. Creamer *et al.* (1961)	13. Sherman *et al.* (1961)
4. Fabrikant (1968)	14. Simnet and Heppleston (1966)
5. Fry *et al.* (1962)	15. Spencer and Shorter (1962)
6. Hanna and O'Brien (1960)	16. Toto and Ojha (1962)
7. Iverson *et al.* (1968)	17. Walker and Rennels (1961)
8. Koburg (1962)	18. Blenkinsopp (1969)
9. Meyer zum Gottesberg and Koburg (1963)	19. Levi *et al.* (1969)
10. Oakberg (1956)	20. Fabrikant (1968)

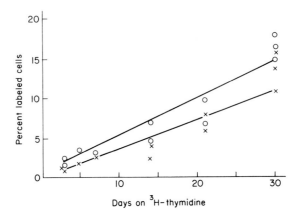

FIG. 6. The percentage of cells with labeled nuclei in radioautographs of the submandibular gland is plotted against time. The mice were given tritiated thymidine in their drinking water. Each mark represents one mouse. The open circles (○) represent the alveolar cell population and the (×) marks represent the glandular tubular cell population. The percentage of labeled cell nuclei appears to be increasing at a roughly linear rate in both cell populations, although perhaps somewhat faster in the case of the alveolar cells. It is estimated that 100% of the alveolar cells would be labeled after about 185 days and 100% of the glandular tubular cells would be labeled in about 210 days.

Cameron (1970) has reclassified the cell populations of the adult nongrowing mouse body based on their proliferative behavior and the reclassification scheme is listed in Table IV. The difference between this classification scheme and prior classification schemes is based on the fact that only adult nongrowing mice or mammals are included in this classification procedure. The categories include *static cell populations; renewal cell populations* broken down into two distinct subcategories: a rapidly renewing category, where cell turnover occurs in less than 30 days, and a slow turnover category, where cell turnover requires more than 30 days but occurs within the average life span of the animal. A third major category includes cell populations which demonstrate *some cell proliferation* but at such a slow rate that not all of the cells renew during the life span of the animal This category includes a goodly number of cell populations which demonstrated some, but so little cell proliferation that they did not seem to fit in the renewal cell category at all. These cell populations included such examples as the glandular cells in the medulla of the adrenal gland, smooth muscles cells of the alimentary tract, the transitional epithelium of the urinary tract, the zymogenic or chief cells in the stomach, the interstitial cells of Leydig in the testis, the glial cells in the

TABLE IV

CLASSIFICATION OF CELL POPULATIONS OF ADULT NONGROWING MICE BASED ON THEIR PROLIFERATIVE BEHAVIOR[a]

Type of population	Examples
1. Static	Neurons of all types Cardiac muscle cells Molar odontoblasts Sertoli cells of the testis
2. Renewing	
A. Rapid (renewal in less than 30 days)	Epidermis Cornea Oral epithelium, tongue, buccal, gingival, esophageal Surface epithelium of stomach, both nonglandular and glandular Intestinal epithelium Seminiferous epithelium Hemopoietic cells Lymphopoietic cells
B. Slow (renewal in more than 30 days but less than the mean life span of the animal)	Respiratory tract epithelium Cell populations in the kidney cortex Hepatocytes and littoral cells Pancreatic acinar and islet cells Salivary gland cells Adrenal cortex cells Dermal connective tissue cells Lamina propria cells of the alimentary tract Parietal cells of the stomach
3. Cell populations which demonstrate some cell proliferation but at such a slow rate that not all of the cells renew during the life span of the animal	Harderian gland cells Smooth muscle cells Glial cells in most areas of the brian Brown fat cells Osteocytes Interstitial cells of Leydig Zymogenic (chief) cells of the stomach Kidney medullary tubule cells Transitional epithelial cells Adrenal medulla cells
4. Neoplastic	Solid tumor cells Metastatic cancer cells

[a] Modified from Cameron (1970).

brain, the brown fat cells, the osteocytes, the Harderian gland cells, and others. A fourth major classification originally proposed by Leblond in 1964 is included for completeness. This category includes *neoplastic cell populations* and includes cell populations which arise after the adult state has been obtained and where cell birth is going on more rapidly than cell death and cell loss occurs. Obviously the net effect is a new growth situation, hence the term neoplastic. This category includes solid tumor cells and metastatic cancer cells.

It is clear from the comparative analysis of Tables II and III that most of the work has been done on mice and rats, and that comparative studies on primates and man in particular would answer a number of interesting and practical questions. For example, are the turnover time values in rats and mice comparable to those in a long-lived animal such as man. Specifically one might ask the question: If the hepatocytes and acinar cells in the pancreas renew more often than every 2 years in mice and rats, do they also renew at this rate in man? If so, one would expect that about 30 renewals of the cell population of the hepatocytes and pancreatic acinar cells would occur during the life span of man.

It is anticipated that the use of the constant labeling techniques either by isotope administration in the drinking water or perhaps by an infusion technique may add a great deal of information to our future knowledge of cell turnover and its control in the body.

V. Regulation of Cell Proliferation

Several adult mammalian tissues have been shown to undergo a daily fluctuation in mitotic activity. The highest rate of mitosis occurs during periods of rest or sleep. The tissues which show this diurnal mitotic cycle include the epidermis, the corneal epithelium, and the oral epithelium. Care should be taken to make sure that variations in mitotic counts are reflecting variation in mitotic rate and not just variations in mitotic duration. Data from colchicine-collected mitotic figures are perhaps the most reliable in such diurnal experiments. Bullough (1965) believes that the diurnal rhythm is related to epinephrine concentration in the bloodstream which is high during periods of wakefulness and low during sleep periods. Indeed, Bullough considers epinephrine the most potent epidermal mitotic inhibitor known.

Table V lists a number of examples of tissues and organs which respond to proliferative stimuli of one sort or another. Several generalizations and conclusions can be drawn from an analysis of the data of Table V. First of

TABLE V

SOME EXAMPLES OF STIMULATED CELL PROLIFERATION RESPONSES IN THE TISSUES AND ORGANS OF MAMMALS[a]

Tissue or organ	Species	Type of stimulus	Time before proliferative response (hr)		Ref.[b]
			DNA synthesis	Mitosis	
Skin, ear epidermis	Mouse	Incision wound >0.1 mm	4	12	7
Cornea epithelium	Rabbit	Superficial wound CO_2 laser, 2 mm	<6		10
Tympanic membrane	Guinea pig	Perforation with blunt probe		10–12	14
Lens epithelium	Rabbit	Incision wound	14–16	~23	6
Tongue epithelium		Incision wound	<12		3
Liver, hepatocytes	Rat	Partial hepatectomy	15	22	5
Littoral cells		Partial hepatectomy	20	30	5
Gall bladder mucosa	Cat	Scraping		24	13
Gall bladder mucosa	Guinea pig	Ligation of the bile duct		24	9
Trachea epithelium	Rat	Scraping		24	17
Kidney, tubules	Rat	Unilateral nephrectomy	24	36	15
Connective tissue	Rat	Unilateral nephrectomy	~48	57	15
Kidney tubules	Rat	Ischemia	20–30		16
Bladder mucosa	Mouse	Carcinogen (ENS) injection	14–16	24–36	11
Bladder mucosa	Cat	Scraping, 0.75 cm areas		24	12
Uterine epithelium	Castrated female mouse	Estrone		24	4
Spleen	Mouse	Erythropoietin	17		8
Salivary gland	Rat Mouse	Isoproterenol Injection	20		1, 2

[a] Adapted from Baserga (1968).

[b] Key to references:

1. Barka (1965)
2. Baserga (1966)
3. Block et al. (1963)
4. Epifanova (1966)
5. Grisham (1962)
6. Harding and Srinivasan (1961)
7. Hell and Cruickshank (1963)
8. Hodgson (1967)
9. Jacoby (1953)
10. Lehmiller (1970)
11. Levi et al. (1969)
12. McMinn and Johnson (1955)
13. McMinn and Johnson (1957)
14. McMinn and Taylor (1966)
15. Phillips and Leong (1967)
16. Stocker (1966)
17. Wilhelm (1953)
18. Williams (1961)

all, it is apparent that both rapidly renewing as well as slowly renewing cell populations are included in the table. The rapidly renewing tissue cell populations, i.e., epidermis, corneal epithelium, tympanic membrane, and tongue epithelium show the earliest proliferative response to the stimulus. Twelve hours or less is all the time that is required for these cell populations to demonstrate an overt burst of mitotic activity. With the exception of the spleen all of the other tissue cell populations fall into a more slowly renewing class. Most of these slowly renewing cell populations require about 24 hours before they demonstrate a burst of mitotic activity. When one compares those cases where both a stimulation of DNA synthesis and a mitotic response is reported, it becomes apparent that about 10 hours elapse between the beginning of cellular DNA synthesis and the burst of mitosis. This temporal value is in good agreement with most of the combined S and G_2 phase duration values reported in Table I. It appears likely that all of the examples listed in Table V respond to the stimulus by initiating events that lead to cellular DNA synthesis, wihch is inevitably followed by mitosis in about 10 hours. In fact, the table shows that the time period between the stimulus and the DNA response can vary from 4 hours or less to more than half a day. It becomes clear that all types of stimuli cause the cells to initiate events that lead to nuclear DNA synthesis, which then leads to cell division. Once again, this suggests that the control of cell division *in vivo* normally operates at a point prior to nuclear DNA replication.

The control of cellular growth and proliferation is of considerable interest to our understanding of cell renewal and to an understanding of the healing and repair processes. Several individuals and groups of workers have put forth models to explain the control of cell proliferation which operates in the body. Many of these models are based on the assumption that each specific cell population of the body produces a substance which regulates its own proliferative activity. Any model dealing with the control of cell proliferation must take into account several established experimental facts. First, it must account for the fact that cell renewal and differentiation continue in some cell population of the adult organism and that in such cases cell birth is balanced by cell differentiation and eventually by cell loss. It must also explain the fact that increased wear and tear, for instance, in the epidermis, brings about hyperplasia of the germinal cells (Iverson and Elgjo, 1967). Another fact concerns the specificity of compensatory organ regeneration as is known to occur in the liver and in several other organs and tissues. For example, if a portion of the liver is removed, the remaining portion of the liver, and only the liver, begins a compensatory cell proliferation response. The importance of recognizing that the other organs and tissues do not show an increased proliferative response is paramount.

Thus, removal of a portion of the liver causes a specific stimulatory or perhaps, anti-inhibitory response in the remaining portion of liver. Although not all of the factors controlling liver regeneration are known, most authors agree that a specific hormonal factor is involved in compensatory regeneration (see Bucher, 1964). As indicated in Table V the hepatocytes of the liver respond first and only later do the nonhepatocyte (littoral) cell populations of the liver respond to the stimulus. Thus, not only do the parenchymal cells of an organ or tissue respond specifically but the specificity also extends to the stroma and the capillary portion of the particular regenerating organ. This author is concerned that in all too many cases the organ specificity of a regenerative response is assumed rather than experimentally verified.

The most prevalent models of cell proliferation control involve negative feedback circuits where a specific substance is made by an organ and is then constantly released to feed back and inhibit the proliferative cells of that particular cell population. The basis for these models comes from the concept of mechanical governors devised by engineers long ago. The most

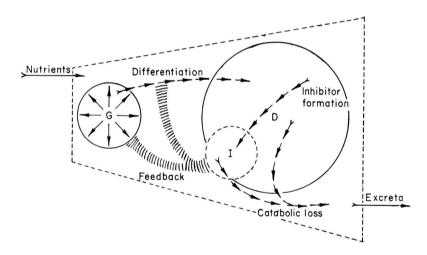

FIG. 7. shows the main features of the Weiss-Kavanau model of growth control (1957). G means generative compartment, D means differentiating compartment, I means inhibiting principle. In this model cells from the generative compartment are transferred to the differentiated compartment, and from there lost by catabolism. The differentiated compartment produces an inhibitor substance which diffuses back and probably regulates both the cell proliferative activity of the generative compartment as well as the rate of cell differentiation. This model can be used to explain the experimental findings concerning the regulation of cell proliferation in the cell populations of the mammalian body. The figure is reproduced by courtesy of the authors and *J. Gen. Physiol.*

comprehensive model of growth and proliferation control is that published by Weiss and Kavanau in 1957. Figure 7 shows the main features of the Weiss-Kavanau model. Cells from a generative compartment eventually differentiate into a functional compartment and may then be lost from this functionally differentiated compartment by processes of migration, death, and/or catabolism. The differentiated compartment produces a specific inhibitor substance which controls cell proliferation in the generative compartment. Several terms have been applied to this specific inhibitor substance, including such names as antitemplate, chalone, and growth inhibitor. Although various authors may have slightly different interpretations for the meaning of the inhibitor substance the principle of action is essentially the same in all cases; hence the differentiated mass produces an inhibitor which diffuses or is transported back and regulates the rate of cell proliferation in the generative compartment and may also regulate the rate of transfer of the generative cells to the differentiated cell compartment. The specific feedback inhibitor substance is organ specific in its action. This model accounts for essentially all the of experimental data including the cell proliferation and differentiation processes which occur in normally renewing epidermis or in epidermis which is subjected to increased wear and tear. The model can also be used to explain the compensatory organ regeneration (as described below) as well as to explain normal organ growth control. In support of the model, Bullough (1967) reports success in extracting from the epidermis an antimitotic chemical messenger which he calls the epidermal chalone. He regards this material to be the specific substance controlling epidermal mitotic activity. He also reports this substance to be epidermal specific but not species specific. The identifying and characterizing of the various types of tissue-specific inhibitor substances in the body is a promising area for future research.

The model of cell proliferation control can also be used to explain neoplastic cell populations. One simply postulates that cancer or tumor cells have lost their ability to respond to the specific inhibitor substance that normally controls their proliferative activity. Thus, it becomes apparent that as our knowledge and understanding of the mechanism which control normal cell proliferation continue to grow, we shall eventually come to understand cancer.

There appear to be two or three major levels of mitogenic control operating in the body. For instance, local trauma by means of an incision made in the epidermis or by means of puncturing an ear drum leads to a local reaction and increased mitotic activity in the local area of trauma. The model of proliferative control can be used to explain such a reaction. For example, the local trauma causes removal, loss, or damage to a portion of the differentiated cell population which normally produces the inhibitor substance; thus the trauma in some way reduces the production of epidermal inhibitor substance which in its turn allows the generative cells to increase their proliferative rate until such time as the differentiated mass has again been regenerated and can produce enough inhibitor substance to reduce the cell proliferative response. If the wounds are small, the reaction is localized and does not involve the epidermis in distant parts of the body. Because the epidermis is normally undergoing some mitotic activity the response to the trauma is comparatively rapid.

A second level of proliferative control acts via the blood stream and appears to operate in cases of compensatory organ regeneration, which, for example, occurs after removal of one member of a pair of organs, i.e., a kidney, an adrenal gland, or a specific salivary gland. By removing one of the paired organs the production of inhibitor has been reduced to about half the original value. In this case the lack of organ-specific inhibitor substance in the bloodstream is sensed by the remaining organ. This organ then responds by increased cell proliferation, eventually leading to more differentiated cells which then produce more inhibitor substance, which eventually slows and stops the proliferative response.

A third level of proliferative control includes general systemic control factors. This level of control would generally operate through the *milieu interieur* and might include such conditions as general body temperature, level of epinephrine in the blood, hormones which operate at the systemic level (e.g., stromatotropic hormone), as well as the general nutritional state of the animal.

In summary it is clear that overall control of growth and cell proliferation is brought about by a complex series of interactions. It should always be kept in mind that several levels of mitogenic control may operate simultaneously in the mammalian body.

REFERENCES

Abercrombie, M. (1946). Estimation of nuclear populations from microtome sections. *Anat. Rec.* **94,** 239.

Barka, T. (1965). Stimulation of DNA synthesis by isoproterenol in the salivary gland. *Exp. Cell Res.* **39,** 355.

Baserga, R. (1965). The relationship of the cell cycle to tumor growth and control of cell division: A review. *Cancer Res.* **25,** 581.

Baserga, R. (1966). Inhibition of stimulation of DNA synthesis by isoproperenol in submandibular glands of mice. *Life Sci.* **5,** 2033.

Baserga, R. (1968). Biochemistry of the cell cycle: A review. *Cell Tissue Kinet.* **1,** 167.

Beagrie, G. S., and Skougaard, M.R. (1962). Observations on the life cycle of the gingival epithelial cells of mice as revealed by autoradiography. *Acta Odontol. Scand.* **20,** 15.

Bertalanffy, F. D. (1957). Mitotic activity and renewal rate of sebaceous gland cells in the rat. *Anat. Rec.* **129,** 231.

Bertalanffy, F. D. (1960). Mitotic rates and renewal times of the digestive tract epithelia in the rat. *Acta Anat.* **40**, 130.

Bertalanffy, F. D., and Lau, C. (1962a). Cell renewal. *Int. Rev. Cytol.* **13**, 357.

Bertalanffy, F. D., and Lau, C. (1962b). Mitotic rate and renewal time of the corneal epithelium in the rat. *Arch. Ophthalmol.* **68**, 546.

Bertalanffy, F. D., and Lau, C. (1963). Mitotic rates, renewal times, and cytodynamics of the female genital tract epithelia in the rat. *Acta Anat.* **54**, 39.

Bertalanffy, F. D., and Leblond, C. P. (1953). The continuous renewal of the two types of alveolar cells in the lung of the rat. *Anat. Rec.* **115**, 515.

Bertalanffy, F. D., and Nagy, K. P. (1961). Mitotic activity and renewal rate of the epithelial cells of human duodenum. *Acta Anat.* **45**, 362.

Betts, A., Sewall, E. L., and Taguay, R. (1966). The effect of necrosis and tumor on the cell kinetics of small bowel. *Cancer Res.* **26**, 898.

Bizzozero, G. (1892). Über die Schlauchförmigen Drüsen des Magendarmkanals und ihr Vertoltnis zum Oberflächenepithel. *Arch. Mikrosk. Anat. Entwicklungsmech.* **40**, 325.

Bizzozero, G. (1894). *Brit. Med. J.* **1**, 728. cited by R. J. Goss *in* "Control of Cellular Growth in Adult Organisms" (H. Teir and T. Rytömaa, eds.), p. 4. Academic Press, New York, 1967.

Blenkinsopp, W. K. (1967). Proliferation of respiratory tract epithelium in the rat. *Exp. Cell Res.* **46**, 144.

Blenkinsopp, W. K. (1969). Cell proliferation in the epithelium of the esophagus, trachea and ureter in mice. *J. Cell Sci.* **5**, 393.

Block, P., Seiter, I., and Oehlert, W. (1963). Autoradiographic studies of the initial cellular responses to injury. *Exp. Cell Res.* **30**, 311.

Bucher, N. L. R. (1964). Regeneration of mammalian liver. *Int. Rev. Cytol.* **15**, 245.

Bullough, W. S. (1965). Mitotic and functional homeostasis: A speculative review. *Cancer Res.* **25**, 1683.

Bullough, W. S. (1967). "The Evolution of Differentiation," p. 103. Academic Press, New York.

Cairnie, A. B., Lamerton, L. F., and Steel, G. G. (1965). Cell proliferation studies in the intestinal epithelium of the rat. *Exp. Cell Res.* **39**, 528.

Cameron, I. L. (1964). Is the duration of DNA synthesis in somatic cells of mammals and birds a constant? *J. Cell Biol.* **20**, 185.

Cameron, I. L. (1966). Cell proliferation, migration and specialization in the epithelium of the mouse tongue. *J. Exp. Zool.* **163**, 271.

Cameron, I. L. (1968). A method for the study of cell proliferation and renewal in the tissues of mammals. *In* "Methods in Cell Physiology" (D. M. Prescott, ed.), Vol. III p. 261. Academic Press, New York.

Cameron, I. L. (1970). Cell renewal in the organs and tissues of nongrowing adult mouse. *Tex. Rep. Biol. Med.* In press.

Cameron, I. L. and Greulich, R. C. (1963). Evidence for an essentially constant duration of DNA synthesis in renewing epithelia of the adult mouse. *J. Cell Biol.* **18**, 31.

Chigasaki, H. (1963). *Brain and Nerve* **15**, 767. cited *in* J. E. Cleaver, "Thymidine Metabolism and Cell Kinetics," p. 128. Wiley, New York, 1967.

Cleaver, J. E. (1967). "Thymidine Metabolism and Cell Kinetics." Wiley, New York.

Clermont, Y., Leblond, C. P., and Messier, A. (1959). Duree du cycle de l'epithelium seminal du rat. *Arch. Anat. Microsc. Morphol. Exp.* **48**, 37.

Cole, J. W., and McKalen, A. (1961). Observations of cell renewal in human rectal mucosa *in vivo* with thymidine-H^3. *Gastroenterology* **41**, 122.

Cole, J. W., and McKalen, A. (1963). Studies on the morphogenesis of adenomatous polyps in the human colon. *Cancer* **16**, 998.

Creamer, B., Shorter, R. G., and Bamforth, J. (1961). The turnover and shedding of epithelial cells. I. The turnover in the gastro-intestinal tract. *Gut* **2**, 110.

Cutright, D. E., and Bauer, H. (1967). Cell renewal in the oral mucosa and skin of the rat. I. Turnover time. *Oral Surg. Oral Med. and Oral Path.* **23**, 249.

Defendi, V., and Manson, L. A. (1963). Analysis of the life cycle in mammalian cells. *Nature (London)* **198**, 359.

Edwards, J. L., Kloch, A. L., Youcis, P., Freese, H. L., Latte, M. B., and Donaldson, J. T. (1960). Some characteristics of DNA synthesis and the mitotic cycle in Ehrlich ascites tumor cells. *J. Biophys. Biochem. Cytol.* **7**, 273.

Enesco, M., and Leblond, C. P. (1962). Increase in cell number as a factor in the growth of the organs and tissues of the young male rat. *J. Embryol. and Exp. Morphol.* **10**, 530.

Epifanova, O. I. (1966), Mitotic cycles in estrogen-treated mice: A radioautographic study. *Exp. Cell Res.* **42**, 562.

Everett, N. B., and Tyler (Caffrey), R. W. (1967) Lymphopoiesis in the thymus and other tissues: Functional implications. *Int. Rev. Cytol.* **22**, 205.

Fabrikant, J. I. (1968). Cell proliferation during lymphopoiesis in the thymus of normal and continuously irradiated mice. *In* "Effects of Radiation on Cellular Proliferation and Differentiation," p. 369. International Atomic Energy Agency, Vienna.

Feinendegen, L. E. (1967). "Tritium-Labeled Molecules in Biology and Medicine." Academic Press, New York.

Fliedner, T. M., Keese, M., Cronkite, E. P., and Robertson, J. S. (1964). Cell proliferation in germinal centers of the rat spleen. *Ann. N.Y. Acad. Sci.* **113**, 578.

Frindel, E., Malaise, E. P., Alpen, E. and Tubiana, M. (1967). Kinetics of cell proliferation of an experimental tumor. *Cancer Res.* **27**, 1122.

Frindel, E., Valleron, A. J., Vassort, F., and Tubiana, M. (1969). Proliferation kinetics of an experimental ascites tumour of the mouse. *Cell Tissue Kinet.* **2**, 51.

Fry, R. J. M., Lesher, S., and Kohn, H. I. (1961). Estimation of time generation of living cells. *Nature (London)* **191**, 290.

Fry, R. J. M., Lesher, S., and Kohn, H. I. (1962). Influence of age on the transit time of cells of the mouse intestinal epithelium. *Lab. Invest.* **11**, 289.

Gaetani, M., Silvestrini, R., and Bellini, O. (1964). La proliferazione cellulare del'epatoma ascite AH 130 di Yoshida. *Sperimentale* **114**, 293.

Galand, P. (1967). Comparison de deux methodes autoradiographiques bases sur l'emploi de thymidine tritiee, pour la mesure de la duree de la phase S (phase de synthese d'acide desoxyribonucleique) et de l'interphase des cellules de differents tissus de la souris. *Arch. Biol.* **78**, 167.

Goldfeder, A. (1965a). Biological properties and radiosensitivity of tumours: Determination of the cell-cycle and time of synthesis of deoxyribonucleic acid using tritiated thymidine and autoradiography. *Nature (London)* **207**, 612.

Goldfeder, A. (1965b). *In* "Cellular Radiation Biology," p. 537. Williams & Wilkins, Baltimore.

Greulich, R. C., and Leblond, C. P. (1953). Radioautographic visualization of radiocarbon in the organs and other tissues of newborn rats following administration of C^{14} labeled bicarbonate. *Anat. Rec.* **115**, 559.

Griem, M. L. (1966). Use of multiple biopsies for the study of the cell cycle of the mouse hair follicle. *Nature (London)* **210**, 213.

Grisham, J. W. (1962). A morphologic study of deoxyribonucleic acid synthesis and cell proliferation in regenerating rat liver; autoradiography with thymidine-H-3. *Cancer Res.* **22**, 842.

Hanna, C., and O'Brien, J. E. (1960). Cell production and migration in the epithelial layer of the cornea. *Arch. Opthalmol.* **64**, 536.

Hanna, C., Bicknell, D. S., and O'Brien, J. E. (1961). Cell turnover in the adult human eye. *Arch. Ophthalmol.* **65**, 695.

Harding, C. V., and Srinivasan, B. D. (1961). A propagated stimulation of DNA synthesis and cell division. *Exp. Cell Res.* **25**, 326.

Hell, E. A., and Cruickshank, C. N., D. (1963). The effect of injury upon the uptake of ³H-thymidine by guinea pig epidermis. *Exp. Cell Res.* **31**, 128.

Heller, C. G., and Clermont, Y. (1963). Spermatogenesis in man: An estimate of its duration. *Science* **140**, 184.

Henry, J. L., Meyer, J., Weinmann, J. P., and Schour, I. (1952). Pattern of mitotic activity in oral epithelium of rabbits. *Arch. Pathol.* **54**, 281.

Hodgson, G. (1967). Synthesis of RNA and DNA at various intervals after erythropoietin injection in transfused mice. *Proc. Soc. Exp. Biol. Med.* **124**, 1045.

Iverson, O. H., and Elgjo, K. (1967). The effect of chalone on the mitotic rate and on the mitotic duration in hairless mouse epidermis. *In* "Control of Cellular Growth in Adult Organisms" (H. Teir and T. Rytömaa, eds.) p. 83. Academic Press, New York.

Iverson, O. H., Bjerknes, R., and Devik, F. (1968). Kinetics of cell renewal, cell migration and cell loss in the hairless mouse dorsal epidermis. *Cell Tissue Kinet.* **1**, 351.

Jacoby, F. (1953). Mitotic activity in the gall bladder epithelium of the guinea-pig after ligation of the common duct. *J. Physiol. (London)* **119**, 21.

Johnson, H. A., Haymaker, W. E., Rubini, J. R., Fliedner, T. M., Bond, V. P., Cronkite, E. P., and Hughes, W. L. (1960). A radioautographic study of a human brain and glioblastoma multiforme after the *in vivo* uptake of tritiated thymidine. *Cancer* **13**, 636.

Katzberg, A. A. (1952). The influence of age on the rate of desquamation of the human epidermis. *Anat. Rec. (Suppl.)* **112**, 418.

Kauffman, S. L. (1966). An autoradiographic study of the generation cycle in the ten-day mouse neural tube. *Exp. Cell Res.* **42**, 67.

Knowlton, N. P., Jr. and Widner, W. R. (1950). The use of x-rays to determine the mitotic and intermitotic time of various mouse tissues. *Cancer Res.* **10**, 59.

Knudtson, K. P., Priest, R. E., Jacklin, A. J., and Jesseph, J. E. (1962). Effect of partial resection on mammalian small intestine. I. Initial autoradiographic study. *Lab. Invest.* **11**, 433.

Koburg, E. (1962). Autoradiographische Untersuchungen zur Zellneubildungsrate an der Epithelian des oberen Respirations—und Verdauungstraktes. *Arch. Ohren Nasen Kehlkopfheilk.* **180**, 616.

Lala, P. K., Unpublished results cited *In* J. E. Cleaver, "Thymidine Metabolism and Cell Kinetics," p. 129. Wiley, New York, 1967.

Lala, P. K., and Patt, H. M. (1966). Cytokinetic analysis of tumor growth. *Proc. Nat. Acad. Sci. U.S.* **56**, 1735.

Lala, P. K., Patt, H. M., and Maloney, M. A. (1966). An evaluation of erythropoiesis in canine marrow. *Acta Haematol.* **35**, 311.

Leblond, C. P. (1959). Classical techniques for the study of the kinetics of cellular proliferation. *In* "The Kinetics of Cellular Proliferation" (F. Stohlman, ed.), p. 31. Grune and Stratton, New York.

Leblond, C. P. (1964). Classification of cell populations on the basis of their proliferative behavior. *Nat. Cancer Inst. Monogr.* **14,** 119.

Leblond, C. P., Vulpe, M., and Bertalanffy, F. D. (1955). Mitotic activity of epithelium of urinary bladder in albino rat. *J. Urol.* **73,** 311.

Leblond, C. P., Greulich, R. C., and Periera, J. P. M. (1964). Relationship of cell formation and cell migration in the renewal of stratified squamous epithelia. *Advan. Biol. Skin* **5,** 39.

Leblond, C. P., and Stevens, C. E. (1948). The constant renewal of the intestinal epithelium in the albino rat. *Anat. Rec.* **100,** 357.

Leblond, C. P., and Walker, B. E. (1956). Renewal of cell populations. *Physiol. Rev.* **36,** 255.

Lehmiller, D. J. (1970). Cell migration and proliferation during repair of superficial wounds produced by a carbon dioxide laser. Tech. Rep. School of Aerospace Medicine, Brooks Air Force Base, 70–29.

Lennartz, K. J., and Maurer, W. (1964). Autoradiographische Bestimmung der Dauer der DNA-Verdopplung und der Generationzeit beim Ehrlich-Ascites tumar der Maus durch Doppel Markierung mit ¹⁴C-und ³H-Thymidin. *Z. Zellforsch. Mikrosk. Auat.* **63,** 478.

Lesher, S., Fry, R. J. M., and Kohn, H. I. (1961). Age and the generation time of the mouse duodenal epithelium cell. *Exp. Cell Res.* **24,** 334.

Levi, P. E., Cowen, D. M., and Cooper, E. H. (1969). Induction of cell proliferation in the mouse bladder by 4-ethylsulphonylnaphthalene-1-sulphonamide. *Cell Tissue Kinet.* **2,** 249.

Lipkin, M., Sherlock, P., and Bell, B. M. (1962). Generation time of epithelial cells in the human colon. *Nature (London)* **195,** 175.

Loran, M. R., and Crocker, T. T. (1963). Population dynamics of intestinal epithelial in the rat two months after partial resection of the ileum. *J. Cell Biol.* **19,** 285.

Lord, B. I. (1968). Distribution of cell cycle times of normoblasts in the bone marrow of normal and continuously irradiated rats. *In* "Effects of Radiation on Cellular Proliferation and Differentiation," p. 247. International Atomic Energy Agency, Vienna.

MacDonald, R. A. (1961). "Lifespan" of liver cells. *Arch. Int. Med.* **107,** 335.

McMinn, R. M. H. (1964). The rate of renewal of intestinal epithelium in the cat. *J. Anat.* **88,** 527.

McMinn, R. M. H., and Johnson, F. R. (1955). The repair of artificial ulcers in the urinary bladder of the cat. *Brit. J. Surg.* **43,** 99.

McMinn, R. M. H., and Johnson, F. R. (1957). Wound healing in the gall-bladder of the cat. *Brit. J. Surg.* **45,** 76.

McMinn, R. M. H., and Taylor, M. (1966). The cytology of repair in experimental perforations of the tympanic membrane. *Brit. J. Surg.* **53,** 222.

Matsuzawa, T., and Wilson, R. (1964). *In* "Mammalian Radiation Lethality" (V. P. Bond, T. M. Fleidner, and J. O. Archambeau, eds.), p. 43. Academic Press, New York.

Maurer, W., Pilgrim, C., Wegener, K., Hollweg, S., and Lennartz, J. (1965). Messung der Dauer der DNA Verdopplung und der Generationszeit bei verschiedenen Zellarten von Maus und Ratte durch Doppel-Markierung mit ³H und ¹⁴C-Thymidin. *In* "Radioaktive Isotope in Klinik und Forschung" (K. Fellinger and R. Hofer, eds.), p. 96. Urban und Schwarzenberg, Berlin.

Mendelsohn, M. L., Dohan, F. C., and Moore, H. A. (1960). Autoradiographic analysis of cell proliferation in spontaneous breast cancer of C^3H mouse. I. Typical cell cycle and timing of DNA synthesis. *J. Nat. Cancer Inst.* **25**, 447.

Messier, B. (1960). Renewal of the colonic epithelium of rat. *Amer. J. Dig. Dis.* **5**, 833.

Meyer zum Gottesberge, A., and Koburg, E. (1963). Autoradiographische Untersuchungen zur Zellneubildung im Respirationstrakt, in der Tube, im~Mittelohr und ausseren Gehorgang. *Acta Oto Laryngol.* **56**, 353.

Monesi, V. (1962). Autoradiographic study of DNA synthesis and the cell cycle in spermatogonia of mouse testis using H^3-thymidine. *J. Cell. Biol.* **14**, 1.

Nachtwey, D. S., and Cameron, I. L. (1968). Cell cycle analysis. *In* "Methods in Cell Physiology" (D. M. Prescott, ed.), Vol. III, p. 214. Academic Press, New York.

Oakberg, E. F. (1956). Duration of spermatogenesis in the mouse and timing of stages of the cycle of the seminiferous epithelium. *Amer. J. Anat.* **99**, 507.

Odell, T. T., Jr., Burch, E. A., Jackson, C. W., and Friday, T. J. (1969). Megakaryocytopoiesis in mice. *Cell Tissue Kinet.* **2**, 363.

Oehlert, W., and Buchner, T. (1961). Mechanismus und zeitlicher Ablauf der physiologischen Regneration im mehrschichtigen Plattenepithel und in der Schleimhaut des Magen-Darmtraktes der weissen Maus. *Beitr. Pathol. Anat. Allg. Pathol.* **125**, 374.

Patt, H. M., and Quastler, H. (1963). Radiation effects on cell renewal and related systems. *Physiol. Rev.* **43**, 357.

Phillips, T. L., and Leong, G. F. (1967). Kidney cell proliferation after unilateral nephrectomy as related to age. *Cancer Res.* **27**, 286.

Pilgrim, C., Lang, W., and Maurer, W. (1966). Autoradiographische Untersuchungen der Dauer der S-Phase und des Generationzykeus der Basal Epithelien des Ohres der Maus. *Exp. Cell Res.* **44**, 129.

Post, J., and Hoffman, J. (1964). Changes in the replication times and patterns of the liver cell during the life of the rat. *Exp. Cell Res.* **63**, 111.

Reiskin, A. B., and Mendelsohn, M. L. (1964). A comparison of the cell cycle in induced carcinomas and their normal counterpart. *Cancer Res.* **24**, 1131.

Richart, R. M. (1963). A radioautographic analysis of cellular proliferation in dysplasia and carcinoma *in situ* of the uterine cervix. *Amer. J. Obstet. Gynecol.* **86**, 925.

Sado, T., and Makinodan, T. (1964). The cell cycle of blast cells involved in secondary antibody response. *J. Immunol.* **93**, 696.

Sasaki, T. (1965). Cell cycle and effects of X-irradiation on germ cells of rat incisors (Part I) *Bull. Tokyo Med. Dent. Univ.* **12**, 379.

Shea, S. N. (1964). Kinetics of hepatocyte proliferation in the early stages of liver regeneration. *Exp. Cell Res.* **36**, 325.

Sherman, F. G., Quastler, H., and Wimber, D. R. (1961). Cell population kinetics in the ear epidermis of mice. *Exp. Cell Res.* **25**, 114.

Simnet, J. D., and Heppleston, A. G. (1966). Cell renewal in the mouse lung; the influence of sex, strain and age. *Lab. Invest.* **15**, 1793.

Spencer, H., and Shorter, R. G. (1962). Cell turnover in pulmonary tissues. *Nature (London)* **194**, 880.

Steel, G. G., Adams, K., and Barrett, J. C. (1966). Analysis of the cell population kinetics of transplanted tumours of widely-differing growth rate. *Brit. J. Cancer* **20**, 784.

Stevens, C. E., and Leblond, C. P. (1953). Renewal of the mucous cells in the gastric mucosa of the rat. *Anat. Rec.* **115**, 231.

Stevens-Hooper, C. E. (1961). Use of colchicine for the measurement of mitotic rate in the intestinal epithelium. *Amer. J. Anat.* **108**, 231.

Stocker, E. (1966). Der Proliferationsmodus in Niere und Leber. *Verh. Deut. Ges. Pathol.* **50**, 53.

Stocker, E., and Pfeifer, U. (1967). Autoradiographische Untersuchungen mit ^{3}H-Thymidin an der regenerierenden Rattenleber. *Z. Zellforsch. Mikrosk. Anat.* **79**, 374.

Storey, W. F., and Leblond, C. P. (1951). Measurement of the rate of proliferation of epidermis and associated structures. *Ann. N.Y. Acad. Sci.* **53**, 537.

Thrasher, J. D. (1966). Analysis of renewing epithelial cell populations. *In* "Methods in Cell Physiology" (D. M. Prescott, ed.), Vol. II, p. 323. Academic Press, New York.

Thrasher, J. D., and Greulich, R. C. (1965). The duodenal progenitor population. I. Age related increase in the duration of the cryptal progenitor cycle. *J. Exp. Zool.* **159**, 39.

Thrasher, J. D., Clark, F. I., and Clarke, D. R. (1967). Changes in the vaginal epithelial cell cycle in relation to events of the estrous cycle. *Exp. Cell Res.* **45**, 232.

Toto, P. D., and Ojha, G. (1962). Generation cycle of oral epithelium in mice. *J. Dent. Res.* **41**, 388.

Trott, J. R., and Gorenstein, S. L. (1963). Mitotic rates in the oral and gingival epithelium of the rat. *Arch. Oral Biol.* **8**, 425.

Vendrely, R., and Vendrely, C. (1956). The results of cytophotometry in the study of deoxyribonucleic acid (DNA) content of the nucleus. *Int. Rev. Cytol.* **5**, 171.

Vincent, P. C., Borner, G., Chanana, A. D., Cronkite, E. P., Greenberg, M. L., Joel, D. D., Shiffer, L. M., and Stryckmans, P. A. (1969). Studies on lymphocytes. XIV. Measurement of DNA synthesis time in bovine thoracic duct lymphocytes by analysis of labeled mitoses and by double labeling, before and after extracorporeal irradiation of the lymph. *Cell Tissue Kinet.* **2**, 235.

von Volksman, R. (1950). Versuche zue Feststellung der Erneuerungsdauer geschichteter Plattenepithelien. *Anat. Nachr.* **1**, 86.

Walker, B. E. (1960). Renewal of cell populations in the female mouse. *Amer. J. Anat.* **107**, 95.

Walker, B. E., and Rennels, E. G. (1961). Adrenal cortical cell replacement in the mouse. *Endocrinology* **68**, 365.

Weiss, P., and Kavanau, J. L. (1957). A model of growth and growth control in mathematical terms. *J. Gen. Physiol.* **41**, 1.

Widner, W. R., Storer, J. B., and Lushbaugh, C. C. (1951). The use of x-ray and nitrogen mustard to determine the mitotic and intermitotic time in normal and malignant rat tissues. *Cancer Res.* **11**, 877.

Wilhelm, D. L. (1953). Regeneration of tracheal epithelium. *J. Pathol. Bacteriol.* **65**, 543.

Williams, G. E. G. (1961). Some aspects of compensatory hyperplasia of the kidney. *Brit. J. Exp. Pathol.* **42**, 386.

Wimber, D. E. (1963). *In* "Cell Proliferation" (L. F. Lamerton and R. J. M. Fry, eds.), p. 1. Blackwell, London.

Wolfsberg, M. F. (1964). Cell population kinetics in the epithelium of the fore-stomach of the mouse. *Exp. Cell Res.* **35**, 119.

Young, R. W. (1962). Cell proliferation and specialization during endochondral osteogenesis in young rats. *J. Cell Biol.* **14**, 357.

CHAPTER 4

Cellular Content and Cellular Proliferation Changes in the Tissues and Organs of the Aging Mammal*

D. E. Buetow

I. Introduction.. 87
II. Changes in Numbers of Cells and Nerve Fibers......................... 88
    A. Nervous System.. 88
    B. Other Tissues and Organs...................................... 89
III. Changes in Mitotic Rates... 97
IV. Changes in Mucosal Cells of the Intestine.......................... 97
    V. Discussion... 101
    References.. 104

I. Introduction

The probability of death increases with age. Why this should be so forms the subject matter of the field of gerontology. It is difficult, however, at this stage of knowledge concerning senescence, to give a precise definition of "aging." Shock (1960, 1962) has measured age changes in physiological functions (e.g., renal blood flow, basal metabolism, cardiac output, nerve conduction velocity, and pulmonary function) in the human and has shown that *on the average* these decline linearly with age starting at age 30–40 years. In spite of rather large variations among individuals, these studies make clear that the functional capacity of the individual as well as the functional capacities of his organs and tissues tend to diminish with age.

Research aimed at elucidating basic mechanisms underlying the aging process has extended the field of gerontology into the areas of cellular

* This presentation was supported in part by Grant HD 03163 from the National Institute of Child Health and Human Development.

structure and function, as discussed by Andrew (1952), Shock (1960), Strehler (1962), Kohn (1965), and Goss (1967). All these authors have commented on the degeneration and loss of cells in mammalian tissues and organs with age. It is the purpose of this chapter to summarize the known data on cell number and on the incidence of mitosis as a function of age in a variety of tissues and organs in various mammals.

Some of the literature on "age-related" changes in anatomy, physiology, and biochemistry is somewhat misleading since it is restricted to developmental processes in individuals from birth *to* adulthood. No data on the very old individual is given in these papers. The literature also contains many references which do consider the very old individual from anatomical, histochemical, and cytochemical viewpoints. As a whole, this latter literature suggests that many degenerative changes accompany old age, but individually, however, these papers frequently present information on only a few subjects (particularly in the case of humans). Therefore, the reader is often left somewhat in doubt as to just which changes are due to age and which are due to the previous medical history of the individual. The data summarized in Tables I, II, and III of this chapter were extracted from the rather large literature on gerontology on the following bases: (1) The data include subjects which are beyond early adulthood and, preferably, include subjects which are very old; (2) the total data include enough subjects and/or cell counts, etc., so that any differences between different age groups are, at least, suggested; and (3) the ages of the subjects are known. Some of the literature on rats and mice uses weight, for example, as a criterion of age. Such references are not included here.

II. Changes in Numbers of Cells and Nerve Fibers

A. Nervous System

Changes in the number of cells and in the number of nerve fibers in certain nerves with age are given in Table I. Data on nerve fibers are included since they form the basis of measurement in many studies on aging. In many cases, the number of nerve cells and number of nerve fibers appear to decrease on the average with age in the human, both male and female. Any such decreases are mainly noted in the oldest subjects. For example, in the study by Gardner (1940), the total number of cells in the VIII and IX thoracic spinal ganglia averaged about 69,700 in eight human subjects aged 30–58 years and about 56,000 in twelve subjects aged 63–85 years.

Some studies on the human, however, do not report decreases with age (Table I). The number of glial cells per neuron (Brownson, 1955) and the number of cells in some areas of the cerebral cortex (Brody, 1955) increase with age, whereas the number of normal Gasserian ganglion cells does not change with age in the human (Truex, 1940).

Interestingly, in contrast to the human data, rats, mice, and cats show loss of cells with age in the nervous system in only a few cases, at least in the studies done so far (Table I). On the average, loss of cells appears to occur in the mouse in the case of large anterior horn cells in the spinal cord (Wright and Spink, 1959), in the rat in the case of Purkinje cells in the cerebellar cortex (Inukai, 1928), and in both the mouse and the rat in the case of the number of glial cells per neuron in the motor cortex (Brownson, 1955). In all the other animal studies on the nervous system in Table I, cell number as well as nerve fiber number on the average either does not change with age or actually increases.

The data on the nervous system shows that a great degree of variation exists among subjects even of the same chronological age (Table I). Also as noted, the animal data do not suggest as much loss of cells with age as the human data suggest. It is possible that there is a species difference as regards changes in the nervous system with age. However, the animal data were collected on animals reared under *controlled* conditions. It is also possible, therefore, that the tendency of the human nervous system to lose cells may be more a reflection of the medical history of the human than a reflection of aging. Before a loss of cells in the nervous system of the human can be attributed to aging only, more studies on large numbers of subjects should be done. Such studies will help sort out the effect of disease as well as, perhaps, reduce some of the variability in the human data.

B. OTHER TISSUES AND ORGANS

Loss of cells in several other tissues and organs including spleen, muscle, cartilage, and the exorbital lacrimal gland of the eye appears to occur in the rat and bovine animals (Table I). In the human, the percent red blood cells appears reduced after age 50 (Shock and Yiengst, 1950). Loss of cells with age does not occur in other tissues, however. For example, gingival epithelial cells increase in the human with age (Meyer *et al.*, 1956). In the mouse, reticular fibers in the myocardium increase up to about 5–13 weeks of age and then remain constant or only slightly decrease by 20–24 months of age (Bacon, 1948). The number of macrophages in the spleen, in contrast, declines early in the life of the rat and then remains constant through old age (Andrew, 1946). In these latter studies on the spleen, however, the variation in individuals of the same age is quite large (Table I); therefore, the exact pattern of any cell changes with age may not be established.

TABLE I

NUMBER OF CELLS OR FIBERS VERSUS AGE IN VARIOUS TISSUES AND ORGANS

Tissue or organ	Type	Subjects			Cells or fibers		Measure	Reference
		(number)	Age	Sex	Total or mean	Range		
Nervous system								
VIII and IX thoracic spinal ganglia	Human	(2)	30–36 years	M	66,947	61,559–72,335	Total cells	Gardner (1940)
		(2)	41–49	M,F	75,648	68,890–82,424		
		(4)	51–58	M,F	66,694	58,086–74,197		
		(5)	63–68	M	52,930	42,818–65,780		
		(5)	72–78	M	52,635	46,171–59,349		
		(2)	80–85	M	52,715	45,415–60,015		
VIII and IX thoracic, dorsal root	Human	(2)	26–27 years	M	11,181	11,058–11,304	Total number of myelinated fibers	Corbin and Gardner (1937); Gardner (1940)
		(2)	34–36	M	10,530	9,665–11,396		
		(8)	41–49	M,F	9,844	8,180–11,757		
		(14)	50–59	M,F	9,250	7,098–11,829		
		(13)	61–69	M,F	8,346	6,432–10,930		
		(16)	71–79	M	8,442	6,262–9,748		
		(5)	80–89	M	8,710	7,923–9,710		
VIII and IX thoracic, ventral root	Human	(2)	26–27 years	M	6,204	6,204–6,205	Total number of myelinated fibers	Corbin and Gardner (1937); Gardner (1940)
		(2)	34–36	M	5,732	5,648–5,816		
		(9)	41–49	M,F	5,500	4,997–5,971		
		(14)	50–59	M,F	5,327	4,309–6,370		
		(13)	61–69	M,F	4,825	3,942–5,611		
		(16)	71–79	M	4,524	3,487–5,258		
		(5)	80–89	M	5,004	3,924–5,517		
II cervical, ventral root	Rat	(4)	7 days	M,F	367	360–372	Total number of myelinated fibers	Dunn (1912)
		(4)	14	M,F	554	518–594		

Location	Animal	(No.)	Age or weight	Sex	Mean	Range	Measurement	Reference
VIII cervical, ventral root	Cat	(4)	36	M,F	633	536–689	Total number of fibers (axis cylinders)	Moyer and Kaliszewski (1958)
		(4)	75	M,F	614	505–726		
		(4)	132	M,F	655	569–731		
		(4)	180	M,F	564	510–662		
		(4)	270	M,F	697	576–853		
		(3)	640	M	864	758–934		
I thoracic, ventral root	Cat	(37)	1 day–14 weeks	M,F	5,404	4,889–6,358	Total number of fibers (axis cylinders)	Moyer and Kaliszewski (1958)
		(16)	1 yr.–5 yrs.	M,F	5,671	4,970–6,387		
		(16)	10 yr.–18 yrs.	M,F	5,844	4,850–6,441		
		(32)	1 day–14 weeks	M,F	4,542	3,664–5,522		
		(16)	1–5 years	M,F	4,981	4,403–5,926		
		(16)	10–18 years	M,F	5,194	4,181–5,746		
VIII thoracic, ventral root	Rat	(12)	18–50 days	M	1,107	1,005–1,351	Total number of fibers (axis cylinders)	Duncan (1934)
		(4)	170–300	M	1,268	1,190–1,364		
		(4)	548–864	M	1,099	1,013–1,229		
	Rat	(5)	14–50 days	F	944	908–992		
		(4)	150	F	986	904–1,079		
		(4)	730–1060	F	1,023	930–1,200		
IV or V lumbar, largest, ventral root	Rat	(8)	18–40 days	M	1,900	1,753–2,011	Total number of fibers (axis cylinders)	Duncan (1934)
		(6)	136–300	M	1,935	1,637–2,142		
		(4)	548–864	M	1,799	1,726–1,930		
	Rat	(9)	14–50 days	F	1,620	1,439–1,891		
		(2)	95–142	F	1,794	1,783–1,805		
		(2)	856–1,060	F	1,632	1,500–1,764		
Spinal cord, large anterior horn cells	Mouse	(5)	25 weeks	M	6,412	5,647–7,745	Total cells	Wright and Spink (1959)
		(3)	50	M	7,032	6,557–7,342		
		(2)	110	M	5,614	5,246–5,981		
	Mouse	(3)	25 weeks	F	6,267	5,688–6,634		
		(3)	50	F	6,064	5,505–6,571		
		(4)	110	F	4,905	4,225–5,589		

TABLE I

NUMBER OF CELLS OR FIBERS VERSUS AGE IN VARIOUS TISSUES AND ORGANS—Continued

Tissue or organ	Type	Subjects (number)	Age	Sex	Total or mean	Range	Measure	Reference
Nervous system (Continued)								
Olfactory nerve	Human	(27)	16–30 years	M,F	20%	0–100%	Number of nerve fibers (mean percent loss from value at birth)	Smith (1942)
		(20)	31–45	M,F	33	0–100		
		(45)	46–60	M,F	57	0–100		
		(55)	61–75	M,F	68	0–100		
		(30)	76–91	M,F	73	0–100		
Optic nerve	Human	(2)	47–51 years	M,F	1.11×10^6	1.02–1.20×10^6	Total number of nerve fibers	Breuch and Arey (1942)
		(6)	61–68	M,F	1.02×10^6	0.92–1.14×10^6		
		(2)	70–71	F	0.89×10^6	0.87–0.90×10^6		
Sciatic nerve	Rat	(9)	50–250 days	—	61%	50–69%	Proportion of nerve occupied by fibers	Birren and Wall (1956)
		(8)	250–650	—	64	51–70		
		(7)	650–850	—	60	46–65		
Cerebellum, Purkinje cells	Human	(4)	22–42 years	M	607	591–624	Right and left hemisphere; number of cells per equivalent unit area anterior to primary sulcus and anterior to great horizontal sulcus	Ellis (1919, 1920)
		(5)	50–65	M	575	509–667		
		(5)	73–100	M	466	403–500		
	Human	(6)	19–32 years	F	543	511–612		
		(3)	50–65	F	478	462–499		
		(5)	71–94	F	418	334–505		
Cerebellar cortex, Purkinje cells	Rat	(1)	200 days	M	506,922	—	Total cells	Inukai (1928)
		(1)	730	M	447,505	—		
		(1)	1,017	M	367,166	—		
	Rat	(1)	200 days	F	471,156	—		
		(1)	730	F	448,841	—		
		(1)	1,085	F	404,733	—		

Region	Species	(n)	Age	Sex	Value	Range	Measure	Reference
Cerebral cortex, Superior temporal gyrus	Human	(4)	16–48 years	M,F	2,079	1,950–2,187	Total cells	Brody (1955)
		(6)	70–78	M,F	1,140	1,055–1,271		
		(3)	80–95	M	949	887–991		
Cerebral cortex, area striata	Human	(7)	16–48 years	M,F	2,355	1,740–2,648	Total cells	Brody (1955)
		(5)	70–78	M,F	1,704	1,243–1,840		
		(3)	80–95	M	1,691	1,489–1,810		
Cerebral cortex, precentral gyrus, fourth quarter	Human	(7)	16–48 years	M,F	1,429	1,215–1,701	Total cells	Brody (1955)
		(5)	73–78	M,F	1,036	977–1,206		
		(3)	80–95	M	937	886–1,016		
Cerebral cortex, post-central gyrus, third quarter	Human	(7)	16–48 years	M,F	1,363	1,126–1,512	Total cells	Brody (1955)
		(6)	73–95	M,F	1,540	1,241–1,932		
Cerebral cortex, microglia	Rat	(6)	109–113 days	M	6,700	—	Cells per mm³ per 20 depth levels	Brizzee et al. (1968)
		(6)	763–972	M	6,700	—		
Cerebral cortex, oligodendroglia plus astrocytes	Rat	(6)	109–113 days	M	42,000	—	Cells per mm³ per 20 depth levels	Brizzee et al. (1968)
		(6)	763–972	M	53,000	—		
Cerebral cortex, neurons	Rat	(6)	109–113 days	M	97,000	—	Cells per mm³ per 20 depth levels	Brizzee et al. (1968)
		(6)	763–972	M	98,000	—		
Precentral primary motor cortex, glial cells	Rat	(3)	17 days	—	1.06	1.02–1.12	Average number of glial cells per large neuron	Brownson (1955)
		(2)	210	—	0.72	0.68–0.76		
		(3)	720	—	0.50	0.34–0.62		
	Mouse	(2)	21 days	—	0.63	0.56–0.70	Average number of glial cells per large neuron	Brownson (1955)
		(2)	129	—	0.70	0.64–0.76		
		(6)	200–700	—	0.47	0.32–0.56		
	Human	(5)	49–59 years	—	0.49	0.38–0.58	Average number of glial cells per large neuron	Brownson (1955)
		(5)	64–70	—	0.64	0.52–0.76		

TABLE I

Number of Cells or Fibers versus Age in Various Tissues and Organs—*Continued*

Tissue or organ	Subjects				Cells or fibers		Measure	Reference
	Type	(number)	Age	Sex	Range	Total or mean		
Nervous system (Continued)								
Gasserian ganglion cells	Human	(8)	36–81 years	M,F	65–74	69	Percent normal unipolar cells	Truex (1940)
Eye								
Exorbital lacrimal gland, mast cells	Rat	(8)	15 days	M	—	278	Average density per mm² of surface area	Bolden (1967)
		(7)	30	M	—	104		
		(7)	60	M	—	155		
		(5)	90	M	—	134		
		(7)	150	M	—	108		
		(7)	300	M	—	123		
		(7)	500	M	—	107		
Blood								
Red blood cells	Human	(39)	20–29 years	M	—	0.475 (±0.005)	Percent red blood cells, estimated from volume of 1 cc capillary blood occupied by red blood cells	Shock and Yiengst (1950)
		(10)	40–49	M	—	0.478 (±0.022)		
		(26)	50–59	M	—	0.441 (±0.007)		
		(54)	60–69	M	—	0.448 (±0.004)		
		(45)	70–79	M	—	0.434 (±0.005)		
		(17)	80–89	M	—	0.415 (±0.007)		

	Species	(N)	Age	Sex	Value	Range	Description	Reference
Spleen								
Macrophages	Rat	(8)	21 days	M,F	0	0	Average number of cells in 0.30 mm² section, 8μ thickness	Andrew (1946)
		(19)	50–150	M,F	90	0–431		
		(13)	200	M,F	325	170–325		
		(25)	300–726	M,F	429	121–684		
		(35)	800–1170	M,F	343	4–692		
Megakaryo-cytes	Rat	(8)	21 days	M,F	59	44–105	Average number of cells in 0.0676 mm² area	Andrew (1946)
		(19)	50–150	M,F	19	4–38		
		(13)	200	M,F	16	4–26		
		(25)	300–726	M,F	22	2–90		
		(35)	800–1170	M,F	16	4–90		
Muscle								
Myocardium, reticular fibers	Mouse	(4)	1 hour	—	15	—	Average number of fibers in 10 oil immersion fields (970 ×)	Bacon (1948)
		(5)	1 day	—	23	—		
		(5)	1 week	—	23	—		
		(4)	3 weeks	—	29	—		
		(6)	5	—	37	—		
		(6)	13	—	37	—		
		(6)	7 months	—	40	—		
		(4)	9	—	38	—		
		(5)	14	—	33	—		
		(4)	20	—	31	—		
		(2)	24	—	30	—		
Myocardium, muscle fibers	Mouse	(4)	1 hour	—	37	—	Average number of fibers in 10 oil immersion fields (970 ×)	Bacon (1948)
		(5)	1 day	—	35	—		
		(5)	1 week	—	26	—		
		(4)	3 weeks	—	18	—		
		(6)	5	—	19	—		
		(6)	13	—	14	—		
		(6)	7 months	—	10	—		
		(4)	9	—	12	—		

TABLE I

Number of Cells or Fibers versus Age in Various Tissues and Organs—*Continued*

Tissue or organ	Subjects				Cells or fibers			Reference
	Type	(number)	Age	Sex	Total or mean	Range	Measure	
Muscle Myocardium, muscle fibers (Continued)	Mouse	(5)	14	—	13	—		
		(4)	20	—	14	—		
		(2)	24	—	14	—		
Muscle mass of hind limb thigh	Rat	(10)	12–14 months	M	28.05 (±2.01)	—	Mass (gm), freed of fat and connective tissue, used as measure of muscle fiber mass	Yiengst *et al.* (1959)
		(10)	24–27	M	18.45 (±1.83)	—		
	Rat	(10)	12–14 months	F	14.56 (±0.67)	—		
		(10)	24–27	F	13.90 (±0.50)	—		
Cartilage Metatarso-phalangeal and metacarpal-phalangeal articulations	Bovine	(4)	Up to 0.5 year	—	133×10^3 ($\pm23 \times 10^3$)	—	Number of cells per mm³ fixed tissue	Rosenthal *et al.* (1941)
		(3)	1–7 years	—	47.2×10^3 ($\pm3.7 \times 10^3$)	—		
		(11)	8–11	—	34.0×10^3 ($\pm5.9 \times 10^3$)	—		
Epithelium Gingival epithelium	Human	(30)	25–34 years	M	55	42–73	Number of cells per $10^4 \mu^2$	Meyer *et al.* (1956)
		(30)	50–78	M	73	50–98		

III. Changes in Mitotic Rates

The number or percent of mitoses declines with age in various tissues and organs of both male and female rats, mice, and guinea pigs (Table II). In the rat there is a decline in mitosis with age in liver cells (Post and Hoffman, 1964), in the proximal convoluted tubules of the kidney (McCreight and Sulkin, 1959), and in the exorbital lacrimal gland of the eye (Walker, 1958). In the mouse, there is a decline in mitosis with age in the epithelial cells of the ear (Whiteley and Horton, 1963). In the guinea pig, a decline occurs in the thyroid, parathyroid, and adrenal cortex (Blumenthal, 1945) but considerable variation is noted in these data.

The only extensive data on humans are those studies on abdominal skin epidermis (Thuringer and Katzberg, 1959) and gingival epithelial cells (Meyer et al., 1956). Both these studies suggest an increased mitotic rate with age.

IV. Changes in Mucosal Cells of the Intestine

Tritiated thymidine has been used to determine generation times, duration of phases of the cell cycle, DNA synthetic indices, and mitotic indices in mucosal cells of the mammalian small intestine as a function of age (Table III).

The generation time of the progenitor cells in the crypts of the colon and the duodenum, jejunum, and ileum of the mouse increases with age (Lesher et al., 1961b,c; Thrasher, 1967; Thrasher and Greulich, 1965a,b). The time it takes the differentiated epithelial cell to move out of the crypt and traverse the villus (transit time, Table III) increases with age in the duodenum and jejunum, but not in the ileum (Lesher et al., 1961a; Fry et al., 1961, 1962). The DNA synthetic index decreases with age in the duodenum and colon, but the length of the DNA-synthetic phase (S-phase, Table III) does not (Thrasher and Greulich, 1965a,b; Thrasher, 1967). Since the G_2 phase and prophase do not change with age, the increased turnover time (generation time) of the stem cells observed with age is most likely due to an increased time spent in the G_1 phase (Thrasher and Greulich, 1965a). A small decrease in the mitotic index occurs in duodenal crypt cells in mice of 579–638 days of age compared to younger animals (Thrasher and Greulich, 1965a).

As summarized by Thrasher (1967), these observations as a whole indicate that the changes occurring in the intestinal mucosal cells of the aging animal are threefold: (1) a decreased rate of cell production, (2) an increased

TABLE II

MITOSIS VERSUS AGE IN VARIOUS TISSUES AND ORGANS

Tissue or organ	Type	(number)	Age	Sex	Number or percent	Range	Measure	Reference
Liver	Rat	—	1 day	—	3.8	—	Percent mitoses; 2000 or more random nuclei	Post and Hoffman (1964)
		—	3 weeks	—	1.1	—		
		—	8	—	0.6	—		
		—	24-156	—	0.1	—		
Kidney proximal convoluted tubules	Rat	(6)	120-125 days	—	2.00(±0.37)	—	Number of mitoses per 2000 cells	McCreight and Sulkin (1959)
		(4)	1160-1170	—	0.50(±0.28)	—		
Skin								
Abdominal skin epidermis	Human	(8)	2 days–19 years	M,F	24.5	8-64	Number of mitoses per 10^5 cells	Thuringer and Katzberg (1959)
		(21)	23-39 years	M,F	36.8	14-106		
		(13)	41-60	M,F	49.7	17-88		
		(12)	61-77	M,F	48.9	19-84		
Ear epithelium	Mouse	(10)	1-3 months	M	16.9(±4.3)	—	Number of mitoses per cm	Whiteley and Horton (1963)
		(9)	3-6	M	17.3(±4.3)	—		
		(9)	6-9	M	15.8(±3.4)	—		
		(10)	9-12	M	14.7(±4.5)	—		
		(10)	15-18	M	13.7(±3.1)	—		
		(9)	18-24	M	12.2(±9.6)	—		
		(10)	27-30	M	11.0(±7.9)	—		
		(4)	30-33	M	2.4(±2.1)	—		
Ear epithelium	Mouse	(9)	1-3 months	F	8.9(±2.8)	—	Number of mitoses per cm	Whiteley and Horton (1963)
		(10)	3-6	F	18.9(±2.5)	—		
		(10)	6-9	F	16.6(±3.7)	—		
		(10)	9-12	F	12.8(±4.0)	—		
		(10)	15-18	F	13.5(±3.1)	—		
		(10)	18-24	F	10.0(±2.9)	—		

	Species	(n)	Age	Sex	Value	Range	Units	Reference
Eye								
Exorbital lacrimal gland	Rat	(10)	27–30	F	15.4(±2.9)	—	Number of mitoses per mm²	Walker (1958)
		(3)	30–33	F	5.6(±4.1)	—		
		(3)	33–36	F	1.9(±0.6)	—		
	Rat	(6)	21 days	M	8.5	—		
		(2)	50	M	1.4	—		
		(2)	100	M	0.23	—		
		(6)	300	M	0.29	—		
		(12)	700	M	0.07	—		
		(9)	900	M	0.05	—		
		(6)	1000	M	0.01	—		
Exorbital lacrimal gland	Rat	(6)	21 days	F	12.2	—	Number of mitoses per mm²	Walker (1958)
		(2)	50	F	6.3	—		
		(2)	100	F	0.01	—		
		(2)	300	F	0.04	—		
		(6)	700	F	0.06	—		
		(13)	700	F	0.06	—		
		(16)	900	F	0.03	—		
		(6)	1000	F	0.02	—		
Epithelium								
Gingival epithelium	Human	(30)	25–34 years	M	0.098	—	Number of mitoses per 1000 cells	Meyer *et al.* (1956)
		(30)	50–78	M	0.156	—		
Thyroid	Guinea pig	(23)	4 days–1 month	M	217	80–960	Number of mitoses per gland, both lobes	Blumenthal (1945)
		(26)	1–4 months	M	134	40–420		
		(24)	4–8	M	96	40–180		
		(16)	8–12	M	48	0–140		
		(13)	12–18	M	23	0–100		
		(9)	1.5–3 years	M	20	0–60		
	Guinea pig	(23)	4 days–1 month	F	560	120–1600	Number of mitoses per gland, both lobes	Blumenthal (1945)
		(23)	1–4 months	F	380	100–1480		
		(31)	4–8	F	225	0–1080		
		(21)	8–12	F	135	20–330		
		(19)	12–18	F	76	0–280		
		(20)	1.5–3 years	F	58	0–170		

TABLE II

Mitosis versus Age in Various Tissues and Organs—*Continued*

Tissue or organ	Subjects				Mitoses			Reference
	Type	(number)	Age	Sex	Number or percent	Range	Measure	
Parathyroid	Guinea pig	(26)	4 days–1 month	M	3.0	0–8.0	Number of mitoses per 10^5 cells	Blumenthal (1945)
		(26)	1–4 months	M	1.6	0–3.7		
		(21)	4–8	M	0.8	0–2.0		
		(18)	8–12	M	0.7	0–4.0		
		(12)	12–18	M	0.6	0–2.3		
		(4)	1.5–3 years	M	0.3	0–1.0		
	Guinea pig	(26)	4 days–1 month	F	4.1	0.9–16.8	Number of mitoses per 10^5 cells	Blumenthal (1945)
		(22)	1–4 months	F	2.8	0.4–8.8		
		(25)	4–8	F	1.3	0–3.3		
		(27)	8–12	F	1.2	0–8.5		
		(21)	12–18	F	0.7	0–3.6		
		(19)	1.5–3 years	F	0.6	0–2.6		
Adrenal cortex	Guinea pig	(26)	4 days–1 month	M	3.3	1.2–9.6	Average number of mitoses per longitudinal section	Blumenthal (1945)
		(26)	1–4 month	M	2.8	0.8–10.0		
		(31)	4–8	M	2.3	0–7.4		
		(24)	8–12	M	1.5	0–8.7		
		(6)	12–18	M	1.2	0.2–1.8		
		(9)	1.5–3 years	M	0.9	0–2.5		
	Guinea pig	(28)	4 days–1 month	F	5.9	1.0–16.6	Average number of mitoses per longitudinal section	Blumenthal (1945)
		(20)	1–4 months	F	4.7	1.1–7.6		
		(20)	4–8	F	2.8	0–10.0		
		(17)	8–12	F	2.1	0–8.4		
		(19)	12–18	F	2.0	0–6.8		
		(25)	1.5–3 years	F	1.1	0–3.8		

turnover time (generation time), and (3) a gradual lengthening of the progenitor (stem) cell cycle due to an increased G_1 phase.

V. Discussion

A striking fact arising from studies on aging is the great degree of variation observed among individuals of the same chronological age. This great variation is observed seemingly irrespective of the parameter being measured, be it physiological, anatomical, or biochemical (e.g., Shock, 1962). This high degree of variation is also seen in the data given in Tables I and II. A very large number of subjects may be needed, therefore, to ascribe a change to aging alone. Otherwise, as discussed in the case of the nervous system of the human, (Section II,A) it may be difficult to determine whether an apparent change or even a tendency toward change is due to aging or due to the medical history of a subject.

Another point of interest is that degenerative changes observed in a tissue with age do not occur uniformly in all cells of that tissue (e.g., Cowdry, 1942; Andrew, 1952; Bourne, 1960). The changes are not uniform even in all cells of the same type in a tissue. Some cells degenerate, but are still surrounded by cells which appear normal even in very old individuals. Further, measurements of the weight of an organ or tissue may not give a true reflection of the loss of functional elements with age since functional cells which have degenerated are often replaced by interstitial substances (e.g., collagen) which, with time, increase both in amount and density (Andrew, 1952; Shock, 1960, 1962; Kohn, 1965). Some method of direct enumeration appears necessary in order to determine any changes in quantities of cells, etc., with age.

It has been commonly observed that cells in many tissues and organs (epidermis, endocrine glands, liver) undergo mitosis or remain capable of mitosis throughout the life span of the mammal (e.g., Cowdry, 1942; Goss, 1967). Other tissues contain cells which tend to be static and show little or no mitosis. For example, nerve cells and striated muscle cells, once formed, do not seem to undergo mitosis (Goss, 1967). Table I shows that there appear to be losses in numbers of cells as a function of age in both the "mitotic" and the "static" (e.g., muscle) tissues and organs. Further, the incidence of mitosis declines with age in many of the mitotic tissues (Table II). Also, intestinal mucosal cells, which undergo renewal throughout the life span of the mouse, show age-related changes in rate of cell production, generation time, and lengthening of the G_1 phase of the cell cycle (Table III). It would seem then that the changes summarized in

TABLE III

AGE-RELATED CHANGES IN MUCOSAL CELLS OF THE MAMMALIAN INTESTINE AS DETERMINED BY ³H-THYMIDINE INCORPORATION

Area	Subjects			Generation time (hours)	Transit Time (hours)			DNA synthetic index (%)	Mitotic index (%)	S phase (hours)	G₂ and prophase (hours)	Reference
	Type	Age	Sex		Crypt	Villus	Total					
Duodenum												
Epithelial cells	Mouse	89 days	M,F	—	5.5	3.5	41	—	—	—	—	Lesher et al. (1961a)
		362	M,F	—	6.5	41.5	48	—	—	—	—	
		945	M,F	—	>10.0	<43	53	—	—	—	—	
Crypt cells (stem or progenitor cells)	Mouse	93 days	M,F	11–11.5	—	—	—	—	—	—	—	Lesher et al. (1961b,c)
		372	M,F	11–11.5	—	—	—	—	—	—	—	
		940	M,F	13–15	—	—	—	—	—	—	—	
	Mouse	10 days	—	11.4	—	—	—	63.3	5.5	7.2	0.75–2.0	Thrasher and Greulich (1965a,b)
		30–70	—	12.4	—	—	—	57.9	5.9	7.4	0.75–2.0	
		380–399	—	14.0	—	—	—	53.4	5.8	7.5	0.75–2.0	
		579–638	—	15.0	—	—	—	50.2	4.9	7.4	0.75–2.0	
Jejunum												
Epithelial cells	Mouse	93 days	M,F	—	3.2	38.8	42	—	—	—	—	Fry et al. (1961)
		372	M,F	—	5.1	46.9	52	—	—	—	—	
		940	M,F	—	6.8	47.2	54	—	—	—	—	

Crypt cells (stem or progenitor cells)	Mouse	93 days	M,F	11	—	—	—	—	—	—	—	Lesher et al. (1961c)
		372	M,F	11	—	—	—	—	—	—	—	
		940	M,F	13	—	—	—	—	—	—	—	
Ileum												
Epithelial cells	Mouse	93 days	M,F	—	4.4	26.6	31	—	—	—	—	Fry et al. (1962)
		372	M,F	—	5.3	27.7	33	—	—	—	—	
		940	M,F	—	8.0	23	31	—	—	—	—	
Crypt cells (stem or progenitor cells)	Mouse	93 days	M,F	11	.	—	—	—	—	—	—	Lesher et al. (1961c)
		372	M,F	11	—	—	—	—	—	—	—	
		940	M,F	13	—	—	—	—	—	—	—	
Colon												
Crypt cells (stem or progenitor cells)	Mouse	10 days	—	15	—	—	—	23.9(±3.3)	—	7.3	1–2	Thrasher (1967)
		30–70	—	19	—	—	—	22.1(±4.1)	—	8.0	1–2	
		380–399	—	19	—	—	—	20.0(±2.8)	—	8.0	1–2	
		579–638	—	21	—	—	—	15.8(±3.8)	—	7.7	1–2	

Tables I, II, and III are in some fashion correlated with declining physiological function with age; indeed, such a correlation has been postulated (e.g., Shock, 1960, 1962). The exact nature of any such correlation, however, remains to be determined.

REFERENCES

Andrew, W. (1946). Age changes in the vascular architecture and cell content in the spleens of 100 Wistar Institute rats, including comparisons with human material. *Amer. J. Anat.* **79,** 1–73.

Andrew, W. (1952). "Cellular Changes with Age." Thomas, Springfield, Illinois.

Bacon, R. L. (1948). Changes with age in the reticular fibers of the myocardium of the mouse. *Amer. J. Anat.* **82,** 469–485.

Birren, J. E., and Wall, P. D. (1956). Age changes in conduction velocity, refractory period, number of fibers, connective tissue space and blood vessels in the sciatic nerve of rats. *J. Comp. Neurol.* **104,** 1–16.

Blumenthal, H. T. (1945). Aging processes in the endocrine glands of the guinea pig. I. The influence of age, sex and pregnancy on the mitotic activity and the histologic structure of the thyroid, parathyroid and adrenal glands. *Arch. Pathol.* **40,** 264–269.

Bolden, T. E. (1967). Age, a factor in growth of the exorbital lacrimal gland. *In* "Control of Cellular Growth in Adult Organisms" (H. Teir and T. Rytömaa, eds.), pp. 275–296. Academic Press, New York.

Bourne, G. H. (1960). General aspects of aging in cells from a physiological point of view. *In* "The Biology of Aging" (B. L. Strehler, ed.), pp. 133–146. AIBS Publ. No. 6, Washington, D.C.

Breuch, S. R., and Arey, L. B. (1942). The number of myelinated and unmyelinated fibers in the optic nerve of vertebrates. *J. Comp. Neurol.* **77,** 631–665.

Brizzee, K. R., Sherwood, N., and Timiras, P. S. (1968). A comparison of cell populations at various depth levels in cerebral cortex of young adult and aged Long-Evans rats. *J. Gerontol.* **23,** 289–297.

Brody, H. (1955). Organization of the cerebral cortex. III. A study of aging in the human cerebral cortex. *J. Comp. Neurol.* **102,** 511–556.

Brownson, R. H. (1955). Perineuronal satellite cells in the motor cortex of aging brains. *J. Neuropathol. Exp. Neurol.* **14,** 424–432.

Corbin, K. B., and Gardner, E. (1937). Decreases in number of myelinated fibers in human spinal roots with age. *Anat. Rec.* **68,** 63–74.

Cowdry, E. V. (1942). "Problems of Aging." Williams and Wilkins, Baltimore, Maryland.

Duncan, D. (1934). A determination of the number of nerve fibers in the eighth thoracic and the largest lumbar ventral roots of the albino rat. *J. Comp. Neurol.* **59,** 47–60.

Dunn, E. H. (1912). The influence of age, sex, weight and relationship upon the number of medullated nerve fibers and on the size of the largest fibers in the ventral root of the second cervical nerve of the albino rat. *J. Comp. Neurol.* **22,** 131–157.

Ellis, R. S. (1919). A preliminary quantitative study of the Purkinje cells in normal, subnormal and senescent human cerebella, with some notes on functional localization. *J. Comp. Neurol.* **30,** 229–252.

Ellis, R. S. (1920). Norms for some structural changes in the human cerebellum from birth to old age. *J. Comp. Neurol.* **32,** 1–33.

Fry, R. J. M., Lesher, S., and Kohn, H. I. (1961). Age effect on cell-transit time in mouse jejunal epithelium. *Amer. J. Physiol.* **201**, 213–216.

Fry, R. J. M., Lesher, S., and Kohn, H. I. (1962). Influence of age on the transit time of cells of the mouse intestinal epithelium. III. Ileum. *Lab. Invest.* **11**, 289–293.

Gardner, E. (1940). Decrease in human neurones with age. *Anat. Rec.* **77**, 529–536.

Goss, R. J. (1967). The strategy of growth. *In* "Control of Cellular Growth in Adult Organisms" (H. Teir and T. Rytömaa, eds.) pp. 3–27. Academic Press, New York.

Inukai, T. (1928). On the loss of Purkinje cells, with advancing age, from the cerebellar cortex of the albino rat. *J. Comp. Neurol.* **45**, 1–31.

Kohn, R. R. (1965). Aging as a consequence of growth cessation. *In* "Reproduction: Molecular, Subcellular, and Cellular" (M. Locke, ed.), pp. 291–324. Academic Press, New York.

Lesher, S., Fry, R. J. M., and Kohn, H. I. (1961a). Influence of age on transit time of cells of mouse intestinal epithelium. I. Duodenum. *Lab. Invest.* **10**, 291–299.

Lesher, S., Fry, R. J. M., and Kohn, H. I. (1961b). Age and the generation time of the mouse duodenal epithelial cell. *Exp. Cell Res.* **24**, 334–343.

Lesher, S., Fry, R. J. M., and Kohn, H. I. (1961c). Aging and the generation cycle of intestinal epithelial cells in the mouse. *Gerontologia* **5**, 176–181.

McCreight, C. E., and Sulkin, N. M. (1959). Cellular proliferation in the kidneys of young and senile rats following unilateral nephrectomy. *J. Gerontol.* **14**, 440–443.

Meyer, J., Marwah, A. S., and Weinmann, J. P. (1956). Mitotic rate of gingival epithelium in two age groups. *J. Invest. Dermatol.* **27**, 237–247.

Moyer, E. K., and Kaliszewski, B. F. (1958). The number of nerve fibers in motor spinal nerve roots of young, mature and aged cats. *Anat. Rec.* **131**, 681–699.

Post, J., and Hoffman, J. (1964). Changes in the replication times and patterns of the liver cell during the life of the rat. *Exp. Cell Res.* **36**, 111–123.

Rosenthal, O., Bowie, M. A., and Wagoner, G. (1941). Studies in the metabolism of articular cartilage. I. Respiration and glycolysis of cartilage in relation to its age. *J. Cell. Comp. Physiol.* **17**, 221–233.

Shock, N. W. (1960). Age changes in physiological functions in the total animal: The role of tissue loss. *In* "The Biology of Aging" (B. L. Strehler, ed.), pp. 258–264, AIBS Publ. No. 6, Washington, D.C.

Shock, N. W. (1962). The physiology of aging. *Sci. Amer.* **206**, 100–106.

Shock, N. W., and Yiengst, M. J. (1950). Age changes in the acid–base equilibrium of the blood of males. *J. Gerontol.* **5**, 1–4.

Smith, C. G. (1942). Age incidence of olfactory nerves in man. *J. Comp. Neurol.* **77**, 589–595.

Strehler, B. L. (1962) "Time, Cells, and Aging," Academic Press, New York.

Thrasher, J. D. (1967). Age and the cell cycle of the mouse colonic epithelium. *Anat. Rec.* **157**, 621–626.

Thrasher, J. D., and Greulich, R. C. (1965a). The duodenal progenitor population. I. Age related increase in the duration of the cryptal progenitor cycle. *J. Exp. Zool.* **159**, 39–46.

Thrasher, J. D., and Greulich, R. C. (1965b). The duodenal progenitor population. II. Age related changes in size and distribution. *J. Exp. Zool.* **159**, 385–396.

Thuringer, J. M., and Katzberg, A. A. (1959). The effect of age on mitosis in the human epidermis. *J. Invest. Dermatol.* **33**, 35–39.

Truex, R. C. (1940). Morphological alterations in the gasserian ganglion cells and their association with senescence in man. *Amer. J. Pathol.* **16**, 255–268.

Walker, R. (1958). Age changes in the rat's exorbital lacrimal gland. *Anat. Rec.* **132,** 49–69.

Whiteley, H. J., and Horton, D. L. (1963). The effect of age on the mitotic activity of the ear epithelium in the CBA mouse. *J. Gerontol.* **18,** 335–339.

Wright, E. A., and Spink, J. M. (1959). A study of the loss of nerve cells in the central nervous system in relation to age. *Gerontologia* **3,** 277–287.

Yiengst, M. J., Barrows, C. H., and Shock, N. W. (1959). Age changes in the chemical composition of muscle and liver in the rat. *J. Gerontol.* **14,** 400–404.

CHAPTER 5

RNA Molecules in Cells and Tissues, *in Vivo* and *in Vitro*

Jack D. Thrasher

I. Introduction	108
II. Intracellular Sites of RNA Synthesis	108
A. The Nucleus as the Site of RNA Synthesis	108
B. Kinetics of Nuclear and Cytoplasmic RNA in Tissue Culture Cells	109
C. Kinetics of Nuclear and Cytoplasmic RNA *in Vivo*	110
III. Nuclear Sites of RNA Synthesis	112
A. Nucleolar Origin of Ribosomal RNA	112
B. Chromatin Synthesis of mRNA and tRNA	112
C. Ribosomal 5 S and 7 S RNA	113
IV. The Biosynthesis of RNA Molecules	113
A. Introduction	113
B. Pattern of RNA Synthesis following Short- and Long-Term Exposure to Labeled Precursors	113
C. Synthesis of HnRNA (DNA-Like RNA, Giant RNA, or mRNA)	116
D. Ribosomal RNA (45 S, 28 S, 18 S, 7 S, and 5 S)	118
E. tRNA (4 S)	122
F. Other Small Molecular Weight RNA Molecules (4 S to 7 S)	122
V. Nucleic Acids of Mitochondria	124
A. Introduction	124
B. Mitochondrial DNA (mDNA)	125
C. Mitochondrial RNA	127
VI. RNA Synthesis in Special Cell Systems	129
A. Introduction	129
B. DNA, RNA, and Hemoglobin Synthesis during Cytodifferentiation of Mammalian Erythroid Cells	130
C. DNA, RNA, and Hemoglobin Synthesis during Cytodifferentiation of Avian Erythroid Cells	132
D. DNA, RNA, and Protein Synthesis during Cytodifferentiation in the Adult Lens	134
E. RNA Synthesis in the Liver	137
F. RNA Synthesis in the Uterus Stimulated by Estrogen Administration	138

VII. RNA Synthesis over the Cell Cycle.................................... 139
    A. Introduction.. 139
    B. RNA Synthesis in G_0 Cells....................................... 140
    C. RNA Synthesis in Continuously Proliferating Cells.................. 140
    References.. 142

I. Introduction

The nuclear origin of RNA and its role in protein synthesis were first suggested by Caspersson and his associates after they had demonstrated the presence of ribonucleic acid in the cytoplasm of cells actively engaged in protein synthesis (Caspersson and Schultz, 1938, 1939; Caspersson, 1950). Since then knowledge of the cellular sites of RNA synthesis and the functions of various species of RNA has been derived from experiments that have used radioactive precursors of nucleic acids (for review, Prescott, 1964; Darnell, 1968; Lengyel and Söll, 1969). It is the purpose of this chapter to review the current status of knowledge on the synthesis and turnover of RNA molecules in mammalian cells and tissues during the processes of cell division and cytodifferentiation. Further information on the synthesis and biological roles of various RNA molecules can be obtained from the following reviews: (1) mRNA (Geiduschek and Haselkorn, 1969); (2) methylated RNA (Starr, 1969); (3) tRNA (Novelli, 1967); and (4) role in protein synthesis (Lengyel and Söll, 1969).

II. Intracellular Sites of RNA Synthesis

A. THE NUCLEUS AS THE SITE OF RNA SYNTHESIS

The early biochemical experiments on nucleic acid metabolism used inorganic phosphate-32 and were designed to determine the difference in the specific activity of nuclear and cytoplasmic components in normal and tumor cells (Marshak, 1940, 1941). Shortly thereafter, Marshak (1948) and Marshak and Calvert (1949), while investigating the specific activity of ribonucleic acid in normal and regenerating livers, suggested that nuclear RNA (nRNA) is the possible precursor of cytoplasmic RNA (cRNA).

The hypothesis of the nuclear origin of cRNA was further strengthened by a series of investigations that examined the kinetics of labeled RNA after injection of ^{32}P (Smellie et al., 1953a), ^{15}N-glycine (Smellie et al., 1953b), and ^{14}C-adenosine (Fresco and Marshak, 1953) in liver of adult rodents and rabbits. In these studies nRNA was rapidly labeled and reached maximum specific activity at 12 to 15 hours following injection of the isotopes. On the other hand, the specific activity of cRNA did not peak until 24 to 30 hours' labeling. This suggested a possible precursor product relationship between nRNA and cRNA (Fresco and Marshak, 1953; Smellie et al., 1953a).

The confirmation of the nuclear site of RNA synthesis was obtained from investigations that utilized autoradiography and labeled precursors of RNA. Following pulse-labeling times (1 hour or less), autoradiographic observations have demonstrated in a variety of cell types that 90% or greater of the labeled nucleosides are incorporated into the nucleus (Goldstein and Micou, 1959; Feinendegen et al., 1960; Perry et al., 1961; Showacre et al., 1967). If the labeling time is held to 30 minutes or less only radioactive nuclei are observed (Goldstein and Micou, 1959). Finally, Goldstein et al. (1960) demonstrated that enucleated fragments of human amnion cells are not capable of carrying out RNA synthesis, although these same fragments remain viable and actively incorporate labeled amino acids into proteins. Similar observations on the nuclear site of RNA synthesis have also been made in *Neurospora* (Zolokar, 1960), *Tetrahymena* (Prescott, 1962), *Vicia faba* (Woods, 1959), and *Triturus* (Prescott, 1964).

B. KINETICS OF NUCLEAR AND CYTOPLASMIC RNA IN TISSUE CULTURE CELLS

The site and time course of RNA synthesis have been investigated in a variety of mammalian cells *in vitro* by autoradiographic methodologies. Typical results of such studies are given in Fig. 1. Exposure of human amnion cells to labeled precursors of RNA for 2 to 5 minutes results in only nuclear chromosmal labeling. Following a pulse label of 10 minutes with ³H-cytidine, the radioactivity can be detected over the nucleolus as well as nuclear chromatin (Goldstein and Micou, 1959). These results suggest that chromosomal RNA synthesis is distinct and separate from nucleolar RNA synthesis, an observation that has been confirmed in the anucleolate mutant of *Xenopus* and in isolated nucleoli from HeLa cells (see Section III,A). The time that it takes labeled RNA to migrate from its site of synthesis in the nucleus into the cytoplasm is 10 to 30 minutes in HeLa cells (Perry et al., 1961) and Chinese hamster fibroblasts (Taylor, 1960) and 1 hour in human amnion cells (Goldstein and Micou, 1959). Peak incorporation of the labeled nucleosides into nuclear RNA occurs immediately upon removal of the isotopes and declines rapidly over the next 2 to 3 hours. Peak labeling of the nucleolus occurs by 2 hours after exposure of cells to labeled nucleosides, after which the specific activity of

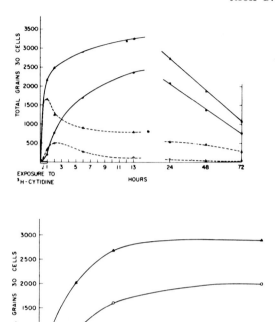

FIG. 1. Distribution of silver grains in autoradiograms of HeLa cells at different times after short-term exposure (1 hour, upper figure; 30 minutes, lower figure) to tritium-labeled cytidine. The grain counts were made over the cells as follows: △, total; ●, cytoplasm; ▲, nucleus; ○, nucleolus. (From Feinendegen *et al.*, 1960.)

the nucleolus falls rapidly. Labeled RNA accumulates in the cytoplasm for the first 24 hours and then begins to fall. The decrease in cytoplasmic labeling over the next 48 hours probably results from a dilution through cell division as well as turnover and degradation of RNA molecules. The label that is found over the nucleus is probably due to labeled DNA rather than chromosomal RNA. Generally, chromosomal RNA is completely diassociated from DNA shortly after division (Prescott and Bender, 1962).

C. KINETICS OF NUCLEAR AND CYTOPLASMIC RNA *in Vivo*

The kinetics of nuclear and cytoplasmic RNA following a single injection of ³H-cytidine have been studied in several tissues of the mam-

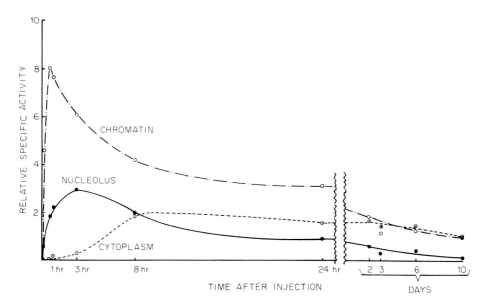

FIG. 2. Time curves of the relative specific activity of RNA calculated as the ratio of the number of silver grains per unit area over the relative RNA concentration in chromatin, nucleolus, and cytoplasm of liver parencyhmal cells following a single subcutaneous injection of tritium-labeled cytidine. (From Amano and Leblond, 1960.)

malian body. Typical curves depicting the time course of label incorporated into chromosomal, nucleolar, and cytoplasmic RNA in the cells of the liver of the mouse are given in Fig. 2. Grain counts over the chromatin, nucleolus, and cytoplasm showed peak nucleolar and chromosomal labeling between 40 to 60 minutes and in the cytoplasm at 8 hours and later (Amano and Leblond, 1960; Leblond and Amano, 1962; Amano et al., 1965). After a few days, the silver grains predominate over the cytoplasm and are still detectable up to 10 days after the initial injection. This long-term cytoplasmic labeling could result from reutilization of labeled breakdown products of RNA (Feinendegen et al., 1964; Feinendegen, 1967). Among the organs of the mammalian body, labeled RNA is most intense over cells actively engaged in protein synthesis. This is particularly evident in pancreatic acinar cells where the rough endoplasmic reticulum is more heavily labeled than the apical portion of the cell with its zymogen granules (Amano et al., 1965). Similarly, chief cells of the gastric mucosa are more intensely labeled than mucous neck cells and parietal cells following injection of ^{3}H-uridine (Berg and Thrasher, 1969, unpublished observations).

112   JACK D. THRASHER

III. Nuclear Sites of RNA Synthesis

A. NUCLEOLAR ORIGIN OF RIBOSOMAL RNA

Considerable evidence has accumulated from biochemical and genetic studies which demonstrate that ribosomal RNA is synthesized in the nucleolus and is then transported to the cytoplasm (Ritossa *et al.*, 1966; Brown, 1966; Birnsteil *et al.*, 1966; Darnell, 1968). In mutants of *Drosophila* that have different numbers of nucleolar organizers, Ritossa and Spiegelman (1965) have demonstrated by RNA–DNA hybridization experiments that the amount of DNA complementary to ribosomal RNA is directly proportional to the number of nucleolar organizers. Furthermore, it has been shown that the anucleolate mutant of *Xenopus laevis* lacks DNA complementary to 28 S and 18 S rRNA (Birnsteil *et al.*, 1966; Brown and Weber, 1968a,b). In addition, developing embryos of the anucleolate toad are incapable of synthesizing rRNA, while mRNA and tRNA continue to be transcribed (Brown, 1967). Finally, it has been shown that the large precursor molecules of rRNA are present in nucleoli isolated from HeLa cells (Penman *et al.*, 1966; Willems *et al.*, 1969b). These observations have been confirmed in rat liver nucleoli, which contain at least 75% of rRNA cistrons as determined by nucleolar DNA–rRNA hybridization experiments (Steele, 1968).

B. CHROMATIN SYNTHESIS OF mRNA AND tRNA

Probably the most convincing evidence for the chromosomal synthesis of mRNA and tRNA has come from observations on RNA synthesis in the embryos of the anucleolate mutant of *Xenopus laevis* and sucrose sedimentation analysis of rapidly labeled nuclear RNA in HeLa cells. In *X. laevis* embryos the cistrons for tRNA are not located with rRNA cistrons. In the anucleolate mutants tRNA synthesis is unaffected although rRNA synthesis is completely absent (Brown, 1967). In addition, tRNA anneals equally with DNA of normal and mutant embryos (Brown and Weber, 1968a,b). The high molecular weight messengerlike RNA is also synthesized in the absence of the nucleolus (Brown, 1967).

The chromosomal site of mRNA and tRNA synthesis has also been established in mammalian cells. Inhibition of nucleolar rRNA synthesis has little or no effect on the synthesis of mRNA (or HnRNA) and tRNA. Thus, the transcription of mRNA and tRNA occurs on extranucleolar DNA (Warner, 1967; Darnell, 1968). Finally, Huberman and Attardi (1967) have shown that rRNA hydridizes with small chromosomes that have a nucleolar organizer, while DNA complementary to cytoplasmic mRNA is distributed among all chromosomes.

C. RIBOSOMAL 5 S AND 7 S RNA

5 S and 7 S RNA are additional ribosomal components. 7 S RNA is presently considered to be a scission product of ribosomal RNA precursor molecules and will be covered below. However, recent evidence on 5 S RNA indicates that its transcription is not coordinated with rRNA cistrons. In the anucleolate mutant of *X. laevis* 5 S rRNA and tRNA anneal with DNA that has a different bouyant density from the DNA for 28 S and 18 S rRNA (Brown and Weber, 1968a,b). The independent transcription of the genes coding for 5 S rRNA has also been confirmed in L-cells (Perry and Kelly, 1968). The synthesis of 5 S RNA continues when 45 S rRNA synthesis is inhibited by actinomycin D. Thus, it appears that in L-cells as well as in *X. laevis* 5 S rRNA is not derived as a scission product of 45 S rRNA.

IV. The Biosynthesis of RNA Molecules

A. INTRODUCTION

The two primary functions of the nucleus are (1) to maintain and when necessary to duplicate the genetic information contained in DNA as a function of cell division and differentiation, and (2) to transcribe the genetic information into various RNA species which are then transported to the cytoplasm where they are translated into proteins. These proteins are then considered to be the phenotypic expression of the information contained in the DNA. This portion of the chapter will present current information and data that are available on the kinetics of RNA synthesis and the rate of transport of the various species of RNA into the cytoplasm of mammalian cells.

B. PATTERN OF RNA SYNTHESIS FOLLOWING SHORT- AND LONG-TERM EXPOSURE TO LABELED PRECURSORS

About 80% of the total cell RNA is represented by the two species of rRNA (28 S and 18 S). The remaining 20% of the cellular RNA is composed of a variety of species of which mRNA comprises only 1% (Table I). If rapidly proliferating cells are continuously exposed to labeled RNA pre-

TABLE I

COMPOSITION AND DISTRIBUTION OF RNA MOLECULES IN HeLa CELLS[a,b]

Cell compartment	RNA species	Total cell RNA (%)	Base composition (%)				
			C	A	G	U	GC
	28 S rRNA	53	32	16	36	16	68
	7 S rRNA	1	28	21	28	23	56
	5 S rRNA	1	26	18	34	22	60
	18 S rRNA	24	27	21	30	22	57
Cytoplasm	tRNA	12	27	22	27	24	54
	Pre-tRNA	1					
	mRNA (polysomes)	3	24	26	21	28	45
	HnRNA (cytoplasmic)[c]	1					
Total		94.5					
Nucleus	45 S pre-rRNA	1	33	13	37	17	70
	32 S pre-rRNA	3	33	14	37	16	70
	HnRNA		22	26	21	31	43

[a] Taken from Darnell (1968).
[b] The base composition of HeLa cell DNA is C, 21; A, 29; G, 22; T, 28.
[c] Heterogeneous RNA not in polysomes.

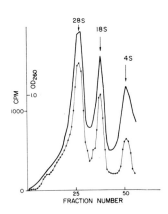

FIG. 3. Sucrose gradient sedimentation analysis of total cell RNA (HeLa cells) after a 24-hour exposure to ^{14}C-uridine. Fraction 1 is the bottom of the gradient; solid line optical density at 260 mμ; $\bigcirc$, counts per minute. (From Scherrer and Darnell, 1962; Darnell, 1968.)

cursors (e.g., ¹⁴C-uridine) and the total cellular RNA is analyzed by sucrose-gradient analysis, the three major classes of RNA (28 S, 18 S, and tRNA) are proportionately labeled (Scherrer and Darnell, 1962; Fig. 3). However, an entirely different pattern of labeled RNA molecules is observed if the

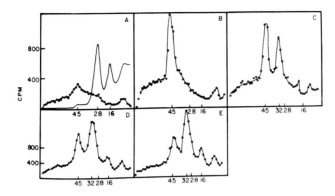

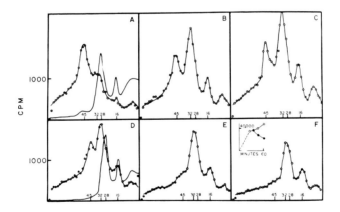

FIG. 4. Sedimentation analysis of radioactivity of total cell RNA (HeLa cells) after exposure to ³H-uridine in the absence (upper figure) and presence (lower figure) of actinomycin D demonstrating the scission of 45 S rRNA into its products. The upper figure shows that at 5 minutes (A) after exposure to the isotope the total cellular RNA is heterodispersed with slight peaks at 45 S and 4 S. With continued exposure (B, 15 minutes) peaks of radioactivity occur at the 45 S and 4 S regions. With longer exposures (C, 30 minutes; D, 45 minutes; and E, 60 minutes) the gradient slowly shifts to 32 S, 28 S, and 18 S rRNA products. In the lower figure A, B, and C were continuously labeled in the absence of actinomycin D, E, and F were sacrified at 10, 20, and 35 minutes after addition of actinomycin D (μg/ml). The treatment with actinomycin D prevents further RNA synthesis and thus illustrates the cleavage of 45 S rRNA into its products (32 S, 28 S, 18 S) with time. (From Darnell, 1968.)

duration of exposure of cells to labeled nucleosides is restricted. Warner et al. (1966) exposed HeLa cells to ^{3}H-uridine and extracted total cell RNA after labeling times of 5, 15, 30, 45, and 60 minutes. Sedimentation analysis and the incorporation of the isotope into various species of RNA at each time interval are presented in Fig. 4. At 5 minutes after exposure to ^{3}H-uridine the UV absorbance of RNA is present in 45 S, 28 S, 18 S, and 4 S peaks. However, the RNA that has incorporated the isotope by 5 minutes sediments from 4 S to about 100 S with slight peaks at 4 S and 45 S. The rapidly labeled RNA sediments in a heterogeneous pattern and therefore has been termed HnRNA. At 15 minutes the 45 S and 4 S peaks are more heavily labeled, indicating the synthesis of these two molecules. By 30 minutes after exposure to the isotope a new peak at 32 S appears. After exposure for 45 to 60 minutes, lighter weight RNA molecules become labeled. These peak between 16 S and 32 S.

In conclusion, it appears that rapidly labeled heterogeneously sedimenting RNA (HnRNA) is the first molecule to be synthesized immediately following exposure of cells to labeled precursors. Shortly thereafter, labeled tRNA and rRNA appear. The rRNA is then cleaved into smaller molecular weight rRNA. These observations are in agreement with the autoradiographic experiments that have shown that nucleolar RNA synthesis lags behind chromosomal RNA synthesis by several minutes.

C. SYNTHESIS OF HnRNA (DNA-LIKE RNA, GIANT RNA, OR mRNA)

The majority of the rapidly labeled RNA, that sediments in sucrose gradients between 17 S and 100 S has recently been termed hetereogeneous RNA (HnRNA) (Darnell, 1968). Others have referred to this RNA as "giant" RNA, mRNA, or dRNA (Attardi et al., 1966; Ellem and Sheridan, 1964). In any event it is characterized by its heterogeneity in size, its rapidity of labeling with isotopic RNA precursors, a guanosine–cytosine composition similar to the average DNA content, its lack of methylated bases that characterizes both rRNA and tRNA; it comprises about 1% of the total cellular RNA and is unassociated with the nucleolus (Warner et al., 1966; Darnell, 1968; Penman et al., 1968).

Attempts have been made to identify the properties and functions of the rapidly labeled HnRNA in HeLa cells (Penman et al., 1968), kidney cells (Willems et al., 1969a), and rat brain (Stévenin et al., 1969). Three species of HnRNA exist that have distinct kinetics of labeling, turnover, and distribution. They have been termed nucleoplasmic, cytoplasmic, and polyribosome-associated messenger fractions (Penman et al., 1968). Nucleoplasmic RNA synthesis is unaffected by doses of actinomycin D that inhibit rRNA synthesis. It remains within the nucleus and turns over with a half-life of approximately 1 hour (Warner *et al.*, 1966; Penman *et al.*, 1968). The cytoplasmic HnRNA is not associated with cellular organelles. It is broadly dispersed in a sucrose gradient from 10 S to 70 S and has no apparent function (Attardi and Attardi, 1967; Penman *et al.*, 1968). The polysome-associated HnRNA comprises a small portion of the total cytoplasmic HnRNA. Under inhibition of rRNA synthesis with actinomycin D, it appears in the polysomes 15 minutes after a pulse label with ^{3}H-uridine. The labeled RNA continues to accumulate in the polysomes for the next 20 minutes (Penman *et al.*, 1968). Apparently, it is this class of HnRNA that may represent true mRNA because of its association with the polysomes. Whether or not the nucleoplasmic and cytoplasmic HnRNA are related to the polysome-associated mRNA must await further clarification. However, it has been suggested that the nuclear restricted HnRNA represent a limited cleavage process for the production of mRNA (Stévenin *et al.*, 1969).

Other evidence suggests that the nucleoplasmic HnRNA may not be the precursor of mRNA. In HeLa cells that have had total RNA synthesis inhibited by actinomycin D without apparent effect upon protein synthesis, labeled HnRNA is not chased into polysomes of the cytoplasm (Latham and Darnell, 1965). Further information on the lability and nuclear turnover of HnRNA has been obtained form experiments on duck erythroblasts. Differentiating avian erythroblasts continue to synthesize hemoglobin and HnRNA, while rRNA synthesis and the formation of new ribosomes do not occur. In these cells HnRNA that sediments from 30 S to 80 S on sucrose gradients turns over with a half-life of 30 minutes. It continues to be resynthesized for almost 2 days after initial labeling of RNA with labeled precursors. During the first few hours following incorporation of labeled nucleosides approximately 60 to 70% of the RNA is degraded and never appears in the cytoplasm. The continued labeling of new RNA over the next 2 days is, therefore, reutilization of breakdown products of RNA (Attardi *et al.*, 1966). In addition, the fact that the long-lived mRNA that has been isolated from these cells sediments at 9 S strongly suggests that a large protion of the HnRNA is not a precursor of mRNA (Scherrer and Marcaud, 1968). Furthermore, when total cellular RNA synthesis is inhibited with actinomycin D in both duck and HeLa cells, about 90% of the HnRNA is degraded into acid-soluble material (Scherrer and Marcaud, 1965; Attardi *et al.*, 1966; Warner *et al.*, 1966). Finally, it has been estimated that the amount of HnRNA synthesized in various cells is approximately 6 times greater than what is needed for protein synthesis on the basis of the quantity of 45 S rRNA precursor in the cell (Darnell, 1968). In conclusion, it appears likely that in both proliferating and differentiating cells a large porportion of the HnRNA is degraded in the nucleus and never enters the cytoplasm. Thus, the exact origin of mRNA, although a small fraction of the HnRNA may be its precursor molecule, still remains to be elucidated.

The biological significance of having a HnRNA that turns over rapidly has not been satisfactorily investigated or discussed. However, several suggestions as to the purpose or possible function of HnRNA have been made. One is that mRNA represents only a small scission product of a large HnRNA molecule, and that the major portion of the molecule is degraded and turns over in the nucleus. This is similar to the nonconservative synthesis of rRNA (see below). Another suggestion has been that many extra copies of each HnRNA are made and only a few of each type of HnRNA become mRNA (Darnell, 1968). In any event, both hypotheses suggest that a large fraction of the genome is transcribed that is never expressed phenotypically. Thus, it may be possible that expression of genetic information is controlled at intermediate or translational levels in addition to transcriptional mechanisms (Scherrer and Marcaud, 1968).

D. Ribosomal RNA (45 S, 28 S, 18 S, 7 S, and 5 S)

The initial event in rRNA synthesis is the appearance of a large precursor molecule in the nucleolus that sediments at 45 S on sucrose gradients and has a molecular weight of about 4.5×10^6 daltons (Penman *et al.*, 1966; Weinberg *et al.*, 1967; Willems *et al.*, 1968; 1969b; McConkey and Hopkins, 1969). Following a pulse label with tritum nucleosides the 45 S RNA remains in the nucleolus for about 16 minutes. The molecule is then cleaved through several intermediate steps into smaller 18 S rRNA (MW = 0.71×10^6 daltons) and 32 S pre-rRNA (MW = 2.4×10^6 daltons). The cellular sites of cleavage, the cleavage stages, and approximate molecular weights of ribosomal 45 S RNA and its products are represented in Figs. 5 and 6.

The scission of the 45 S molecule to its ribosomal products (18 S and 28 S) occurs in a nonconservative manner. Recent evidence from molecular weight determinations (McConkey and Hopkins, 1969), analysis of the ratio of methyl groups to uridine bases (Willems *et al.*, 1968; Weinberg *et al.*, 1967), and base composition (Jeanteur *et al.*, 1968) have shown that approximately 30 to 50% of the 45 S RNA molecule is lost during the cleavage steps to 18 S and 32 S RNA. In addition, approximately 30% of the 32 S rRNA contains nonribosomal bases that are also lost in the cleavage of this molecule to 28 S rRNA (Jeanteur *et al.*, 1968; Willems *et al.*, 1969b).

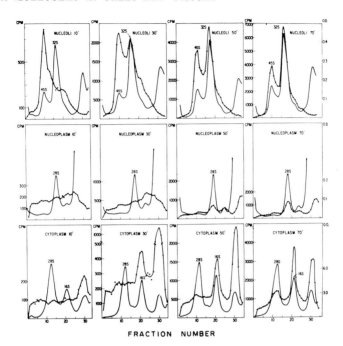

FRACTION NUMBER

FIG. 5. Sucrose gradient analysis of RNA extracted from nucleolar, nuclear, and cytoplasmic fractions from HeLa cells following exposure to ^{14}C-uridine at a concentration of 0.1 μCi/ml. The figure graphically illustrates that 45 S and 32 S rRNA are found only within the nucleolus for up to 70 minutes following the introduction of the label. 28 S and 18 S rRNA appear in the nucleoplasm between 30 to 70 minutes after incorporation of the isotope. 16S to 18 S rRNA first appears in the cytoplasm at 30 minutes, while 28 S rRNA is not found in the cytoplasm until 50 to 70 minutes after labeling. (From Penman *et al.*, 1966.)

18 S rRNA is derived from an intermediate precursor molecule (20 S) that is a product of the cleavage of a 41 S to a 36 S molecule within the nucleolus. The 20 S RNA is detectable in the nucleoplasm within a few minutes following a pulse label with ^{14}C-uridine. Further scission leads to an 18 S rRNA product which is then rapidly transported to the cytoplasm where it appears in the small ribosomal subunit (Penman *et al.*, 1966; Willems *et al.*, 1969b).

The 36 S RNA is cleaved to a smaller 32 S molecule. In contrast to the rapid transport of the 18 S rRNA into the cytoplasm, the 32 S RNA molecule remains associated with the nucleolus for about 40 to 50 minutes (Penman *et al.*, 1966, Willems *et al.*, 1969b). The 28 S rRNA that is cleaved from the 32 S molecule remains in the nucleolus or nucleoplasm for an additional 20 minutes before it appears in the cytoplasm in the larger ribo-

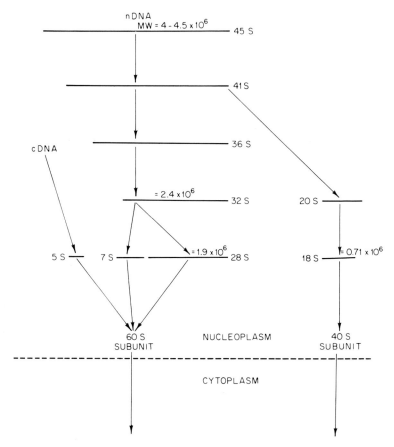

FIG. 6. Schematic representation of the synthesis of rRNA and the possible sites of association of the RNA with ribosome subunits. Abbreviations: cDNA (chromosomal DNA), nDNA (nucleolar DNA), MW (molecular weight in daltons).

somal subunit (60 S). The 28 S rRNA becomes associated with ribosomal proteins within the nucleolus or nucleoplasm (see Chapter 6).

Regulation and processing of nucleolar RNA synthesis has been investigated under inhibition of protein synthesis by puromycin and cycloheximide (Soeiro *et al.*, 1968; Willems *et al.*, 1969b). In cycloheximide-inhibited HeLa cells the synthesis of 45 S rRNA falls rapidly, while the nucleolar content of the molecule remains relatively constant. This results mainly from an increase in the processing time of 45 S RNA. The transformation of 45 S to 32 S RNA, although considerably slower under inhibition of protein synthesis, has a relatively normal efficiency. That is, for every 45 S molecule synthesized one 32 S is cleaved. Moreover, 18 S rRNA is not cleaved and transported to the cytoplasm, while the appearance of 28 S rRNA in the cytoplasm is delayed up to 3 hours. The increased processing time of 45 S rRNA under inhibition of protein synthesis directly contrasts with the rapid decay of 45 S following inhibition of transcription in the presence of actinomycin D. Thus, it appears that protein synthesis is necessary for normal processing of rRNA, although the exact mechanism involved is not known. However, it has been suggested that a decreased RNA polymerase activity may be responsible for the delayed appearance of rRNA in cycloheximide- and puromycin-inhibited cells. The decreased polymerase activity could possibly result from either a nonrenewable–unstable polymerase or an inhibition of polymerase activity in the absence of normal protein synthesis (Willems et al., 1969b).

Two additional small molecular weight rRNA's (7 S and 5 S) have been shown to be associated with the larger 28 S rRNA and the 60 S ribosomal subunit. The 7 S rRNA, which contains about 130 nucleotides, is a cleavage product of 32 S rRNA and, therefore, is synthesized at the same rate as 28 S rRNA. The 7 S molecule is released from isolated 28 S rRNA by heat, 5 M urea, and dimethylsulfoxide, all of which disrupt hydrogen bonds. In addition, a small difference exists between the sedimentation coefficient when untreated 28 S rRNA is compared to 28 S that has been disassociated from the 7 S molecule. Because of this shift in sedimentation values, it has been suggested that the 7 S rRNA may have a confirmational role with 28 S rRNA (Pene et al., 1968; Darnell, 1968).

The 5 S rRNA contains approximately 121 nucleotides (Forget and Weismann, 1967). It is present, like the 7 S molecule, in a 1:1 molar ratio with the 28 S rRNA (Galibert et al., 1965; Knight and Darnell, 1967). The 5 S rRNA appears first associated with subribosomal nuclear particles that contain 28 S rRNA. It is then demonstrable in the large cytoplasmic subunits, monomeric and poly-ribosomes (Knight and Darnell, 1967; Warner and Soeiro, 1967).

Unlike 7 S rRNA, the synthesis and kinetics of 5 S rRNA suggest that its transcription occurs on DNA that is not associated with 45 S rRNA nucleolar cistrons (Knight and Darnell, 1967; Brown and Weber, 1968a,b; Perry and Kelley, 1968). Newly formed 5 S rRNA appears in ribosomal subunits after 28 S rRNA has been synthesized. The delayed appearance of 5 S rRNA into the cytoplasm results from a large nuclear pool of the molecule. This pool accounts for 20 to 25% of the total 5 S RNA in HeLa cells (Knight and Darnell, 1967). These observations have been confirmed in L-cells in which 45 S and subsequently 28 S and 18 S rRNA synthesis were selectively inhibited by actinomycin D. Under these conditions 5 S rRNA continues to be synthesized when the formation of 28 S and 18 S rRNA is reduced to negligible levels for up to 8 hours. Thus, the transcription of 5 S rRNA is independent of 45 S rRNA and is probably not regulated by the 45 S molecule or any of its products (Perry and Kelley, 1968). Finally, Brown and Weber (1968a,b) have shown by DNA–RNA hybridization that a normal complement of 5 S DNA cistrons is present in anucleolate mutants of *X. laevis*.

E. tRNA (4 S)

Recently, Bernhardt and Darnell (1969) have demonstrated a class of small RNA molecules in HeLa cells that appear to be precursors (pre-tRNA) of tRNA. The pre-tRNA migrates between tRNA and 5 S RNA on polyacrylamide gels. Brief exposure of exponentially growing cells to ^{3}H-uridine shows that the pre-tRNA is more rapidly labeled (at least 10 minutes earlier) than tRNA. When RNA synthesis is inhibited by actinomycin D, the pre-tRNA disappears and the label appears in tRNA. In addition, brief exposure of cells to ^{14}C-methionine results in the incorporation of the labeled methyl group into both pre-tRNA and tRNA. There is a slight shift of the label from pre-tRNA to tRNA. Final proof of this precursor–product relationship must await additional data.

F. OTHER SMALL MOLECULAR WEIGHT RNA MOLECULES (4 S TO 7 S)

Small molecular weight RNA that sediment from 4 S to 7 S in sucrose gradients have been described in normal and tumor cells (Watson and Ralph, 1966a,b; Muramastsu *et al.*, 1966; Smith *et al.*, 1967; Nakamura *et al.*, 1968; Weinberg and Penman, 1968; Moriyama *et al.*, 1969). These RNA molecules comprise about 0.4% of the total cellular RNA. They are almost entirely confined to the nucleus and the nucleolus and have a long half-life of about 48 hours in HeLa cells. Estimates have shown that they consist of 100 to 180 nucleotides (Weinberg and Penman, 1968). Their base composition ranges from uridylic acid-rich fractions to G–C-rich molecules with methylated bases (Weinberg and Penman, 1968; Moriyama *et al.*, 1969).

Watson and Ralph (1966a,b) have found a 7 S RNA in mouse liver and sarcoma 180 cells that has apparent template activity. The 7 S RNA is associated with ribosomes in the cytoplasm. It resembles tRNA in base composition but contains no methylated bases or pseudouridylic acid. In addition, no amino acid-accepting activity could be demonstrated. Under conditions in which rRNA synthesis is inhibited, both the 7 S and HnRNA are continually formed. On the other hand, inhibition of total cellular RNA synthesis prevents the synthesis of the 7 S molecule. Finally, the 7 S RNA stimulated the incorporation of ^{14}C-glutamic acid into protein in an *in vitro* protein-synthesizing system. However, the authors have pointed out that the 7 S RNA could be a degradation product of rRNA with a messengerlike template activity.

Nucleolar 4–6 S RNA that is not associated with rRNA function or synthesis has been reported in tumor cells (Nakamura *et al.*, 1967, 1968) and rat liver cells (Muramatsu *et al.*, 1966). Three peaks of RNA were obtained by fractionation with exclusion chromatography on Sephadex G-100 in Novikoff hepatoma ascites cells (Nakamura *et al.*, 1968). The three peaks were then separated on sucrose gradients. Fraction I in the void volume contained approximately one half of the nucleolar 4–6 S RNA. The second fraction obtained from the exclusion volume consisted of 5 S RNA, while a third fraction of 4 S RNA was obtained from the remainder of the column. The 4–6 S RNA has a high template activity, lacks methylated bases (thus excluding tRNA and rRNA), and is resolvable into several minor components on acrylamide gels. The 5 S RNA is characterized by a relatively high G–C content (52%). However, it lacks methylated bases and has neither template nor amino acid-accepting activities. The 4 S RNA accepts amino acids and probably consists of tRNA. In conclusion, it appears that the nucleolus contains several low molecular weight RNA molecules that are rapidly synthesized and appear to be unrelated to rRNA.

Moriyama *et al.* (1969) have also investigated 4–7 S RNA in nuclear preparations from Novikoff hepatoma cells. The RNA can be separated into four main peaks on Sephadex G-100 columns. They are further resolvable by polyacrylamide gel electrophoresis into eleven or more components. The 4–7 S RNA is composed of two fractions rich in uridylic acid (5 S and 7 S) and two G–C-rich (4–5 S) fractions. The 5 S RNA rich in uridylic acid is further resolvable into five bands on polyacrylamide gels. This heterogeneous 5 S fraction and the 7 S RNA are not methylated and can be demonstrated in both the nucleus and cytoplasm. They are not breakdown products of rRNA, appear to be stable, and turn over at a slow rate within the nucleus. A similar fraction of small molecular weight RNA has been found in HeLa cells to turnover with a half-life of 48 hours (Weinberg and Penman, 1968). Although these RNA molecules are not bound to protein, it is possible that they may be part of the nucleoprotein complex involved in gene expression (see Chapter 6). The G–C-rich 4–5 S RNA, on the other hand, is methylated and appears to be tRNA and rRNA. Thus, it appears that further clarification of the functions of the uridylic acid-rich RNA might help to elucidate some aspects of gene expression in mammalian cells.

V. Nucleic Acids of Mitochondria

A. INTRODUCTION

The existence of DNA and RNA and the capability of mitochondria to replicate DNA and to undergo RNA and protein synthesis are now well documented (for review, Roodyn and Wilkie, 1968; Nass, 1969c). This portion of the chapter will briefly discuss the nucleic acids of mitochondria in a variety of cell types. Protein synthesis and the turnover of proteins in mitochondria will be described in Chapter 6.

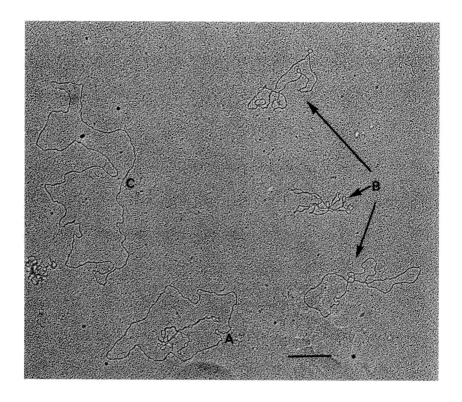

FIG. 7. Electron micrographs of circular DNA molecules isolated from mitochondria of mouse fibroblasts (L-cells). A highly twisted or supercoiled monomer is lying inside an open monomer (A); three lossely twisted monomers (B); one open dimer (C). The molecules have been spread on the surface of a monolayer of protein and subsequently contrasted by shadow casting from all directions with vaporized platinum-iridium. Scale is $0.5\,\mu$. (From Nass, 1969c.)

B. MITOCHONDRIAL DNA (mDNA)

Mitochondrial DNA, on the average, is a double-stranded circle with a perimeter of 4.7 to 5.5 μ and a molecular weight of 9 to 10 $\times$ 10^6 daltons in multicellular animals (Nass, 1969c). Circular molecules of mDNA larger than 5 μ have been reported in some cells (Nass, 1969c). In yeast the bulk of mDNA consists of linear filaments (Shapiro et al., 1968). However, mDNA isolated from all other cell types is circular and upon examination by the electron microscope has multiple forms, i.e., monomer, dimers, and oligomers (Fig. 7). The circles may be opened or supercoiled (Nass, 1969c). The significance of these multiple forms is not known, but they may be a function of replication, genetic information, or even redundancy of cistrons.

TABLE II

CONTENT OF DNA PER MILLIGRAM OF MITOCHONDRIAL PROTEIN[a]

Cell type	DNA (μg/mg protein)	References[b]
Nondividing cell populations		
Rat liver	0.65, 0.8, 0.51	1, 2, 3
Hamster liver	0.58	3
Mouse liver	0.55	3
Chicken liver	0.5	4
Frog oocytes	0.52	5
Rapidly dividing populations		
L-cells (fibroblasts)	1.0–1.2	4
Mouse embryo	1.3	3
Mouse placenta	0.9	3
Rat embryo	1.8	3
Rat placenta	1.7	3
Hamster embryo	1.3	3
Hamster placenta	1.1	3
Tumors		
Ascites tumor	2.5	1
Hepatoma (rat)	5.3	3
Walker carcinoma	4.7, 8.2	2, 3
Jensen sarcoma	4.7, 5.4	2, 3
Sarcoma (mouse)	4.7	3
Sarcoma (hamster)	4.7	3

[a] Modified from Nass (1969c).

[b] Key to references:

1. Nass (1969c)
2. Neubert (1966)
3. Wunderlick et al. (1966)
4. Borst et al. (1967)
5. Dawid (1966)

The amount of mDNA accounts for only 0.15% of total nuclear DNA in most cell types (Nass, 1969c). However, in *Physarum polycephalum* cytoplasmic DNA accounts for 10% of the total cellular DNA (Holt and Gurney, 1969). Estimates of the DNA content per mitochondrion and per milligram of mitochondrial protein have been made in several cell types and are summarized in Table II. In general, mitochondria from rapidly proliferating cells (tissue culture, embryos) contain more DNA than nonproliferating cells (liver). Tumor cells contain considerably more mDNA per microgram of mitochondrial protein than normal cell types. The purpose of this multiplicity of mDNA in tumor cells is not presently understood. However, it may be related to the rate of turnover or the need of multiple genetic information.

Nass (1969a,b) has investigated with electron microscopy (EM) the intramiochondrial arrangement of mDNA in serial sections of fixed mitochondria and in hyoptonic spreads of lysed single mitochondria. Examination of serial EM sections of branched mitochondria in embryonic chick muscle has shown that up to 6 "nucleoid" areas are present in each mitochondrion. At least one such aggregation of DNA filaments occurs in each branch of the mitochondrion. Similar observations on mouse fibroblasts have revealed from 2 to 6 nucleoids per mitochondrion. Examination of mDNA isolated by lysing of mitochondria has also confirmed that from 2 to 6 circular molecules are present with in a single mitochondiron. Frequently, these are in dimer and oligomer configurations. Further examination of either sectioned material or mitochondrial spreads by electron microscopy has shown that the DNA filaments are frequently attached to the inner mitochondrial membrane. This latter observation is analogous to the attachment of bacterial DNA filaments to the mesosome, the site of respiratory enzymes in bacteria (Ryter and Landman, 1964). In conclusion, it appears that mitochondria contain from 2 to 6 circular molecules of DNA in the form of a nucleoid. In addition, the mDNA may be attached to the inner mitochondrial membrane in much the same manner as the nucleoid of bacteria.

It is now evident that mDNA is self-replicating and that the mitochondrial DNA polymerase is distinct from nuclear DNA polymerase (Neubert *et al.*, 1967; Meyer and Simpson, 1968). Recently, Gross and Rabinowitz (1969) have shown that mDNA probably undergoes semiconservative replication, an observation that has also been made with chloroplast DNA (Chiang and Sueoka, 1967).

Mitochondrial DNA in nonproliferating cell populations turns over at a higher rate and has a higher specific activity than nuclear DNA of the same cell type. Estimates of the turnover time of mDNA have shown it to be most rapid in heart (half-life = 6.7 days), with liver, kidney, and brain mDNA having half-lives of 9.4, 10.4, and 31 days, respectively (Gross et al., 1969). The mDNA synthesis in these tissues reflects mitochondrial turnover rather than repair of damaged DNA (Gross and Rabinowitz, 1969).

DNA synthesis in mitochondria has been investigated in several types of dividing cells. The bulk of evidence suggests that mDNA is synthesized independently of nuclear DNA in yeast (Smith et al., 1968), *Tetrahymena pyriformis* (Stone and Miller, 1965; Parsons, 1965), *Physarum polycephalum* (Guttes et al., 1967; Holt and Gurney, 1969), chick fibroblast (Meyer and Ris, 1966), and mouse L-cells (Nass, 1969a,b,c). Periodicity of mDNA synthesis occurs in yeast and L-cells, but does not seem to happen in the synchronous cell cycle of *P. polycephalum*. Finally, Stone and Miller (1965) have observed mitochondria that were labeled with ^{3}H-thymidine in *T. pyriformis* over three consecutive cell cycles. Their results show that one half of the radioactivity in the mitochondria is transmitted to each daughter cell at division.

The most obvious role that can be assigned to mDNA is that of extranuclear genes. This can be concluded from its ubiquity, its semiconservative replication, and its ability to direct mitochondrial RNA (see below) and protein (see Chapter 6) synthesis. Recent estimates suggest that the amount of genetic information stored in mDNA is sufficient to code for approximately 5000 amino acids or about 30 proteins with a molecular weight of 20,000 each (Sinclair and Stevens, 1966; Roodyn and Wilkie, 1968; Nass, 1969c). Thus, it is probable that structural proteins of the inner mitochondrial membrane as well as some of the cytochromes are encoded in mDNA, while outer membrane proteins and most of the mitochondrial enzymes arise from nuclear-directed mRNA (Roodyn and Wilkie, 1968; see Chapter 6).

C. MITOCHONDRIAL RNA

Several discrete species of RNA have been isolated from mitochondria in a variety of cell types. These include a messengerlike RNA (Comorosan et al., 1968; Attardi and Attardi, 1968; Vesco and Penman, 1969), ribosomes and ribosomal RNA (Dubin and Brown, 1967; O'Brien and Kalf, 1967a,b; Küntzel, 1969), several species of tRNA, mitochondrial-specific aminoacyl-tRNA synthetases (Barnett and Brown, 1967; Barnett et al., 1967) and N-formylmethionyl-tRNA (Smith and Marcker, 1968; Galper and Darnell, 1969; Knight and Sugiyama, 1969).

RNA with sedimentation coefficients that suggest mRNA has been isolated from mitochondria of HeLa cells (Attardi and Attardi, 1968; Vesco and Penman, 1969) and mouse liver (Comorosan et al., 1968). In

HeLa cells the RNA is membrane associated and is synthesized at a high rate on mitochondrial DNA (Attardi and Attardi, 1968). Its base composition is similar to that of mitochondrial DNA. The RNA is labeled after 3 minutes' exposure of mitochondria to ^{3}H-uridine. Its specific activity increases linearly and reaches a maximum after about 100 minutes. The RNA is rapidly transported from the mitochondria into the cytoplasm where it becomes associated with ribosomes. It is not clear whether or not this RNA functions in either or both the cytoplasmic and mitochondrial protein-synthesizing system. Two additional species of mitochondrial RNA that are associated with mitochondrial cytochrome oxidase-containing structures have also been described (Vesco and Penmen, 1969). They have sedimentation coefficients of 12 S and 21 S and a G–C content of 43%. However, no functional role has been ascribed to these two species. In mouse liver a rapidly labeled RNA has been isolated and characterized from mitochondria. The RNA has a molecular weight of 1.5×10^5 (9.7 S) and is continuously synthesized for 120 minutes both *in vivo* and *in vitro*. The RNA slightly stimulates amino acid incorporation into mitochondria. In addition, it hybridizes with mitochondrial DNA to a greater extent than with nuclear DNA. Finally, estimates of its codon length suggest that the RNA can code for nearly 150 amino acids corresponding to a polypeptide with a molecular weight of 17,000 (Comorosan *et al.*, 1968).

Eighteen species of tRNA have been identified in purified mitochondrial preparations from *Neurospora* (Barnett and Brown, 1967; Barnett *et al.*, 1967; Epler and Barnett, 1967). Of these eighteen, three (aspartyl, phenlyalanyl, and leucyl) have mitochondrial-specific aminoacyl-tRNA synthetases. Buck and Nass (1968, 1969) have extended these observations in rat liver to include tRNA for leucine, tyrosine, aspartate, valine, and serine. The existence of leucyl-tRNA and its synthetase has also been confirmed in *Tetrahymena pyriformis* (Suyuma and Eyer, 1967). In rat liver mitochondria both leucyl- and tyrosyl-tRNA cannot be acetylated by cytoplasmic tRNA synthetase and, therefore, appear to be specific to rat liver mitochondria (Nass and Buck, 1969). Moreover, mitochondrial leucyl-tRNA anneals with mitochondrial DNA, while under identical conditions almost no hybridization occurs between cytoplasmic leucyl-tRNA and mitochondrial DNA (Nass and Buck, 1969).

Recently, it has been suggested that tRNA of mitochondria in HeLa cells, rat liver, and *Neurospora* may be similar to bacterial tRNA (Smith and Marcker, 1968; Galper and Darnell, 1969; Knight and Sugiyama, 1969). N-formylmethionyl-tRNA (f-met tRNA), which initiates bacterial protein synthesis, has been isolated from mitochondria of these three cell types. The RNA specifically incorporates ^{14}C-methionine and the uptake of the isotope is inhibited by aminopterin, an inhibitor of folic acid reductase. Although it remains to be demonstrated that protein synthesis in mitochondria is initiated by f-met tRNA, there is evidence that suggests that protein synthesis in mitochondria may be similar to bacteria. In addition chloramphenicol, an inhibitor of bacterial protein synthesis, also inhibits *in vitro* mitochondrial protein synthesis (Clark-Walker and Linnane, 1966). Furthermore, Knight and Sugiyama (1969) have shown that mitochondria of HeLa cells probably contain two species of tRNA that are electrophoretically similar to *Escherichia coli* tRNA. They have been designated type A (the bulk of tRNA) and type B (migrates between type A and 5 S RNA). Although type B has amino acid-accepting activity in *E. coli*, no function has been demonstrated for it in HeLa mitochondria.

The presence of ribosomes and rRNA in mitochondria have also been demonstrated in various eucaryotic cells (Dubin and Brown, 1967; O'Brien and Kalf, 1967a,b; Künztel, 1969). The monomeric ribosomes of mitochondria have sedimentation values of 55 S (rat liver) and 73 S (*Neurospora*) and are similar to the monomers of bacterial ribosomes (approximately 70 S). The monomeric forms of cytoplasmic ribosomes of eucaryotic cells, on the other hand, sediment between 77 S and 80 S in sucrose gradients (Elson, 1967). In addition, sedimentation analysis of mitochondrial rRNA has given values of 12.7 S to 18 S for the small subunit, and 22.4 S to 27 S for the large rRNA in *Neurospora* (Wood and Luck, 1969; Künztel, 1969), *Saccharomyces cerevisiae* (Rogers *et al.*, 1967; Steinschneider, 1969) and chinese hamster cells (Dubin and Brown, 1967). These values are similar to those obtained for rRNA of bacterial ribosomes (16 S and 23 S) and are lower than cytoplasmic rRNA of eucaryotes (mammals, 18 S and 28 S; *Neurospora*, 17 S and 25 S (Peterman, 1964; Künztel, 1969). Finally, recent hybridization studies have shown that mitochondrial rRNA anneals with mitochondrial DNA to such an extent that approximately 18% of the nucleotides of one mDNA strand may code for mitochondrial rRNA (Wood and Luck, 1969). In conclusion, it appears that both the biochemical and physical properties of mitochondria (ribosomes, rRNA, tRNA, f-met-tRNA, and mitochondrial DNA) do permit the speculation that mitochondria could possibly have arisen from a symbiotic relationship between a primitive procaryotic cell and a protomitochondrion (Sagan, 1967; Roodyn and Wilkie, 1968).

VI. RNA Synthesis in Special Cell Systems

A. INTRODUCTION

The rates of turnover of RNA in cells and whole tissues have been reported. In general, the turnover rate of total tissue RNA is shortest in rapidly renewing cell populations such as intestinal epithelia (3.6 to 4.6 days), testis (4.0 days), and spleen (5 days), while the RNA of nonproliferating skeletal muscle turnsover in 17 days. Intermediate values have been demonstrated for the kidney (8.7 days) and liver (7.2 days), which are considered to be slowly renewing cell populations (Gerber et al., 1960).

Measurements of the turnover of different species of RNA have been made both in vivo and in vitro. Amano et al. (1965) have shown from autoradiographic observations that three pools of RNA occur within the nucleolus, nucleoplasm, and cytoplasm. Apparently, these correspond to mRNA, tRNA, and rRNA with turnover times of approximately 4 hours, 16 hours, and 1 week, respectively. These estimates are very close to the values obtained by biochemical methods. Thus, in poliovirus-infected HeLa cells nuclear RNA turns over with a half-life of 15 to 20 minutes, while cytoplasmic mRNA turnover occurs in about 3 hours. Similarly, Wilson and Hoagland (1967) have shown that most of the mRNA of liver cells decays with a half-life of 3 to 4 hours. Calculations on the turnover of rRNA have produced half-life values that range from 5 to 115 days in a variety of tissues (Erdos and Bessada, 1966). These estimates, however, only reflect average values for the turnover of RNA molecules. They do not account for long-lived mRNA's that are involved in cytodifferentiation as well as the synthesis of specific proteins. Thus, in this portion of the chapter special attention will be given to RNA synthesis during cytodifferentiation and in mature cell populations undergoing sequential gene activation. For detailed account of the molecular events of early embryogenesis the following reviews are recommended (Moscona and Monroy, 1966–1969); Davidson, 1968).

B. DNA, RNA, AND HEMOGLOBIN SYNTHESIS DURING CYTODIFFERENTIATION OF MAMMALIAN ERYTHROID CELLS

The erythroid lineage is an excellent cell system in which to follow the relationship between DNA and RNA synthesis and the subsequent appearance of a specific end product, hemoglobin, during cytodifferentiation. For descriptive purposes the terminology used by Marks and Kovach (1966) will be adhered to: stem cell → proerythrolblast → basophilic erythroblast → polychromatic erythroblast → orthrochromatic erythroblast → reticulocyte → erythrocyte.

On the basis of autoradiographic studies utilizing ^{3}H-thymidine in fetal hepatic and adult bone marrow in a variety of animals, DNA synthesis occurs in stem cells through baspohilic erythroblast. Cell division probably does not occur beyond the polychromatic erythrobalst stage (Cronkite, 1964; Lajtha, 1964; Lala et al., 1966). In the latter stages of cytodifferentiation the nucleus becomes pyknotic and is lost by extrusion at the orthrochromatic erythroblast stage, after which maturation through reticulocytes to erthrocytes takes place (Bro-Rasmussen and Henriksen, 1964). Estimates for the maturation time for orthrochromatic erythroblasts are 40 to 50 hours, reticulocytes from 48 to 72 hours, and the live span of erythrocytes at 62 (rat) to 120 (man) days (Finch, 1959; Cronkite, 1964; Cleaver, 1967).

RNA synthesis as measured by the incorporation of ^{3}H-cytidine in autoradiographs of rat bone marrow occurs most intensely in the immature cells (proerythroblast to polychromatic erythroblast) (Feinendegen et al., 1964). Similarly, the concentration of RNA as measured by microspectrophotometric techniques decreases during this period of cytodifferentiation (Grasso et al., 1963). Orthochromatic erythroblasts are not labeled initially with ^{3}H-cytidine, but become labeled one day following the incorporation of the isotope by more immature cells. In addition, reticulocytes and erythrocytes do not synthesize RNA (Borsook et al., 1962; Feinendegen et al., 1964; Marks and Kovach, 1966). Thus, it appears that intense RNA synthesis is restricted to early stages of erythrocytic cytodifferentiation and ceases by the time that the nucleus becomes pyknotic at the orthrochromatic erythroblast stage (Grasso et al., 1963; Feinendegen et al., 1964).

The incorporation of ^{3}H-leucine, on the other hand, into the hemoglobin of rabbit erythroid cells is first detectable in basophilic erythroblast and continues through late reticulocyte stages (Borsook et al., 1962). In mouse fetal hepatic erythroid cells hemoglobin is synthesized at a greater rate in circulating reticulocytes as compared to erythroblast (Marks and Kovach, 1966). Thus, hemoglobin continues to be synthesized for almost 120 hours after the cessation of RNA synthesis in the orthochromatic erythroblast stage.

It is now evident that RNA synthesis takes place in the early stages of erythroid cytodifferentiation, while hemoglobin synthesis continues through late reticulocytes. The RNA, apparently, is packaged in polyribosomes that decrease in quantity from the erythroblast to the late reticulocyte (Marks and Kovach, 1966). In rabbit reticulocytes the total cellular RNA is distributed as follows: rRNA (80%) mRNA (1%), and tRNA-like RNA (19%) (Laycock and Hunt, 1969).

The mRNA of mouse and rabbit reticulocytes has been isolated and the α- and β-chains of hemoglobin have been synthesized in cell-free systems. In mice, the RNA sediments at 9 S in a sucrose gradient and is capable of directing the synthesis of β- chains in a protein-synthesizing system obtained from rabbit reticulocytes (Lockard and Lingrel, 1969). A similar mRNA (8 S) with a G–C content of 42% has been obtained from rabbit reticulocytes. It is capable of directing the synthesis of N-acetyl globin in an *E. coli* cell-free system (Laycock and Hunt, 1969). Recently, Hunt *et al.* (1969) showed in rabbit reticulocytes that the α-chain is translated at a faster rate than the β-chain. This strongly suggests that the two chains are translated from two different mRNA molecules.

In conclusion, a long-lived mRNA that sediments between 8 S and 9 S in a sucrose gradient is present in reticulocytes. This mRNA is probably preassociated with polyribosomes before the orthochromatic erythroblast stage. Its exact time of synthesis, its relationship to the appearance of heme synthesis of hemoglobin, and the means of translational control as well as degradation remain to be elucidated.

C. DNA, RNA, and Hemoglobin Synthesis during Cytodifferentiation of Avian Erythroid Cells

The cessation of RNA synthesis in mammalian erythrocytes generally occurs in the orthochromatic erythroblast stage coincident with the time that the nucleus is extruded. However, this leaves open the question as to whether nuclear extrusion acts to suppress RNA synthesis or if the phenomenon is an actual repression of transcription. Observations on nucleated erythrocytes of birds and other lower vertebrates indicate that enucleation is not the event that produces loss of transcription during erythroid cytodifferentiation.

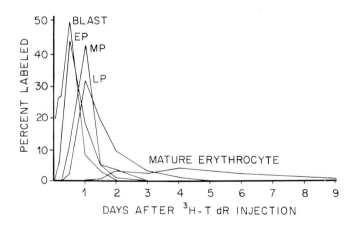

Fig. 8. Chickens were injected with ³H-thymidine and blood samples were taken at times after injection. The figure shows the appearance of labeled red blood cells for each of the developmental stages of erythrocyte maturation. Blast = basophilic erythroblast; EP = early polychromatic erythrocyte; MP = mid-polychromatic erythrocyte; LP = late polychromatic erythrocyte. (From Cameron and Kastberg, 1969.)

The stages of cytodifferentiation in avian erythrocytes have been described by Lucas and Jamroz (1961). These are erythroblast → early polychromatic erythrocytes → mid-polychromatic erythrocytes → late polychromatic erythrocytes → erythrocytes. Hemoglobin appears in the cytoplasm in the last portion of the late polychromatic erythrocyte stage.

Figure 8 demonstrates the appearance of each stage of the chick erythroid lineage following a single injection of ³H-thymidine. Erythroblast are labeled at 1 hour and reach maximum labeling at 12 hours after the injection. Labeled early polychromatic erythrocytes appear at 4 hours, reaching a peak at 12 hours and then approach zero labeling by 3 days postinjection. Mid- and late polychromatic erythrocytes follow a similar labeling pattern, but with a delay in maximum labeling at 24 hours and disappearing by 3 to 5 days following ³H-thymidine injection. Labeled mature erythrocytes appear in significant numbers by 2 days after thymidine administration (Cameron and Prescott, 1963; Cameron and Kastberg, 1969).

The patterns of RNA and protein synthesis during cytodifferentiation of chick erythrocytes is similar to that observed in mammalian cells. RNA synthesis (Fig. 9) is most intense in the erythroblast and early to mid-polychromatic erythrocyte stages. It is almost negligible in late polychromatic erythrocytes and is not found in mature erythrocytes. The majority of protein synthesis (Fig. 8) occurs in the erythroblast through the late polychromatic erythrocyte stages. It decreases at a linear rate to

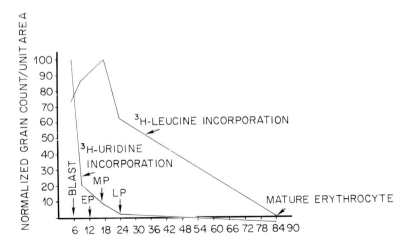

Fig. 9. The incorporation of ³H-uridine and ³H-leucine into developmental stages of chicken erythocytes. The data are plotted against the post-³H-thymidine injection time that each developmental erythrocyte stage required to reach its median percent labeled value. The abbreviations are the same as in Fig. 8. (From Cameron and Kastberg. 1969.)

almost 84 hours after the blast stage, i.e., at the beginning of the mature erythrocyte stage. Comparison of the two curves shows that 29 hours elapse between the time that ^{3}H-uridine incorporation into RNA decreases to 50% of its maximum value and the uptake of ^{3}H-leucine into protein decreases to 50% of its maximum (Cameron and Kastberg, 1969). In chick and turtle erythrocytes protein synthesis continues for 24 hours after mRNA synthesis has been inhibited with actinomycin D (Scott and Malt, 1965). In duck erythrocytes, on the other hand, the majority of mRNA decays with a half-life of 6 to 8 hours (Scherrer *et al.*, 1966). Thus, nucleated erythrocytes of lower vertebrates contain a long-lived mRNA that directs translation for as much as 29 hours after nuclear RNA has stopped. The predominant species of mRNA sediments at 9 S in duck erythrocytes and appears, therefore, to be similar to the long-lived mRNA of mammalian erythrocytes (Scherrer and Marcaud, 1965, 1968).

D. DNA, RNA, AND PROTEIN SYNTHESIS DURING CYTODIFFERENTIATION IN THE ADULT LENS

The ocular lens is unique in that it is composed of a single epithelial cell type. In the fetal lens, DNA synthesis and cell division occur over the entire surface epithelium. As the lens approaches adult morphology the proliferative cells become restricted to a circumferential zone (proliferative zone) just anterior to the equator of the lens (Mikulicich and Young, 1963; Hanna, 1965; Riley and Devi, 1967). The newly formed cells migrate posteriorly toward the equator where eventually they elongate into the lens fibers of the cortex (Mikulicich and Young, 1963). During this migration the lens fibers undergo intense RNA and protein synthesis (Hanna, 1965; Young and Fulhorst, 1966; Fulhorst and Young, 1966). The cortical lens fibers are then transformed into the proteinaceous material of the nucleus (Fulhorst and Young, 1966).

RNA synthesis during lens cell cytodifferentiation has been investigated by autoradiography after administration of ^{3}H-uridine in immature and adult lens of a variety of animals (Hanna, 1965). The results are graphicially presented in Fig. 10. Radioactivity has been observed over the cells of the lens epithelium, cortex, and early differentiating lens fibers. In the adult lens the incorporation of ^{3}H-uridine is three times higher in the cortical cells than in the epithelial cells. As the cortical cells in the Bow region begin to elongate into lens fibers the amount of RNA synthesis diminishes. In the inner cortical regions where the nuclei of the lens fibers undergo progressive disintegration, RNA synthesis is no longer detectable. Similarly, protein synthesis in the lens has almost an identical distribution (for more

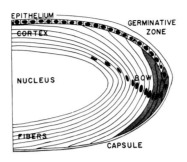

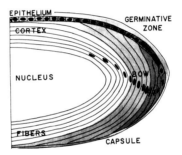

FIG. 10 Schematic representation of the sites of RNA synthesis (upper figure) and protein synthesis (lower figure) as determined by silver grain distribution following exposure to tritium-labeled uridine and amino acids, respectively, in adult rat lenses. (From Hanna, 1965.)

detail see Chapter 6). However, the degree of intense protein synthesis that occurs in the cytoplasm of the Bow cortical cells with respect to the small amount of RNA synthesis suggests that long-lived mRNA is probably synthesized in the cortical cells and is carried in the cytoplasm of lens fibers during cytodifferentiation.

Additional evidence for the existence of long-lived mRNA has also been obtained from autoradiographic observations on the developing chick lens (Fig. 11). Chick lens cells that synthesize DNA are located in a small zone anterior to the annular pad. The newly formed cells then migrate posteriorly through the annular pad, elongate to form lens fibers, and eventually become part of the cortex. The cells most active in RNA synthesis are located in the epithelium with a line of intense incorporation of ^{14}C- and ^{3}H-uridine extending through the annular zone into the nuclei of the lens

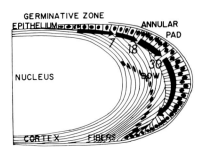

FIG. 11. Graphic illustration of the developing lens of chickens. The distribution of silver grains following administration of tritium-labeled uridine and amino acids is similar to that observed in the rat lens. For more detailed description see text. (From Hanna, 1965.)

fibers in the Bow region of the cortex. Protein synthesis, as determined by incorporation of labeled amino acids, is very intense over the epithelial through the Bow regions. In addition, significant but considerably less labeling of proteins occurs in the remainder of the cortex where no RNA synthesis is detectable (Hanna, 1965; Reeder and Bell, 1965).

The existence of short- and long-lived mRNA in chick and mammalian lens has been confirmed by observing protein synthesis while total RNA synthesis is inhibited by actinomycin D. In the developing chick lens that has had RNA synthesis inhibited for 8 hours the protein synthesis of the epithelial through the Bow regions drops to the level of cortical protein synthesis. In a lens that has had RNA synthesis inhibited for 24 hours protein synthesis continues at a low level in both the cortex and epithelium. These patterns of protein synthesis suggest that a stable mRNA exists throughout the lens, while an mRNA with a relatively short half-life is present in the cells of the epithelium and Bow regions (Scott and Bell, 1964; Reeder and Bell, 1965). A stable mRNA has also been found in the lenses of young rats (Zigman and Lerman, 1968) and calves (Stewart and Papaconstantinou, 1967). In the calf lens that has had RNA synthesis inhibited for 24 hours with actinomycin D crystalline proteins are synthesized in the latter stages of fiber cell formation, while the same treatment totally inhibits their synthesis during earlier stages of lens fibrogenesis (Stewart and Papaconstantinou, 1967). It appears, therefore, the stabilization of mRNA occurs in the transition between early and late stages of lens fiber cell formation. Similarly, rRNA is synthesized in the dividing epithelial cells of calf and adult lenses. However, in epithelial cells in stationary phase and in fiber cells, 45 S and 30 S rRNA precursors are synthesized but are not cleaved to 28 S and 18 S rRNA (Papaconstantinou and Julku, 1968). Thus, it appears that the synthesis and packaging of long-lived mRNA may be connected in some manner with the altered rRNA synthesis during lens cell fibrogenesis.

E. RNA SYNTHESIS IN THE LIVER

Contrary to the popular belief, the liver does not consist of a homogeneous population of cells. Protein metabolism within individual liver cells is at a relatively high rate in a zone of parenchyma that immediately surrounds the terminal portal venule, while those liver cells adjacent to the central vein (terminal hepatic venule) are least active in protein synthesis (LeBouton, 1968, 1969). For clarification of the discussion on protein synthesis in liver cells to be given in Chapter 6, it is necessary to discuss briefly RNA synthesis of liver cells.

Synthesis of rRNA and tRNA in liver cells follows the same general kinetics as discussed for HeLa cells. Estimates have been made for the turnover of rRNA and tRNA in fed and starved animals. In fed animals degradation of ribosomes and rRNA approximates synthesis. In fasting animals degradation exceeds synthesis and production of rRNA and ribosomes. In either physiological state rRNA and ribosomes have a half-life of about 5 days (Loeb et al., 1965; Hirsch and Hiatt, 1966; Erdos and Bessada, 1966). Similar values for the half-life of tRNA have been reported (Erdos and Bessada, 1966).

Rapidly labeled high molecular weight RNA has been investigated in rat livers (Schutz et al., 1968). It has a G–C composition close to rat liver DNA. The RNA is labeled within 4 minutes following administration of radioactive precursors and it sediments from 10 S to 80 S in sucrose gradients. Following treatment with actinomycin D there is a shift of labeled RNA from heavier than 45 S values to lighter coefficients. This suggests a very rapid turnover of the 10 S to 80 S RNA similar to that observed for the HnRNA of HeLa cells. However, the physiological significance of this RNA is unknown, but the giant RNA molecules may represent polycistronic RNA.

Estimates of the decay rate of polysomes following starvation and refeeding have shown the existence of both short- and long-lived messengers in the rat liver. Starvation of rats for 5 days leads to a marked decrease in cytoplasmic polysomes and, therefore, the appearance of monomers and dimers. Refeeding of starved rats for 10 to 30 hours leads to a rapid reassembly of polysomes. The newly formed polysomes in the presence of actinomycin D decay in a biphasic manner. Approximately two thirds have a half-life of 3 to 3 1/2 hours, while the remaining one third appear to be stable up to 80 hours (Wilson and Hoagland, 1967). Similarly, short-

and long-lived mRNA's in the rat liver have been reported by others (Trakatellis *et al.*, 1964; Revel and Hiatt, 1964). In starved, refed rats, when only the stable messenger is present in the cytoplasm of liver cells, albumin synthesis is increased from 27 to 63% of the total protein synthesis in the liver (Wilson *et al.*, 1967) LeBouton (1970, in press) has suggested from autoradiographic observations that this long-lived mRNA is found in the paryenchyma immediately surrounding the terminal portal venule. Thus, as in reticulocytes and lens epithelium, liver cells synthesize their specific end product, albumin, on a stable mRNA. It should prove interesting to determine if other liver proteins destined for export are synthesized in a similar manner.

F. RNA Synthesis in the Uterus Stimulated by Estrogen Administration

The early actions of estradiol on the uterus of immature and ovariectomized adult rodents have been investigated by several individuals. The first detectable event is the association of estrogen with cytoplasmic and nuclear receptors (uterine cytosol) within a few minutes after injection of ³H-estradiol-17β (Toft and Gorski, 1966; Toft *et al.*, 1967). The cytosol molecules sediment at 9.5 S and 5 S in sucrose gradients and have a molecular weight of about 200,000 (Toft and Gorski, 1966). The proteins are acidic and contain protein-bound phosphate (King *et al.*, 1969). Approximately 20,000 binding sites per cell for estradiol exist (Gorski *et al.*, 1969). Estradiol first associates with the extranuclear 9 S protein. It appears that the 9 S-hormone complex is then transferred to the nucleus where it is either cleaved or undergoes a conformational change into a 5 S-hormone complex (Jensen *et al.*, 1968). The uptake of estrogen into the nucleus is rapid. ³H-estradiol is bound with uterine chromatin by 2 minutes and reaches maximum association with the chromatin by 4 hours after injection of the hormone (Teng and Hamilton, 1968). The significance of the binding of estrogen to the chromatin may be to open up and regulate new cistrons for transcription. RNA synthesis is detectable within 15 minutes, while the synthesis of acidic proteins increases during the first 4 hours following estrogen administration. In addition, the histone content of uterine chromatin falls in parallel with the increase in RNA and total uterine proteins (Teng and Hamilton, 1968, 1969). The causal relationships could be a 5 S-estrogen initiation of transcription and an acidic protein synthesis. The increase in acidic proteins could then counter the inhibitory action of histones on transcription (Teng and Hamilton, 1969).

The early appearance of RNA synthesis in hormone-treated uteri correlates with the biphasic increase in the activities of two DNA-dependent

RNA polymerases. Within 20 minutes after estrogen treatment, RNA synthesis that is dependent upon the increase activity of a Mg^{++}-activated RNA polymerase commences (Hamilton et al., 1965, 1968). The polymerase activity is dependent upon continuous protein synthesis and its activity appears to be temperature sensitive (Nicolette and Mueller, 1966; Nicolette et al., 1968). This RNA polymerase is most active at the time that both rRNA and tRNA synthesis occur (Billing et al., 1969). The second RNA polymerase, which is activated by Mn^{++} $(NH_4)_2SO_4$, has maximum synthetic activity from 12 to 72 hours following estrogen treatment (Hamilton et al., 1965, 1968).

Changes in the patterns of synthesis of various species of RNA also occur on a temporal basis. The earliest detectable event is an increase in the synthesis of rRNA within 30 minutes after administration of estrogen (Billings et al., 1969). The rRNA rapidly appears in the cytoplasm as ribonucleoprotein, which is presumably new ribosomes (Hamilton et al., 1968). Coincidental with the synthesis of rRNA is the production of new 7 S RNA and tRNA. The 7 S RNA is probably a rRNA cleavage product. tRNA synthesis increases greatly between 1 to 6 hours and, therefore, lags slightly behind the synthesis of rRNA. The synthesis of mRNA is not measurable during the first 6 hours, but appears to increase slightly beginning with the sixth hour following hormone treatment (Billings et al., 1969). The significance of this mRNA is not known, but could it play an essential role in the temporal biochemical events initiated by estrogen.

It is interesting to note that cells of the uterine epithelium generally enter DNA synthesis between 12 to 18 hours following injection of estrogen in ovariectomized mice (Perrotta, 1962, 1966). The causal relationships of the hormone-initiated RNA and acid protein syntheses and the subsequent burst of synchronized cell division have yet to be elucidated. However, the cytoplasmic–receptor–gene activation system of the uterus may well be a classic example of cytoplasmic and extracellular control of nuclear activity in a differentiated tissue.

VII. RNA Synthesis over the Cell Cycle

A. INTRODUCTION

The cell cycle of mammalian cells has been described in detail in Chapter 3. For convenience RNA synthesis over the cell cylce will be discussed as the molecular events of G_0 (cells stalled in G_1 that can be called forth to enter DNA synthesis and undergo mitosis with the proper stimulus, e.g., liver regeneration, estrogen-stimulated uterus), G_1 (the time between the end of mitosis and the beginning of S phase of rapidly proliferating cells, e.g., tissue culture cells), S (period of DNA synthesis), G_2 (the time between the end of DNA synthesis and the beginning of mitosis), and D (mitosis).

B. RNA Synthesis in G_0 Cells

A large number of cell populations exhibit the state of G_0. Normally, these epithelia do not undergo DNA synthesis and divide. But under the proper stimulus most of the cell systems enter DNA synthesis between 12 to 24 hours. Examples of these are (1) regenerating liver (18 hours), (2) PHA-stimulated lymphocytes (18 to 24 hours), (3) estrogen-stimulated uterus (18 hours), and (4) lens epithelium after injury (14 hours) (for review see Baserga, 1968).

The earliest molecular event is exemplified in the estrogen-stimulated uterus of immature and ovariectomized rodents. Within 20 minutes after treatment the activity of a DNA-dependent RNA polymerase increases (Hamilton et al., 1965; 1968). This is followed by intense rRNA synthesis beginning at 1/2 to 1 hour later in the uterus (Billings et al., 1969), regenerating liver (Church and McCarthy, 1967a,b), serum-fed stationary mouse fibroblasts (Bloom et al., 1966), and PHA-stimulated lymphocytes (Rubin and Cooper, 1965). The increased RNA synthesis occurs in a coordinate fashion with rRNA appearing first, followed within a few hours by tRNA and eventually mRNA. It is reasonable to assume that this intense period of RNA synthesis is in preparation for cell growth and DNA synthesis prior to cell division. Inhibition of this RNA synthesis by actinomycin D inhibits the subsequent appearance of enzymes responsible for DNA synthesis such as DNA polymerase (Fausto and Van Lancker, 1965), thymidine kinase (Lieberman et al., 1963; Maley et al., 1965), and deoxycytidylate deaminase (Maley et al., 1965). However, the mechanism that permits a three- to fourfold increase in RNA and protein synthesis during the calling forth of a G_0 cell into an actively proliferating cell is yet to be fully understood. Possibly, the phosphorylation of acidic proteins and the acetylation of histones may be fundamental in this presumed initiation (see Chapter 6). It should be cautioned, on the other hand, that these molecular events of G_0 could be a release of inhibition rather than an initiation of temporal molecular events that eventually culminate in cell division (Baserga, 1968).

C. RNA Synthesis in Continuously Proliferating Cells

The temporal molecular events of the cell cycle are best understood through investigations using synchronous populations of continuously proliferating cells. Methods employed for synchrony involve isolation of cells in mitosis in Ca^{++}-free medium (Robbins and Marcus, 1964), inhibitors of DNA synthesis to collect cells in S (Stubblefield, 1968), or by arresting cells in mitosis with mitotic inhibitors (Stubblefield, 1968). Subsequent subculturing of isolated mitotic cells permits biochemical analyses during synchronized G_1 and S, while rescuing amethopterin-blocked cells, allows investigations on synchronized S and to a lesser degree G_2 (for detailed information on synchrony methods see Stubblefield, 1968). However, interpretation of data obtained from metabolically (amethopterin, colcemid) synchronized cells must be circumspect because such cells continue to synthesize RNA and proteins during the periods of blockage (Rueckert and Mueller, 1960; Stubblefield and Mueller, 1965; Stubblefield and Murphree, 1967; Stubblefield, 1968).

RNA synthesis commences about 30 minutes following nuclear reconstruction in a variety of cell types (Scharff and Robbins, 1965; Klevecz and Stubblefield, 1967; Pfeiffer and Tolmach, 1968). In HeLa cells where G_1 lasts for 5 to 6 hours, RNA synthesis continues at a linear rate for 4 to 5 hours, (Terasima and Tolmach, 1963; Scharff and Robbins, 1965). At the time of transition from G_1 to S an accelerated increase in RNA synthesis occurs. The rate of total nuclear RNA synthesis at least doubles during the first half of DNA synthesis (Terasima and Tolmach, 1963; Kim and Perez, 1965; Klevecz and Stubblefield, 1967; Pfeiffer and Tolmach, 1968). If the initiation of DNA synthesis is blocked by metabolic inhibitors, the accelerated rate of RNA synthesis is reduced and sometimes totally eliminated (Pfeiffer and Tolmach, 1968). This suggests a gene–dosage effect. Similarly, the rate of synthesis of each major class of RNA (rRNA, tRNA, mRNA) is linear during G_1 and then doubles during late G_1 and the first half of the S phase (Enger et al., 1968; Pfeiffer, 1968). This doubling of the rate of synthesis of each class of RNA is also eliminated when the cells are prevented from entering DNA synthesis (Pfeiffer, 1968).

The DNA that is replicated during the first half of the S phase is responsible for the gene–dosage effect on RNA synthesis. That is, as transcribable DNA is replicated more cistrons become available for transcription and, therefore, the rate of RNA synthesis increases. In addition, replication and transcription of early replicating DNA are necessary for the survival of the cell. Thus, if 5-bromodeoxyuridine (BdeU) is given to cells that are in early S (first one half) a striking decrease in cloning efficiency ensues, where as introduction of BdeU during late S has no effect upon clone production (Kajiwara and Mueller, 1964). Similar observations have been made with chromomycin succinate and actinomycin D treatments during early S (Fujiwara, 1967; Elkind et al., 1969). Thus, it appears that early replicating DNA plays a more important role in RNA synthesis and cell division than does late replicating DNA (Pfeiffer, 1968).

RNA synthesis continues at an increased rate through the remainder of S and G_2. However, it abruptly ceases during mitosis (Prescott and Bender, 1962; Salb and Marcus, 1965; Johnson and Holland, 1965). The absence of RNA synthesis during mitosis results from the condensation of DNA in the chromosomes, making the DNA unavailable for transcription (Johnson and Holland, 1965). However, the initiation of macromolecular events in G_1 of the next cell cycle does not require new RNA synthesis (Steward et al., 1968; Hodge et al., 1969). In mitotically synchronized HeLa cells that have had RNA synthesis inhibited after subculturing, protein synthesis commences and increases in rate for 45 minutes after mitosis without new RNA synthesis. This protein synthesis involves at least six different polypeptides (Hodge et al., 1969). This suggests the persistence of at least six mRNA molecules that cause a re-formation of polyribosomes in the G_1 of a new cell cycle. These may be responsible for the initiation of a new round of transcription and replication. It would be of interest to determine if persistent mRNA molecules are present during cytodifferentiation in rapidly renewing cell populations.

REFERENCES

Amano, M., and Leblond, C. P. (1960). Comparison of the specific activity time curves of ribonucleic acid in chromatin, nucleolus and cytoplasm. *Exp. Cell Res.* **20**, 250.

Amano, M., Leblond, C. P., and Nadler, N. J. (1965). Radioautographic analysis of nuclear RNA in mouse cells revealing three pools with different turnover times. *Exp. Cell Res.* **38**, 314.

Attardi, G., and Attardi, B. (1967). A membrane-associated RNA of cytoplasmic origin in HeLa cells. *Proc. Nat. Acad. Sci. U.S.* **58**, 1051.

Attardi, G., and Attardi, B. (1968). Mitochondrial origin of membrane-associated heterogeneous RNA in HeLa cells. *Proc. Nat. Acad. Sci. U.S.* **61**, 261.

Attardi, G., Parnas, H., Hwang, M. L. H., and Attardi, B. (1966). Giant size rapidly labeled nuclear ribonucleic acid and cytoplasmic messenger ribonuleic acid in immature duck erythrocytes. *J. Mol. Biol.* **20**, 145.

Barnett, W. E., and Brown, D. H. (1967). Mitochondrial transfer ribonucleic acid *Proc. Nat. Acad. Sci. U. S.* **57**, 452.

Barnett, W. E., Brown, D. H., and Epler, J. L. (1967). Mitochondrial-specific aminoacyl–RNA synthetase. *Proc. Nat. Acad. Sci. U. S.* **57**, 1775.

Baserga, R. (1968). Biochemistry of the cell cycle. *Cell Tissue Kinet.* **1**, 167.

Berg, N., and Thrasher, J. D. (1969). Protein and RNA synthesis in the differentiating gastric mucosa (unpublished observations).

Bernhardt, D., and Darnell, J. E. (1969). tRNA synthesis in HeLa cells: a precursor to tRNA and the effects of methionine starvation on tRNA synthesis. *J. Mol. Biol.* **42**, 43.

Billing, R. J., Barbiroli, B., and Smellie, R. M. S. (1969). Changes in the patterns of synthesis of ribonucleic acid species in immature rat uterus in response to oestradiol–17β. *Biochem. J.* **112**, 563.

Birnstiel, M. L., Wallace, H., Sirlin, J. L., and Fischberg, M. (1966). Localization of ribosomal DNA complements in the nucleolar organizer region of *Xenopus laevis*. *Nat. Cancer Inst. Monogr.* **23**, 431.

Bloom, S., Todaro, G. J., and Green, H. (1966). RNA synthesis during preparation for growth in a resting population of mammalian cells. *Biochem. Biophys. Res. Commun.* **24**, 412.

Borsook, J. L., Lingrel, J. B., Scaro, J. L., and Millette, R. L. (1962). Synthesis of haemoglobin in relation to the maturation of erythroid cells. *Nature (London)* **196**, 347.

Borst, P., Ruttenberg, G. J. C. M., and Kroon, A. (1967). Mitochondrial DNA I. Preparation and properties of mitochondrial DNA from chick liver. *Biochim. Biophys. Acta* **149**, 140.

Bro–Rasmussen, F., and Henriksen, O. (1964). Foetal erythropoiesis in the mouse. *Scand. J. Hematol.* **1**, 26.

Brown, D. D. (1966). The nucleolus and synthesis of ribosomal RNA during oogenesis and embryogenesis of *Xenopus laevis*. *Nat. Cancer Inst.* Monogr. **23**, 297.

Brown, D. D. (1967). The genes for ribosomal RNA and their transcription during amphibian development. *Curr. Topics Develop. Biol.* **2**, 48.

Brown, D. D., and Weber, C. S. (1968a). Gene linkage by RNA–DNA hybridization I. Unique DNA sequences homologous to 4S RNA, 5S RNA and ribosomal RNA *J. Mol. Biol.* **34**, 661.

Brown, D. D., and Weber, C. S. (1968b). Gene Linkage by RNA–DNA hybridization II. Arrangement of the redundant gene sequences for 28S and 18S ribosomal RNA. *J. Mol. Biol.* **34**, 681.

Buck, C. A., and Nass, M. M. K. (1968). Differences between mitochondrial and cytoplasmic transfer RNA and aminoacyl transfer RNA synthetases from rat liver. *Proc. Nat. Acad. Sci. U. S.* **60**, 1045.

Buck, C. A., and Nass, M. M. K. (1969). Studies on mitochondrial tRNA from animal cells. I. A. comparison of mitochondrial and cytoplasmic tRNA and aminoacyl-tRNA synthetases. *J. Mol. Biol.* **41**, 67.

Cameron, I. L., and Kastberg, M. L. (1969). DNA, RNA and protein synthesis during cytodifferentiation of two types of chick cells. *Cytobios* **3**, 229.

Cameron, I. L., and Prescott, D. M. (1963). RNA and protein metabolism in the maturation of the nucleated chicken erythrocyte. *Expt. Cell Res.* **30**, 609.

Caspersson, T. O. (1950). "Cell Growth and Cell Function." Norton, New York.

Caspersson, T., and Schultz, J. (1938). Nucleic acid metabolism of the chromosomes in relation to gene reproduction. *Nature (London)* **142**, 294.

Caspersson, T., and Schultz, J. (1939). Pentose nucleotides in the cytoplasm of growing tissues. *Nature (London)* **143**, 602.

Chiang, K. S., and Sueoka, N. (1967). Replication of chloroplast DNA in *Chlamydomonas reinhardi* during vegetative cell cycle: Its mode and regulation. *Proc. Nat. Acad. Sci. U. S.* **57**, 1506.

Church, R. B., and McCarthy, B. J. (1967a). Ribonucleic acid synthesis in regenerating and embryonic liver. I. The synthesis of new species of RNA during regeneration of mouse liver after partial hepatectomy. *J. Mol. Biol.* **23**, 459.

Church, R. B., and McCarthy, B. J. (1967b). Ribonucleic acid synthesis in regenerating and embryonic liver. II. The synthesis of RNA during embryonic liver development and its relationship to regenerating liver. *J. Mol. Biol.* **23**, 477.

Clark-Walker, B. F. C., and Linnane, A. W. (1966). *In vivo* differentiation of yeast cytoplasmic and mitochondrial protein synthesis with antibiotics. *Biochem. Biophys. Res. Commun.* **25,** 8.

Cleaver, J. E. (1967). "Thymidine Metabolism and Cell Kinetics." North-Holland Publ., Amsterdam.

Comorosan, S., Gaspar, A., and Sandru, D., (1969). Isolation and characterization of a rapidly labelled RNA from mouse liver mitochondria. *Biochim. Biophys. Acta* **166,** 394.

Cronkite, E. P. (1964). Erythropoietic cell proliferation in man. *Medicine* **43,** 635.

Darnell, J. E. (1968). Ribonucleic acids from animal cells. *Bacteriol. Rev.* **32,** 262.

Davidson, E. H. (1968). "Gene Activity in Early Development." Academic Press, New York.

Dawid, I. B. (1966) Evidence for the mitochondrial origin of frog egg cytoplasmic DNA. *Proc. Nat. Acad.Sci. U. S.* **56,** 269.

Dubin, D. T., and Brown, R. E. (1967). A novel ribosomal RNA in hamster cell mitochondria. *Biochim. Biophys. Acta* **145,** 538.

Elkind, M. M., Kano, E., and Sutton-Gilbert, H. (1969). Cell killing by actinomycin D in relation to the growth cycle of Chinese hamster cells. *J. Cell Biol.* **42,** 366.

Ellem, K. A. O., and Sheridan, J. W. (1964). Tenacious binding of the bulk of the DNA-like RNA of metazoan cells to methylated columns. *Biochem. Biophys. Res. Commun.* **16,** 505.

Elson, D. (1967). Ribosomal enzymes. *In* "Enzyme Cytology" (D B. Roodyn, ed.) p. 407. Academic Press, New York.

Enger, M. D., Tobey, R. A., and Saponara, A. G. (1968). RNA synthesis in Chinese hamster cells. I. Differential rate for ribosomal RNA in early and late interphase. *J. Cell Biol.* **36,** 583.

Epler, J. L., and Barnett, W. E. (1967). Coding properties of *Neurospora* mitochondrial and cytoplasmic leucine transfer RNA. *Biochem. Biophys. Res. Commun.* **28,** 328.

Erdos, T., and Bessada, R. (1966). The turnover of ribosomal RNA and soluble RNA in the rabbit uterus. *Biochim. Biophys. Acta* **129,** 628.

Fausto, N., and Van Lancker, J. L. (1965). Molecular mechanisms of liver regeneration. *J. Biol. Chem.* **240,** 1247.

Feinendegen, L. E. (1967). Tritium Labeled Molecules in Biology and Medicine." Academic Press, New York.

Feinendegen, L. E., Bond, V. P, Shreeve, W. W., and Painter, R. B. (1960). RNA and DNA metabolism in human tissue culture cells studied with tritiated cytidine. *Exp. Cell Res.* **19,** 443.

Feinendegen, L. E., Bond, V. P., Cronkite, E. P., and Hughes, W. L. (1964). RNA turnover in normal rat bone marrow. *Ann. N. Y. Acad. Sci.* **113,** 727.

Finch, C. A. (1959). Some quantitative aspects of erythropoiesis. *Ann. N. Y. Acad. Sci.* **77,** 410.

Forget, B. G., and Weissman, S. M. (1967). Nucleotide sequence of KB cell 5S RNA. *Science* **158,** 1695.

Fresco, J. R., and Marshak, A. (1953). On the biosynthesis of nucleic acids in the livers of adult mice. *J. Biol. Chem.* **205,** 585.

Fujiwara, Y. (1967). Role of RNA synthesis in DNA replication of synchronized populations of cultured mammalian cells. *J. Cell. Physiol.* **70,** 291.

Fulhorst, H. W., and Young, R. W. (1966). Conversion of soluble lens protein to albuminoid. *Invest. Opthalmol.* **5,** 298.

Galibert, F., Larsen, C. L., Lelong, J. C., and Boiron, M. (1965). RNA of low molecular weight in ribosomes of mammalian cells. *Nature (London)* **207**, 1039.

Galper, J. D., and Darnell, J. E. (1969). The presence of N-formyl-methionyl-tRNA in HeLa cell. *Biochem. Biophys. Res. Commun.* **34**, 205.

Geiduschek, E. P., and Haselkorn, R. (1969). Messenger RNA. *Annu. Rev. Biochem.* **38**, 647.

Gerber, G., Gerber, G., and Altman, K. I. (1960). The catabolism of tissue specific nucleic acid in the rat. II. Turnover time of ribonucleic acid and free nucleotides. *J. Biol. Chem.* **235**, 2682.

Goldstein, L., and Micou, J. (1959). On the primary sites of nuclear RNA systhesis. *J. Biophys. Biochem. Cytol.* **6**, 301.

Goldstein, L., Micou, J., and Crocker, T. T. (1960). Nuclear–cytoplasmic relationships in human cells. IV. A study of some aspects of nucleic acid and protein metabolism in enucleate cells. *Biochim. Biophys. Acta* **45**, 82.

Gorski, J., Shyamala, G., and Toft, D. (1969). Interrelationships of nuclear and cytoplasmic estrogen receptors. *Curr. Topics Develop. Biol.* **4**, 149.

Grasso, J. A., Woodward, J. W., and Swift H. (1963). Cytochemical studies of nucleic acids and proteins in erythrocytic development. *Proc. Nat. Acad. Sci., U. S.* **50**, 134.

Gross, M. J., and Rabinowitz, M. (1969). Synthesis of new strands of mitochondrial and nuclear deoxyribonucleic acid by semiconservative replication. *J. Biol. Chem.* **244**, 1563.

Gross, N. J., Getz, G. S. and Rabinowitz, M. (1969). Apparent turnover of mitochondrial deoxyribonucleic acid and mitochondrial phospholipids in the tissues of the rat. *J. Biol. Chem.* **244**, 1552.

Guttes, E. W., Hanawalt, P. C., and Guttes, S. (1967). Mitochondrial DNA synthesis and the mitotic cycle in *Physarum polycephalum*. *Biochim. Biophys. Acta* **142**, 181.

Hamilton, T. H., Widnell, C. C., and Tata, J. R. (1965). Sequential stimulation by oestrogen of nuclear RNA synthesis and DNA-dependent RNA polymerase activities in rat uterus. *Biochim. Biophys. Acta* **108**, 168.

Hamilton, T. H., Teng, C. S. and Means, A. P. (1968). Early estrogen action: Nuclear synthesis and accumulation of protein correlated with enhancement of two DNA-dependent RNA polymerase activities. *Proc. Nat. Acad. Sci. U. S.* **59**, 1265.

Hanna, C (1965). Changes in DNA, RNA and protein synthesis in the developing lens. *Invest. Opthalmol.* **4**, 480.

Hirsch, C. A., and Hiatt, H. H. (1966). Turnover of liver ribosomes in fed and in fasted rats. *J. Biol. Chem.* **241**, 5936.

Hodge, L. D., Robbins E., and Scharff, M. D. (1969). Persistence of messenger RNA through mitosis in HeLa cells. *J. Cell Biol.* **40**, 497.

Holt, C. E., and Gurney, E. G. (1969). Minor components of the DNA of *Physarum polycephalum*. *J. Cell Biol.* **40**, 484.

Huberman, J. A., and Attardi, G. (1967). Studies of fractionated HeLa cell chromosomes I. The chromosomal distribution of DNA complementary to 28S and 18S ribosomal RNA and to cytoplasmic messenger RNA. *J. Mol. Biol.* **29**, 487.

Hunt, T., Hunter, T., and Munro, A. (1969). Control of haemoglobin synthesis: Rate of translation of the messenger RNA for the α and β chains. *J. Mol. Biol.* **43**, 123.

Jeanteur, P., Amaldi, F., and Attardi, G. (1968). Partial sequence analysis of ribosomal RNA II. Evidence for sequences of non-ribosomal type in 45S and 32S ribosomal RNA precursors. *J. Mol. Biol.* **33**, 757.

Jensen, E. V., Suzuki, T., Kawashima, T., Stumpf, W. E., Jungblut, P. W., and De-
    Sombre, E. R. (1968). A two-step mechanism for the interaction of estradiol
    with rat uterus. *Proc. Nat. Acad. Sci. U. S.* **59,** 632.
Johnston, T. C., and Holland, J. J. (1965). Ribonucleic acid and protein synthesis in
    mitotic HeLa cells. *J. Cell Biol.* **27,** 565.
Kajiwara, K., and Mueller, G. C. (1964). Molecular events in the reproduction of
    animal cells III. Fractional synthesis of deoxyribonucleic acid with 5-bromo-
    deoxyuridine and its effect on cloning efficiency. *Biochim. Biophys. Acta* **91,** 486.
Kim, J. H., and Perez A. G. (1965). Ribonucleic acid synthesis in synchronously dividing
    populations of HeLa cells. *Nature (London)* **207,** 974.
King, R. J. B., Gordon, J., and Steggles A. W. (1969). The properties of a nuclear
    acidic protein fraction that binds [6, 7-³H] oestradiol-17β. *Biochem. J.* **114,** 649.
Klevecz, R. R., and Stubblefield, E. (1967). RNA synthesis in relation to DNA replica-
    tion in synchronized Chinese hamster cell cultures. *J. Exp. Zool.* **165,** 259.
Knight, E., and Darnell, J. E. (1967). Distribution of 5S RNA in HeLa cells. *J. Mol.
    Biol.* **28,** 491.
Knight, E., and Sugiyama, T. (1969). Transfer RNA: A comparison by gel electro-
    phoresis of tRNA in HeLa cytoplasm, HeLa mitochondrial fraction and *E. coli.
    Proc. Nat. Acad. Sci. U. S.* **63,** 1383.
Küntzel, H. (1969). Mitochondrial and cytoplasmic ribosomes from *Neurospora crassa:*
    Characterization of their subunits. *J. Mol. Biol.* **40,** 315.
Lajtha, L. G. (1964). Recent studies in erythroid differentiation and proliferation.
    Medicine **43,** 625.
Lala, P. K., Patt, H. M., and Maloney, M. A. (1966). An evaluation of erythropoiesis in
    canine marrow. *Acta Haematol.* **35,** 311.
Latham, H., and Darnell, J. E. (1965). Distribution of mRNA in the cytoplasmic
    polyribosomes of the HeLa cell. *J. Mol. Biol.* **14,** 1.
Laycock, D. G., and Hunt, J. A. (1969). Synthesis of rabbit globin by a bacterial cell
    free system. *Nature (London)* **221,** 1118.
Leblond, C. P., and Amano, M. (1962). Synthetic processes in the cell nucleus IV.
    Synthetic activity in the nucleolus as compared to that in the rest of the cell.
    J. Histochem. Cytochem. **10,** 162.
LeBouton, A. V. (1968). Heterogeneity of protein metabolism between liver cells as
    studied by radioautography. *Curr. Mod. Biol.* **2,** 111.
LeBouton, A. V. (1969). Relations and extent of the zone of intensified protein me-
    tabolism in the liver cells. *Curr. Mod. Biol.* **3,** 4.
LeBouton, A. V. (1970). Protein synthesis in the rat liver acinus after injection of
    actinomycin D: A radioautography study *Curr. Mod. Biol.* (in press).
Lengyel, P., and Soll, D. (1969). Mechanism of protein biosynthesis. *Bacteriol. Rev.* **33,**
    264.
Lieberman, I., Abrams, R., Hunt, N., and Ove, P. (1963). Levels of enzyme activity and
    deoxyribonucleic acid synthesis in mammalian cells cultured from the animal.
    J. Biol. Chem. **238,** 3955.
Lockard, R. E., and Lingrel, J. B. (1969). The synthesis of mouse hemoglobin β-chains
    in a rabbit reticulocyte cell-free system programmed with mouse reticulocyte 9S
    RNA. *Biochem. Biophys. Res. Commun.* **37,** 204.
Loeb, J. N., Howell, R. R., and Tompkins, G. T. (1965). Turnover of ribosomal RNA in
    rat liver. *Science* **149,** 1093.
Lucas, A. M., and Jamroz, C. (1961). "Atlas of Avian Histology." U. S. Dept Agric.
    Monogr. No. 25, Washington, D. C.

McConkey, E. H., and Hopkins, J. W. (1969). Molecular weights of some HeLa ribosomal RNA. *J. Mol. Biol.* **39**, 545.

Maley, G. F., Lorenson, M. G., and Maley, F. (1965). Inhibitors of protein synthesis: Effect on the levels of deoxycytidylate deaminase, thymidylate synthetase and thymidine kinase in regenerating liver. *Biochem. Biophys. Res. Commun.* **18**, 364.

Marks, P. A., and Kovach, J. S. (1966). Development of mammalian erythroid cells. *Curr. Topics Develop. Biol.* **1**, 213.

Marshak, A. (1940). Uptake of radioactive phosphorous by nucleic of liver and tumors. *Science* **92**, 460.

Marshak, A. (1941). P^{32} uptake by nuclei. *J. Gen. Physiol.* **25**, 275.

Marshak, A. (1948). Evidence for a nuclear precursor of ribo- and desoxyribonucleic acid. *J. Cell. Comp. Physiol.* **32**, 381.

Marshak, A., and Calvert, F. (1949). Specific activity of P^{32} in cell constituents of rabbit liver. *J. Cell. Comp. Physiol.* **34**, 451.

Meyer, R. R., and Ris, H. (1966). Incorporation of tritiated thymidine and tritiated deoxyadenosine into mitochondrial DNA of chick fibroblasts. *J. Cell Biol.* **31**, 76A.

Meyer, R. R., and Simpson, M. V. (1968). DNA biosynthesis in mitochondria: partial purification of a distinct DNA polymerase from isolated rat liver mitochondria. *Proc. Nat. Acad. Sci. U. S.* **61**, 130.

Mikulicich, A. G., and Young, R. W. (1963). Cell proliferation and displacement in the lens epithelium of young rats injected with tritiated thymidine. *Invest. Opthalmol.* **2**, 344.

Moriyama, Y., Hodnett, J. L., Prestayko, A. W., and Busch, H. (1969). Studies on the nuclear 4 to 7S RNA of the Novikoff hepatoma. *J. Mol. Biol.* **39**, 335.

Moscona, A. A., and Monroy, A., eds. (1966–1969). "Current Topics in Developmental Biology," Vols. 1–4. Academic Press, New York.

Muramatsu, M., Hodnett, J. L., and Busch, H. (1966). Base composition of fractions of nuclear and nucleolar ribonucleic acid obtained by sedimentation and chromatography. *J. Biol. Chem.* **241**, 1544.

Nakamura, T., Rapp, F., and Busch, H. (1967). Common features of the base composition of rapidly labeled RNA of nucleoli in a number of experimental tumors. *Cancer Res.* **27**, 1084.

Nakamura, T., Prestayko, A. W., and Busch H. (1968), Studies on nucleolar 4 to 6S ribonucleic acid of Novikoff hepatoma cells. *J. Biol. Chem.* **243**, 1368.

Nass, M. M. K. (1969a). Mitochondrial DNA I. Intramitochondrial distribution and structural relations of single- and double-length circular DNA. *J. Mol. Biol.* **42**, 521.

Nass, M. M. K. (1969b). Mitochondrial DNA II. Structure and physicochemical properties of isolated DNA. *J. Mol. Biol.* **42**, 529.

Nass, M. M. K. (1969c). Mitochondrial DNA: Advances, problems and goals. *Science* **165**, 25.

Nass, M. M. K., and Buck, C. A. (1969). Comparative hybridization of mitochondrial and cytoplasmic amino-acyl transfer RNA with mitochondrial DNA from rat liver. *Proc. Nat. Acad. Sci. U. S.* **62**, 506.

Neubert, D. (1966). Vergleiche Untersuchungen uber die Nucleinsaure-synthese in Zellkernen und Mitochondrien und ihre Beeinflussbarkeit durch Pharmaka. *Naunyn-Schmiedebergs Arch. Pharmakol. Exp. Pathol.* **253**, 152.

Neubert, D., Oberdisse, E., Schmieder, M., and Reinsch, I. (1967). Solubilization and some properties of vertebrate mitochondrial DNA polymerase. *Hoppe-Seyler's Z. Physiol. Chem.* **348**, 1709.

Nicolette, J. A., and Mueller, G. C. (1966). *In vitro* regulation of RNA polymerase in estrogen-treated uteri. *Biochem. Biophys. Res. Commun.* **24**, 851.

Nicolette, J. A., Lemahieu, M. A., and Mueller, G. C. (1968). A role of estrogens in the regulation of RNA polymerase in surviving rat uteri. *Biochim. Biophys. Acta* **166**, 403.

Novelli, G. D. (1967). Amino acid activation for protein synthesis. *Annu. Rev. Biochem.* **36**, 449.

O'Brien, T. W., and Kalf, G. F. (1967a). Ribosomes from rat liver mitochondria I. Isolation procedure and contamination studies. *J. Biol. Chem.* **242**, 2172.

O'Brien, T. W., and Kalf, G. F. (1967b). Ribosomes from rat liver mitochondria II. Partial characterization. *J. Biol. Chem.* **242**, 2180.

Papaconstantinou, J., and Julku, E. J. (1968). The Regulation of ribosomal RNA synthesis and ribosomal assembly in the vertebrate lens. *J. Cell. Physiol.* **72**, 161.

Parsons, J. A. (1965). Mitochondrial incorporation of tritiated thymidine in *Tetrahymena pyriformis*. *J. Cell Biol.* **25**, 614.

Pene, J. J., Knight, E., and Darnell, J. E. (1968). Characterization of a new low molecular weight RNA in HeLa cell ribosomes. *J. Mol. Biol.* **33**, 609.

Penman, S., Scherrer, K., Becker, Y., and Darnell, J. E. (1963). Polyribosomes in normal and polio-virus-infected HeLa cells and their relationship to messenger RNA. *Proc. Nat. Acad. Sci. U. S.* **49**, 654.

Penman, S., Smith, I., and Holtzman, E. (1966). Ribosomal RNA synthesis and processing in a particulate site in the HeLa cell nucleus. *Science* **154**, 786.

Penman, S., Vesco, C., and Penman, M. (1968). Localization and kinetics of formation of heterodisperse RNA, cytoplasmic heterodisperse RNA and polyribosome-associated mesenger RNA in HeLa cells. *J. Mol. Biol.* **34**, 49.

Perrotta, C. A. (1962). Initiation of cell proliferation in the vaginal and uterine epithelia of the mouse. *Amer. J. Anat.* **111**, 195.

Perrotta, C. A. (1966). Effect of x-irradiation on DNA synthesis in the uterine epithelium. *Radiat. Res.* **28**, 232.

Perry, R. P., and Kelley, D. E. (1968). Persistent synthesis of 5S RNA when production of 28S and 18S ribosomal RNA is inhibited by low doses of actinomycin D. *J. Cell. Physiol.* **72**, 235.

Perry, R. P., Errera, M., Hell, A., and Durwald, H. (1961). Kinetics of nucleoside incorporation into nuclear and cytoplasmic RNA. *J. Biophys. Biochem. Cytol.* **11**, 1.

Peterman, M. L. (1964). "The Physical and Chemical Properties of Ribosomes." Elsevier, Amsterdam.

Pfeiffer, S. E. (1968). RNA synthesis in synchronously growing populations of HeLa S3 cells II. Rate of synthesis of individual RNA fractions. *J. Cell. Physiol.* **71**, 95.

Pfeiffer, S. E., and Tolmach, L. J. (1968). RNA synthesis in synchronously growing populations of HeLa S3 cells. I. Rate of total RNA synthesis and its relationship to DNA synthesis. *J. Cell. Physiol.* **71**, 77.

Piko, L., Tyler, A., and Vinograd, J. (1967). Amount, location, priming capacity, circularity and other properties of cytoplasmic DNA in sea urchin eggs. *Biol. Bull.* **132**, 68.

Prescott, D. M. (1962). Synthetic processes in the cell nucleus II. Nucleic acid and protein metabolism in the macronuclei of two ciliated protozoa. *J. Histochem. Cytochem.* **10**, 145

Prescott, D. M. (1964). Cellular sites of RNA synthesis. *Progr. Nucl. Acid Res. Mol. Biol.* **3**, 33.

Prescott, D. M., and Bender, M. A. (1962). Synthesis. of RNA and protein during mitosis in mammalian tissue culture cells. *Exp. Cell Res.* **26**, 260.

Reeder, R., and Bell, E. (1965). Short- and long-lived messenger RNA in embryonic chick lens. *Science* **150**, 71.

Revel, M., and Hiatt, H. (1964). The stability of liver messenger RNA. *Proc. Nat. Acad. Sci. U. S.* **51**, 810.

Riley, E. F., and Devi, S. K. (1967). Dynamics of cell populations in the rat lens epithelium. *Exp. Eye Res.* **6**, 383.

Ritossa, F. M., and Spiegelman, S. (1965). Localization of DNA complementary to ribosomal RNA in the nucleolus organizer region of *Drosophila melanogaster. Proc. Nat. Acad. Sci. U. S.* **53**, 737.

Ritossa, F. M., Atwood, K. C., Lindsley, D. L., and Spiegelman, S. (1966). On the chromosomal distribution of DNA complementary to ribosomal and soluble RNA. *Nat. Cancer Inst.* Monogt. **23**, 449.

Robbins, E., and Marcus, P. I. (1964). Mitotically synchronized mammalian cells: A simple method for obtaining large populations. *Science* **144**, 1152.

Rogers, P. J., Preston, B. N., Titchener, E. B., and Linnane, A. W. (1967). Differences between the sedimentation characteristics of the ribonucleic acids prepared from yeast cytoplasmic ribosomes and mitochondria. *Biochem. Biophys. Res. Commun.* **27**, 405.

Roodyn, D. B., and Wilkie, D. (1968). "The Biogenesis of Mitochondria." Methuen, London.

Rubin, A. D., and Cooper, H. L. (1965). Evolving patterns of RNA metabolism during transition from resting state to active growth in lymphocytes stimulated by phytohemagglutinin. *Proc. Nat. Acad. Sci. U. S.* **54**, 469.

Rueckert, R. R., and Mueller, G. C. (1960). Studies on unbalanced growth in tissue culture I. Induction and consequences of thymidine deficiency. *Cancer Res.* **20**, 1584.

Ryter, A., and Landman, O. L. (1964). Electron microscope study of the relationship between mesosome loss and the stable L state (or protoplast state) in *Bacillus subtilis. J. Bacteriol.* **88**, 457.

Sagan, L. (1967). On the origin of mitosing cells. *J. Theoret. Biol.* **14**, 225.

Salb, J., and Marcus, P. (1965). Translational inhibition in mitotic HeLa cells. *Proc. Nat. Acad. Sci. U. S.* **54**, 1353.

Scharff, M. W., and Robbins, E. (1965). Synthesis of ribosomal RNA in synchronized HeLa cells. *Nature (London)* **208**, 464.

Scherrer, K., and Darnell, J. E. (1962). Sedimentation characteristics of rapidly labelled RNA from HeLa cells. *Biochem. Biophys. Res. Commun.* **7**, 486.

Scherrer, K., and Marcaud, L. (1965). Remarques sur less ARN messengers polycistroniques dans les cellules animales. *Bull. Soc. Chim. Biol.* **47**, 1697.

Scherrer, K., and Marcaud, L. (1968). Messenger RNA in avian erythroblasts at the transcriptional and translational levels and the problem of regulation in animal cells. *J. Cell. Physiol.* **72**, 181.

Scherrer, K., Marcaud, L., Zajdela, F., London I. M., and Gros, F. (1966). Patterns of RNA metabolism in a differentiated cell: A rapidly labeled unstable 60S RNA with messenger properties in duck erythroblasts. *Proc. Nat. Acad. Sci U. S.* **56**, 1571.

Schutz, G., Gallwitz, D., and Sekeris, C. E. (1968). Rapidly labelled high molecular weight RNA from rat liver. *Eur. J. Biochem.* **4**, 149.

Scott, R. B., and Bell, E. (1964). Protein synthesis during development: control through messenger RNA. *Science* **145**, 711.

Scott, R. B., and Malt, R. A. (1965). Stable messenger RNA in nucleated erythrocytes. *Nature (London)* **208**, 497.

Shapiro, L., Grossman L. I., Marmur, J., and Kleinshmidt A. K. (1968), Physical studies on the structure of yeast mitochondrial DNA. *J. Mol. Biol.* **33**, 907.

Showacre, J. L., Copper, W. G. and Prescott D. M. (1967). Nucleolar and Nuclear RNA synthesis during the cell life cycle in monkey and pig kidney cells *in vitro*. *J. Cell Biol.* **33**, 273.

Sinclair, J. H., and Stevens, B. J. (1966). Circular DNA filaments from mouse mitochondria. *Proc. Nat. Acad. Sci. U. S.* **56**, 508.

Smellie, R. M. S., McIndoe, W. M., and Davidson J. N. (1953a). The incorporation of ^{15}N, ^{35}S and ^{14}C into nucleic acids and proteins of rat liver. *Biochim. Biophys. Acta* **11**, 559.

Smellie, R. M. S., McIndoe, W. M., Logan, R., and Davidson, J. N. (1953b). Phosporous compounds in the cell. 4. The incorporation of radioactive phosphorous into live cell fractions. *Biochem. J.* **54**, 280.

Smith, A. E., and Marcker, K. A. (1968). *N*-formylmethionyl transfer RNA in mitochondria from yeast and rat liver. *J. Mol. Biol.* **38**, 241.

Smith, D., Tauro, P., Schweizer, E. and Halvorson, H. O. (1968). The replication of mitochondrial DNA during the cell cycle in *Saccharomyes lactis*. *Proc. Nat. Acad. Sci. U. S.* **60**, 936.

Smith, S. J., Higoshi, K., and Busch, H. (1967). Studies on nucleolar RNA fractions of the Walker and Novikoff tumors. *Cancer Res.* **27**, 49.

Soeiro, R., Vaughn, M., and Darnell, J. E. (1968). The effect of puromycin on intranuclear steps in ribosome biosynthesis. *J. Cell Biol.* **36**, 91.

Starr, J. L. (1969). Methylated ribonucleic acids. *Physiol. Rev.* **49**, 623.

Steele, W. J. (1968). Localization of deoxyribonucleic acid complementary to ribosomal ribonucleic acid and preribosomal ribonucleic acid in the nucleous of rat liver. *J. Biol. Chem.* **243**, 3333.

Steinschneider, A. (1969). Isolation and sucrose density gradient centrifugation of ribosomal and mitochondrial RNA from yeast. *Biochim. Biophys. Acta* **186**, 405.

Stevenin, J., Mandel, P., and Jacob, M. (1969). Relationship between nuclear giant-size dRNA and microsomal dRNA of rat brain. *Proc. Nat. Acad. Sci. U. S.* **62**, 490.

Steward, D. L., Shaeffer, J. R., and Humphrey, R. M. (1968). Breakdown and assembly of polyribosomes in synchronized Chinese hamster cells. *Science* **161**, 791.

Stewart, J. A., and Papaconstantinou, J. (1967). A stabilization of RNA templates in lens cell differentiation. *Proc. Nat. Acad. Sci. U. S.* **58**, 95.

Stone, G. E., and Miller, O. L. (1965). A stable mitochondrial DNA in *Tetrahymena pyriformis*. *J. Exp. Zool.* **159**, 33.

Stubblefield, E. (1968). Synchronization methods for mammalian cell cultures. *Methods Cell Physiol.* **3**, 25.

Stubblefield, E., and Mueller, G. C. (1965). Thymidine kinase activity in synchronized HeLa cell cultures. *Biochem. Biophys. Res. Commun.* **20**, 535.

Stubblefield, E., and Murphree, S. (1967). Synchronized mammalian cell cultures II. Thymidine kinase activity in colcemid synchronized fibroblasts. *Exp. Cell Res.* **48**, 652.

Suyama, Y., and Eyer, J. (1967). Leucyl tRNA and leucyl tRNA synthetase in mitochondria of *Tetrahymena pyriformis*. *Biochem. Biophys. Res. Commun.* **28**, 746.

Taylor, J. N. (1960). Nucleic acid synthesis in relation to the cell division cycle. *Ann. N. Y. Acad. Sci.* **90**, 409.

Teng, C–S., and Hamilton, T. H. (1968). The role of chromatin in estrogen action in the uterus I. The control of template capacity and chemical composition and the binding of H^3-estradiol-17β. *Proc. Nat. Acad. Sci. U. S.* **60**, 1410.

Teng, C–S., and Hamilton, T. H. (1969). Role of chromatin in estrogen action in the uterus II. Hormone-induced synthesis of nonhistone acidic proteins which restore histone-inhibited DNA-dependent RNA synthesis. *Proc. Nat. Acad. Sci. U. S.* **63**, 465.

Terasima, T., and Tolmach, L. J. (1963). Growth and nucleic acid synthesis in synchronously dividing cell populations of HeLa cells. *Exp. Cell Res.* **30**, 344.

Toft. D., and Gorski, J. (1966). A receptor molecule for estrogens: Isolation from the rat uterus and preliminary characterization. *Proc. Nat. Acad. Sci. U. S.* **55**, 1574.

Toft, D., Shyamala, G. and Gorski, J. (1967). A receptor molecule for estrogens: Studies using a cell-free system. *Proc. Nat. Acad. Sci. U. S.* **57**, 1740.

Trakatellis, A. C., Axelrod, A. E., and Montjar, M. (1964). Studies on liver messenger ribonucleic acid. *J. Biol. Chem.* **239**, 4237.

Tsukada, K., and Liberman, I. (1964). Synthesis of ribonucleic acid by nuclear and nucleolar preparations after partial hepatectomy. *J. Biol. Chem.* **239**, 2952.

Vesco, C., and Penman, S. (1969). The cytoplasmic RNA of HeLa cells: New discrete species associated with mitochondria. *Proc. Nat. Acad. Sci. U. S.* **62**, 218.

Warner, J. (1967). The species of RNA in the HeLa cell. *In* "The Control of Nuclear Activity" (L. Goldstein, ed.), p. 79. Prentice-Hall, Englewood Cliffs, New Jersey.

Warner, J. R., and Soeiro, R. (1967). Nascent ribosomes from HeLa cells. *Proc. Nat. Acad. Sci. U. S.* **58**, 1984.

Warner, J. R., Soeiro, R. Birnboim, H. C. and Darnell, J. E. (1966), Rapidly labeled HeLa cell nuclear RNA I. Identification by zone sedimentation of a heterogeneous fraction separate from ribosomal precursor RNA. *J. Mol. Biol.* **19**, 349.

Watson, J. D., and Ralph, R. K. (1966a). The nature of 7S RNA in mammalian cells. *J. Mol. Biol.* **22**, 67.

Watson, J. D., and Ralph, R. K,. (1966b). Template activity of 7S RNA isolated from mammalian cells. *Biochem. Biophys. Res. Commun.* **24**, 257.

Weinberg, R. A., and Penman, S. (1968). Small molecular weight monodisperse nuclear RNA. *J. Mol. Biol.* **38**, 289.

Weinberg, R. A., Loening, U., Willems, M. and Penman, S. (1967). Acrylamide gel electrophoresis of HeLa cell nucleolar RNA. *Proc. Nat. Acad. Sci. U. S.* **58**, 1088.

Willems, M., Wagner, E., Laing, R., and Penman, S. (1968). Base composition of ribosomal RNA precursors in the HeLa cell nucleolus: Further evidence of non-conservative processing. *J. Mol. Biol.* **32**, 211.

Willems, M., Musilova, H. A., and Malt, R. A. (1969a). Giant nucleoplasmic RNA in the switch-on of compensatory renal growth. *Proc. Nat. Acad. Sci. U. S.* **62**, 1189.

Willems, M., Penman, M., and Penman, S. (1969b). The regulation of RNA synthesis. *J. Cell Biol.* **41**, 177.

Wilson, S. H., and Hoagland, M. B. (1967). Physiology of rat liver polysomes. The stability of messenger ribonucleic acid and ribosomes. *Biochem. J.* **103**, 556.

Wilson, S. H., Hill, H. Z., and Hogland, M. B. (1967). Physiology of rat liver polysomes. Protein synthesis by stable polysomes. *Biochem. J.* **103**, 567.

Wood, D. D., and Luck, J. L. (1969). Hybridization of mitochondrial ribosomal RNA. *J. Mol. Biol.* **41**, 211.

Woods, P. S. (1959). RNA in nuclear-cytoplasmic interaction. *Brookhaven Symp. Biol.* **12**, 153.

Wunderlich, V., Schutt, M., and Graffi, A. (1966). Uber Differenzen im DNS-Gehalt von mitochondrien aus Tumor- und Normalgeweben. *Acta Biol. Med. Ger.* **17**, K27.

Young, R. W., and Fulhorst, H. W. (1966). Regional differences in protein synthesis within the lens of the rat. *Invest. Ophthalmol.* **5,** 288.

Zigman, S., and Lerman, S. (1968). Effect of actinomycin D on rat lens protein synthesis. *Exp. Eye Res.* **7,** 556.

Zolokar, M. (1960). Sites of protein and ribonucleic acid synthesis in the cell. *Exp. Cell Res.* **19,** 559.

CHAPTER 6

Turnover of Intracellular Proteins

Jack D. Thrasher

I. Introduction.. 153
II. Proteins of the Nucleus... 155
  A. Introduction.. 155
  B. Classification of Nuclear Proteins................................ 155
  C. Enzymes of the Nucleus... 156
  D. The Cytonucleoproteins... 158
  E. Protamines... 159
  F. Histones.. 159
  G. Acidic Nuclear Proteins.. 168
III. Turnover of Proteins in Cytoplasmic Systems.......................... 169
  A. Turnover of Mitochondrial Proteins............................... 169
  B. Ribosomes.. 171
  C. Synthesis and Turnover of Membrane Proteins...................... 175
  D. The Soluble Phase of the Cell.................................... 177
IV. Proteins and the Cell Cycle... 178
  A. Introduction... 178
  B. Protein Synthesis over the Cell Cycle............................ 180
  C. Control of Cell Division and Differentiation..................... 182
V. Protein Metabolism in Special Cell Systems............................ 184
  A. Protein Synthesis in the Immature and Adult Lens................. 184
  B. Renewal of Outer Segment in Rods and Cones....................... 186
  C. Synthesis and Transport of Glycoproteins and Mucopolysaccharides.... 190
  D. Synthesis and Transport of Proteins in Zymogenic Cells........... 196
  E. Synthesis and Turnover of Liver Proteins......................... 198
  References... 205

I. Introduction

The dynamic nature of intracellular protein metabolism and the turnover of these macromolecules are no longer doubted. But for the student of biology it is bewildering to pick up a textbook of biochemistry, read it, set it to memory, and then attempt to apply this newly acquired knowledge to the concept of interphase ("resting stage") of modern textbooks of histology and cell biology. The term interphase was originally used to describe a cell that is not engaged in the process of mitosis. This cell, therefore, came to be considered as "resting."

As pointed out by Cameron in this book, the cells of the mammalian body are in two general states of physiological activity. These take the form of either a progenitor cell or a differentiated cell. The progenitor or stem cells of the mammalian body continuously proliferate. Their progeny either return to the progenitor pool and recycle through G_1, S, G_2, and M or migrate out of the birth compartment, differentiate, and become permanently stalled in G_1. Occasionally, some of the progenitor cells are arrested in G_2 or G_0, a stage from which they can be called upon a given stimulus to engage in progenitor pool activities. The remaining cells of the body, which are differentiated, have the function of carrying out almost all of the metabolic activities of the organ in which they form the parenchyma. In either case the cell cannot be considered as resting because of the constant synthesis and degradation of RNA and proteins that take place. This point has recently been emphasized by the estimates of Quincey and Wilson (1969) on the synthetic rates of ribosomes, 5 S RNA, and tRNA in the adult rat liver. According to these authors each liver cell in the adult rat synthesizes 650 ribosomes, 650 molecules of 5 S RNA, and 11,000 molecules of tRNA each minute. Assuming that the numbers of genes per liver cell are 330 (rRNA), 1660 (5 S RNA), and 13,000 (tRNA), then individual genes are transcribed twice a minute (rRNA), once a minute (tRNA), and once every 2.5 minutes (5 S RNA). The magnitude of this transcription activity is even greater when one considers that the half-life of liver ribosomes is 5 days and tRNA 4 to 6 hours. Thus, it should be apparent that the interphase cell of the liver is not resting, but is undergoing continuous metabolic activity to maintain the steady-state equilibrium between the intracellular environment and plasma constituents.

This chapter, therefore, is an attempt to review the literature on the dynamic state of intracellular proteins. To completely review the voluminous literature on this subject is impossible. As a result, I have relied upon recent reviews on the subject and current literature. Thus, oversight of some of the publications is possible, but it is felt that most of the pertinent references are either cited in these reviews or in the current literature used for this chapter. I had intended to include a description on cellular dynamics of neurons. However, this subject has been adequately covered in a recent symposium. For those individuals interested I must refer you to this publication (Barondes, 1969).

In this chapter the turnover of intracellular proteins has been approached through discussions on special cell systems as well as on subcellular fractions. The proteins of the cell have been covered with respect to morphological systems: the proteins of the nucleus, mitochondria, ribosomes, soluble phase of the cell, and cellular membranes. The next section of the chapter deals with proteins of the cell cycle *in vitro* as well as changes in enzymes during cytodifferentiation of the small intestinal epithelium. The special cell systems chosen for this review are the immature and adult lens, photoreceptor cells, zymogenic cells, liver cells, and cells that synthesize and secrete large quantities of glycoproteins and mucopolysaccharides.

II. Proteins of the Nucleus

A. INTRODUCTION

To fully discuss the proteins of the nucleus would occupy several chapters by itself. Therefore, a conscientious attempt will be made to make this review as concise as possible. In addition, papers in the field will be selected on the basis of their contribution as well as for their extensive bibliographies. In this manner it is hoped that the reader will not only obtain an appreciation of this rapidly expanding field, but will also be able to use the cited references for his own literature research.

B. CLASSIFICATION OF NUCLEAR PROTEINS

Hnilica (1967) has reviewed the proteins of the nucleus. They can be classified either according to their solubility properties or by their origin based upon fractionation of morphological substructures of the nucleus.

Proteins soluble in 0.14M NaCl have been termed *nuclear globulins* (Dounce *et al.*, 1950). These are probably a mixture of ribonucleoproteins. However, their amino acid composition is different than histones, which suggests they are not basic proteins (Wang and Wang, 1962; Hnilica, 1967). Another group of proteins that are soluble in tris buffer and deoxycholate have also been isolated from the nucleus. Hnilica (1967), however, regards these as globular proteins. The *acid-soluble proteins* consist of histones, soluble nuclear ribosomal proteins, and nucleolar proteins. A group of proteins that are soluble in alkaline solutions have been referred to as the *acidic nuclear proteins*. This class probably consists of the phosphoproteins, ribonucleoproteins, nuclear enzymes, chromosomal structural proteins, as well as lipoproteins of the nuclear membrane. It is possible that some of these proteins may interact with histones and RNA to derepress gene loci (see

TABLE I
ENZYMES INVOLVED IN DNA METABOLISM

Enzyme	Function	Reference
DNA polymerase	DNA replication	Keir (1965)
Terminal nucleotidyl transferase	Catalyzes nucleoside-5'-triphosphate into 3'-terminal position of DNA	Krakow *et al.* (1961)
Polynucleotide kinase	Catalyzes the transfer of a phosphate of 5'-triphosphate to 5'-OH terminus of a polynucleotide	Novogrodsky *et al.* (1966)
DNA ligases	Catalyzes the synthesis of a phosphodiester bond by esterification of 5'-phosphoryl group to the 3'-OH group of DNA chains	Lindahl and Edelman (1968)
DNase I	Hydrolyzes to yield 5'-mononucleotides	Laskowski (1967)
DNase II	Hydrolyzes to yield 5'-mononucleotides	Richardson (1969)

below). The last group of nuclear proteins is poorly defined and is referred to as the *residual nuclear proteins*. Their origin is obscure, but according to Hnilica (1967) they may arise from cytoplasmic contamination and denatured nuclear proteins.

Probably the most meaningful classification of nuclear proteins for the cell biologists is based upon the association of proteins with morphological structures of the nucleus. It is this classification that will form the basis for the discussion of nuclear proteins in this portion of the chapter. Proteins associated with chromosomes and chromatin consist of protamines of spermatozoa (Felix, 1960), histones (Butler, 1966), acidic proteins (Wang, 1966), and phosphoproteins (Langan, 1968). The proteins of the nucleolus have been shown to resemble nuclear ribosomal proteins, histones, acidic proteins, and residual proteins (Liau *et al.*, 1965; Hnilica *et al.*, 1966a,b). The remaining nuclear proteins are found in ribosomes, the mitotic apparatus (Mazia, 1961), and a variety of nuclear enzymes (Wang and Wang, 1962; Georgiev, 1967; Barnard, 1969; Richardson, 1969; Roeder and Rutter, 1969).

C. ENZYMES OF THE NUCLEUS

Tables I to III list several of the enzymes that have been found in the nucleus of eucaryotic cells. In addition to those enzymes responsible for DNA and RNA synthesis, the enzymes of the glycolytic pathway and the citric acid cycle have also been identified. These proteins are probably continuously synthesized and catabolized within the nucleus. However,

TABLE II
ENZYMES INVOLVED IN RNA METABOLISM

Enzyme	Location	Function	Reference
RNA polymerase			
I	Nucleolus	rRNA synthesis	Roeder and Rutter (1969, 1970)
II	Nucleoplasm	mRNA synthesis (?)	Roeder and Rutter (1969, 1970)
III	?	?	Roeder and Rutter (1969, 1970)
Ribonucleases			
Phosphotransferases (cyclizing RNases)	Extracellular and intra-cellular	Forms 3- or 2- phosphate monoesters	Barnard (1969)
Phosphodiesterases (noncyclizing RNases and nucleases)	Extracellular and intra-cellular	Forms 3- or 5-phosphate monoesters	Barnard (1969)

detailed information on the turnover of these enzymes is lacking. A few of the enzymes, especially those responsible for DNA and RNA synthesis do undergo periodic synthesis during the cell cycle (see below) and during gene activation produced by a variety of stimuli (see Chapter 5). For further information on the function of these enzymes the reader is referred to the cited references.

TABLE III
ENZYMES INVOLVED IN ENERGY PRODUCTION AND INTERMEDIARY METABOLISM

Metabolic pathway	Location	Function of enzymes	Reference
Glycolysis	Nuclear sap	Glucose→lactate	McEwen et al. (1963)
Citric acid cycle	Nuclear sap and ribo-somes	Acetate→CO_2 Pyruvate ↗	McEwen et al. (1963)
Nucleotides			
Kinases	Nuclear sap	Phosphorylation of mononucleotides	Georgiev (1967); Reid et al. (1964)
Phosphatases	Nuclear sap	ATPase Pyrophosphatase	Siebert (1961) Grossman and Lang (1962)
		Polyphosphatases	

D. The Cytonucleoproteins

A group of nuclear proteins, which may be acidic and do contain trypto-phan, have been described in mammalian cells, *Amoeba proteus*, and *Chironomus*. These proteins may be involved in nuclear–cytoplasmic control mechanisms. In mammalian cells exposed to ^{3}H-amino acids the proteins of the interphase nucleus become heavily labeled. Presumably, the amino acids are incorporated into all classes of nuclear proteins, e.g., histones, acidic proteins, enzymes (Prescott and Bender, 1963; Prescott, 1964b, 1966; Sims, 1965). On the other hand, the condensed chromosomes of metaphase, anaphase, and early telophase incorporate very little of the labeled amino acids (Prescott and Bender, 1963; Sims, 1965). Those nuclear proteins that are synthesized during interphase have a very interesting behavior. In the epithelial cells of rat hair and tongue they leave the nucleus at the time of mitosis and enter the cytoplasm. During nuclear reconstruction (late telophase and early G_1) they migrate back into the nucleus and become evenly distributed between daughter cell nuclei (Sims, 1965). In Chinese hamster cells *in vitro* they have a similar migration pat-tern. However, no labeled proteins are detectable in the nucleus or chromo-somes of daughter cells after four division cycles, a time period of 48 hours (Prescott and Bender, 1963; Prescott, 1964b). Thus, the cytonucleoproteins of mammalian cells continuously migrate from the nucleus to the cyto-plasm and back to the nucleus. They also turn over because they are not conserved in dividing cells *in vitro*.

In *Amoeba proteus* two classes of cytonuclear proteins have been found. These two groups are defined upon the basis of their rate of migration and turnover. When a nucleus containing heavily labeled proteins is trans-planted into a nonradioactive host cell, the nucleus of the host cell picks up labeled proteins within 10 minutes following the transplantation (Byers *et al.*, 1963a,b). Further characterization of these proteins has shown that the two classes consist of slow turnover proteins (STP) and rapidly migrating proteins (RMP). The RMP of the nucleus rapidly mi-grate back and forth between the nucleus and the cytoplasm. They com-prise about 40% of the labeled nuclear proteins. The STP are the remaining labeled proteins of the nucleus (Goldstein and Prescott, 1967). More recent observations have shown that the RMP equilibrate between donor:host cell nuclei in about 3 hours after nuclear transplantation. Also, STP leave the nucleus at a rate of 25% of the total labeled proteins per cell genera-tion time. Additional properties of the RMP proteins are (1) they undergo complete turnover as determined by repeated cytoplasmic amputation, (2) there is a cytoplasmic pool of the proteins, and (3) about 95% of the all nuclear proteins are lost to the cytoplasm at division (Goldstein and

Prescott, 1968a,b). Although the functional role of these nuclear proteins has not been determined, it has been suggested that they may be involved in the regulation of DNA synthesis (Goldstein and Ron, 1969).

E. PROTAMINES

The protamines are small (MW averages 3000–5000) basic proteins that are complexed with the DNA of mature sperm of fish and possibly the rooster. Their chemical, physical, and functional properties have been reviewed by several authors (Felix, 1960; Murray, 1965; Busch, 1965; Hnilica, 1967; Stellwagen and Cole, 1969). The protamines are named after the species from which they have been isolated. In general, arginine represents as much as 50% of the total amino acid content. According to Hnilica (1967) they can be classified into three groups with respect to the composition of basic amino acids: *Monoprotamines* contain only arginine (clupeine, salmine, scombrine, fontinine, truttine, galline); *diprotamines* have histidine or lysine in addition to arginine (iridine, lacustrine); and *triprotamines* contain all three of the basic amino acids (sturine). The neutral amino acids consist of serine, proline, alanine, glycine, threonine, valine, etc.

The protamines appear in the latter stages of cytodifferentiation of spermatozoa. The nuclei of cells in the early stages of spermatogenesis have histones (Felix, 1960; Ingles *et al.*, 1966). The histones are replaced by protamines by the spermatid stage. This occurs concomitantly with the condensation of chromatin and the cessation of RNA synthesis in the spermatid (Bloch, 1966). During the early stages of spermatogenesis, the protamines undergo phosphorylation on serine residues. The phosphorylation ceases during the last stages of cytodifferentiation and coincides with the time of cessation of RNA synthesis mentioned above. In mature spermatozoa phosphate residues cannot be detected in protamines (Ingles and Dixon, 1967). It has been suggested that the function of protamines is to inhibit the template activity of DNA of mature sperm. Recently, Suzuki and Ando (1969) have shown that the protamine, clupeine, does inhibit RNA synthesi in an *in vitro* RNA-generating system that consisted of DNA isolated from sperm of the herring, *Clupea pallasii*, and *Escherichia coli* RNA polymerase.

F. HISTONES

1. *Introduction*

Stedman and Stedman (1950) first suggested that histones may be involved in differentiation of cells by suppressing gene activity. The first experimental evidence that demonstrated that histones may express their biological activities through the inhibition of DNA-dependent RNA synthesis was published by Huang and Bonner (1962) in pea seed embryos and by Allfrey *et al.* (1963) with calf thymus nuclei. Since then symposia (Bonner and T'so, 1964; deRueck and Knight, 1966) and reviews (Murray, 1965; Bonner *et al.*, 1968; Allfrey, 1968; Stellwagen and Cole, 1969) have been published. In spite of the early optimism that histones may repress gene activity through binding with DNA, it is now generally accepted that they play only a portion of the role of nuclear proteins in gene expression. It is now believed that mechanisms such as acetlylation, methylation, and phosphorylation (histones as well as acidic proteins) and their interaction with chromosomal RNA may regulate gene expression (for review, Bonner *et al.*, 1968; Stellwagen and Cole, 1969). An attempt will be made to review as briefly as possible the metabolic activity of histones.

2. *Classification of Histones*

The classification of histones is summarized in Table IV. Histones are routinely extracted from chromatin by 0.2 N H_2SO_4 and then precipitated by ethanol. They are then separated on a weak cation-exchange resin

TABLE IV
CLASSIFICATION OF HISTONES[a]

Histone fraction	Synonym	Description	Amino terminal	Carboxy terminal
Pea Iab		Lysine-rich	Blocked	Lysine
Calf thymus Iab	f(1)	Lysine-rich	Blocked	Lysine
Pea IIa$_{1,2}$		Moderately lysine-rich	Proline	Serine and alanine
Peas IIb		Moderately lysine-rich	Blocked	Alanine
Calf thymus IIb$_1$	f2a2	Moderately lysine-rich	Blocked	Lysine
Calf thymus IIb$_2$	f2b	Moderately lysine-rich	Proline	Lysine
Pea III			Alanine	Alanine
Calf thymus III	f(3)	Arginine-rich	Alanine	Alanine
Pea IV		Arginine-rich	Blocked	Glycine
Calf thymus IV	f2a1	Arginine-rich	Blocked	Glycine

[a] From Bonner *et al.* (1968).

(Amberlite GC–50) with a gradient consisting of guanidium chloride buffered at neutral pH (Rasmussen et al., 1962; Bonner et al., 1968). The elution profile consists of an early runoff peak (designated A) that contains a weakly basic protein as well as some ribosomal proteins. The weakly basic proteins may function in a molecular interaction with histones and chromosomal RNA to regulate gene transcription (see below).

The first histones to be recovered after the elution of the runoff peak have been termed Ia and Ib. These are incompletely resolved and have been labeled lysine-rich histones. These are then followed by histone fractions IIa and IIb, which are moderately rich in lysine residues. The final fractions of histones are III and IV and have been shown to be rich in the amino acid, arginine.

The arginine-rich histones are a small class of rather homogeneous proteins. Two classes have been described with molecular weights of 11,000 and 20,000 (Starbuck et al., 1968; Fambrough and Bonner, 1968). They are structurally similar among a variety of species. For example, histones III of pea seed embryos and calf thymus have almost identical amino acid compositions; they differ in only 1 mole of cysteine (Fambrough and Bonner, 1968). In addition, histones IV in these two species are identical in 19 amino acid terminal residues (DeLange et al. 1968a,b). The only difference in fraction IV between the two species results from the fact that calf thymus histones have more residues (one each) of ϵ-N-methyllysine, argininine, isoleucine, and valine, and one less glycine. Finally, it is now apparent that the total amount of arginine-rich histone fractions is independent of phenotype and the physiological state of the tissue (Kischer et al., 1966; Vidali and Neelin, 1968). The possible role of these histones in gene regulation will be discussed below.

The moderately lysine-rich histones also appear to consist of only a few molecular species (for review, Butler et al., 1968). In addition, their proportion from tissue to tissue is remarkably constant. Also, the primary structure as determined by trypsin digest of histones IIa and IIb from different tissues have practically no difference (Hnilica et al., 1963, 1966a,b). Thus, as in the case of the arginine-rich histones, the moderately lysine-rich histones are homogeneous and probably have a minor role in gene regulation (see below).

The very lysine-rich histones, on the other hand, appear to be a heterogeneous group of proteins. They consist of four components (Kinkade and Cole, 1966). Further analysis has revealed that each component has one to several molecular species (Kinkade and Cole, 1966; Bustin and Cole, 1968). In addition, the heterogeneity of this class of histones is reflected in the facts that (1) there are proportional differences between species as well as among organs with in the same species (Bustin and Cole, 1968); (2)

they are absent in yeast (Tonino and Rozijin, 1966); (3) they are initially
low in content before gastrulation in sea urchin embryos (Ord and Stocken
1968, 1969). Similar observations have been made in pea seed embryos,
(Fambrough et al., 1968) and newt embryos (Asao, 1969). Finally, (4) the
very lysine-rich histones are more abundant in the repressed heterochromatin of the male mealybug when compared to the euchromatin of the
female (Stellwagen and Cole, 1969). However, it is interesting to note that
these observations on the accumulation of lysine-rich histones during
embryogenesis and their phenotypic differences among various cells may
not necessarily be universal. Comings (1967) has shown that there is no
difference in the histone fractions of hetero- and euchromatin of the mealybug. These observations have also been extended to include metaphase
chromosomes vs interphase cells as well as phytohemagglutinin-stimulated
lymphocytes. More recently, Thaler et al. (1970) have demonstrated that
the histone pattern of the sea urchin embryo, *Arbacia punctulata*, changes
from lysine-rich to arginine-rich fractions during the time from egg to
gastrulation. Thus, it is quite possible that the specificity for gene expression may not exist in histones, because all histone fractions may be the
same regardless of the state of cytodifferentiation (Comings, 1967). Although histones could be involved in genetic inactivation of a large number
of unrelated genes (e.g., heterochromatin), individual gene regulation is
probably controlled by a variety of molecular interactions. These include
both transcriptional and translational mechanisms (see below).

3. *Metabolism of Histones*

a. Cellular Sites of Histone Synthesis. Evidence in the literature indicates
that histones are synthesized at different sites in different cell types. The
lysine-rich histones of calf thymus nuclei are synthesized in the nucleus
(Reid and Cole, 1964; Reid et al., 1968). In pea seedlings, tobacco cells,
and Novikoff hepatoma it appears that histones are more readily synthesized in the nucleolus, rather than the nucleoplasm and the chromosomes
(Birnstiel and Flamm, 1964; Hnilica et al., 1966a,b). In contrast, histones
of HeLa cells and chicken erythrocytes are synthesized in the cytoplasm
(Freedman et al., 1966; Borun et al., 1967; Robbins and Borun, 1967). In
HeLa cells the synthesis of histones occurs on a small class of cytoplasmic
ribosomes. The mRNA is characterized by being rapidly labeled following
the administration of labeled nucleosides and has a short half-life of approximately 1 hour (Borun et al., 1967). The reason for the different sites
of synthesis in different cell types probably results from the fact that functional ribosomes may not be present in the nucleus of some cells (Allfrey,
1963; Penman, 1966).

b. Time of Histone Synthesis and Turnover. The temporal relationships of histone biosynthesis have been investigated in a variety of cell types over the cell cycle (for review, Stellwagen and Cole, 1969). It is generally accepted that the rate of histone synthesis depends upon the proliferative rate of the tissue. Byvoet (1966, 1968) has reported the relative rates of turnover of histones and DNA in tissues of the rat and Walker carcinosarcoma cells. The results indicate that histones turn over with a half-life value similar to that for the DNA of the particular tissue. Thus, the half-life of lysine-rich histones in days is as follows: liver (5.01), spleen (2.18–4.06), thymus (1.6), small intestine (0.9–1.34), and Walker carcinosarcoma (1.34). In the brain of the adult rat, two fractions of histones turn over with half-lives of 54 and 104 days, while the liver has three fractions that are renewed every 18, 56, and 93 days (Piha *et al.*, 1966). The longer values for liver histones obtained by Piha *et al.* result from the fact that they have considered the contribution of proliferating sinusoidal lining cells to histone metabolism. Histones have also been shown to turn over in Chinese hamster cell *in vitro*. However, they are conserved for at least three generation times before evidence of turnover is observable. Only the f1 histones (lysine-rich) have a relatively short half-life of 74 hours in these cells. The turnover of the other fractions of histones can only be accurately measured after the inhibition of both DNA and RNA synthesis. During inhibition of DNA synthesis the half-life values for histones f2a1, f2a2, f2b, and f3 are 60, 58, 55 and 68 hours, respectively. The time for f1 histones is reduced to 31 hours during inhibition of DNA synthesis and to 47 hours if RNA synthesis is prevented (Gurley *et al.*, 1968; Gurley and Hardin, 1970). Thus, histones are not conserved and do undergo metabolic turnover in both nonproliferating and dividing cell populations. This metabolic activity may or may not reflect changes in gene transcription.

The timing of histone synthesis in relation to DNA synthesis varies among dividing cells. In general, histones are synthesized just before the beginning or during DNA replication. In regenerating liver histones begin synthesis about 3 hours prior to the beginning of the S phase (Orlova and Rodionov, 1970). In *Euplotes, Tetrahymena,* and Chinese hamster cells they accumulate simultaneously with DNA synthesis (Prescott, 1966; Hardin *et al.*, 1967; Gurley and Hardin, 1968). Also, HeLa cells that are undergoing synchronous DNA synthesis incorporate labeled amino acids into histones (Spalding *et al.*, 1966). In conclusion, DNA synthesis is usually accompanied by histone synthesis. However, if DNA synthesis is inhibited, the incorporation of amino acids into histones continues, but at a reduced rate (Spalding *et al.*, 1966; Gurley *et al.*, 1968; Gurley and Hardin, 1970).

c. Methylation, Acetylation, and Phosphorylation of Histones. Histones are methylated (Allfrey *et al.*, 1964, 1966; Kim and Paik, 1965), acetylated (Allfrey *et al.*, 1964, 1966; Allfrey, 1968), and phosphorylated (Kleinsmith *et al.*, 1966; Allfrey *et al.*, 1966, Langan, 1968). The metabolism and turn-over of these added groups have been investigated in attempts to relate them to the role of histones in gene regulation. It has been suggested that these biochemical modifications of histones may probably change the specificity of the molecules at the polymer level. This change in the poly-meric structure and specificity of histones may then permit the opening of new genes for transcription (Allfrey *et al.*, 1966; Allfrey, 1968; Stellwagen and Cole, 1969).

Methylation of histones occurs by way of S-adenosylmethionine. The methyl group is added to the ϵ-amino group of lysine residues. The methyla-tion of the lysine residue has been observed in calf thymus nuclei (Allfrey *et al.*, 1964), rat liver (Sekeris *et al.*, 1967) and Ehrlich ascites cells (Comb *et al.*, 1966). The methylation occurs at the level of the chromatin and, therefore, may result in a change in the DNA–histone complex (Comb *et al.*, 1966; Sekeris *et al.*, 1967). However, the significance of histone methylation has not at the present time been determined. In regenerating liver, the methylation of histones occurs after acetylation and at a time when DNA synthesis has declined (Tidwell *et al.*, 1968). The addition of the methyl group also occurs at a time when gene transcription is reduced. Therefore, it is unlikely that histone methylation results in the opening up of cistronic activity. It is possible that histone methylation may be part of the structural modifications required for the packaging of chromatin into chromosomes in preparation for mitosis. This should be examined in greater detail with synchronous populations of dividing cells.

The phosphorylation of histones appears to coincide with changes in gene activity as well as RNA and DNA synthesis (Stevely and Stocken, 1968; Ord and Stocken, 1968, 1969; Stocken and Ord, 1969). All histone fractions are phosphorylated on both serine and threonine residues. His-tones f1 (lysine-rich) and f2b (moderately lysine-rich) contain more phos-phate than f2a (moderately lysine-rich) and f3 (arginine-rich) of calf thymus nuclei (Langan, 1968). During liver regeneration the f3 histones undergo a 50% increased in phosphorylation by 1 to 2 hours after partial hepatectomy (Ord and Stocken, 1969). This occurs concomitantly to an increase in RNA synthesis. The f1 histones, on the other hand, begin phosphorylation about 3 hours prior to the onset of DNA synthesis (Stevely and Stocken, 1968). Also, f1 histones are phosphorylated to a greater ex-tent in rapidly proliferating tissues (Stevely and Stocken, 1968). Moreover, the phosphate content of this fraction is high in fetal livers, and declines with the decrease in DNA synthesis and cell division during neonatal life (Ord and Stocken, 1969). The significance of the phosphorylation of f1 histones in relation to DNA synthesis and cell division is not clear. But it is known that phosphorylated f1 and f3 histones are less effective in decreasing DNA synthesis by DNA polymerase than the nonphosphorylated counterparts (Ord and Stocken, 1968). Thus, the phosphorylation of f3 histones may be associated with early gene activation in regenerating liver, while the addition of phosphate groups to f1 histones may have a role in DNA synthesis. These possible functions of f1 and f3 histones may result from a change of the polymeric structure of histones through the addition of phosphate to serine and threonine residues. This in return could alter the molecular interactions between DNA and histones to permit more efficient gene transcription and DNA replication.

The acetylation of histones occurs in isolated nuclei with acetyl-CoA as the donor (Allfrey et al., 1966). Histone acetylation is one of the earliest biochemical events to occur prior to the onset of RNA synthesis in a variety of experimental systems (for review, Allfrey, 1968). It is because of this fact that more is known about histone acetylation than either phosphorylation or methylation.

Allfrey (1968) has recently reviewed the literature on histone acetylation. It is known that the classes of histones are acetylated to different extent as well as on various amino acid residue sites. Newly incorporated labeled acetyl groups appear as both N-acetyl and O-acetyl. A large number of the O-acetyl residues occur in the arginine-rich f3 histone (Pogo et al., 1968), while N-acetyl lysine has been found in the f2a1 fraction (Gershey et al., 1968). Byvoet (1968) has investigated the turnover of N-acetyl groups of histones and has compared these values to the turnover of total histones in several cell types. The total histones of liver, spleen, thymus, Walker carcinosarcoma, Jensen sarcoma, and Novikoff hepatomas have half-life values of 380, 87, 47, 58, 36, and 46 hours, respectively. Relative to these times, the N-acetyl groups have half-lives of 2.0, 3.9, 2.5, 4.7, 1.8, and 25.0 hours, respectively. Thus, the N-acetyl groups turn over much more rapidly than total histones and occurs more rapidly in the liver when compared to tumor cells. In addition, the incorporation into lysine-rich histones was only about 10 to 20% of that observed in arginine-rich and moderately lysine-rich histones. The higher rate of acetylation of arginine-rich histones has also been reported for other cell systems (for review, Allfrey, 1968).

The acetylation of arginine-rich histones may, therefore, have an important role in gene activation. This has been deduced from a variety of experimental observations. The acetylation of histones has been shown to lower the capacity of these proteins to inhibit RNA polymerase in *in vitro* systems from calf thymus nuclei (Allfrey et al., 1966). It has also been demonstrated by autoradiography that the incorporation of ³H-acetate is more pronounced in the "diffuse" (euchromatin) chromatin than in the "condensed" (heterochromatin) chromatin of calf thymus nuclei (Allfrey, 1968). This has proved an interesting observation because it is known that euchromatin supports RNA synthesis, while heterochromatin is rather inactive (Allfrey et al., 1966). Other studies have shown that the acetylation of histones is increased 300% within the first hour following partial hepatectomy. During this time of active acetylation, the acetyl groups of histones in the regenerating liver turnover more slowly than normal liver. This increase in the metabolism of acetyl groups in histones takes place just prior to the augmentation of RNA synthesis (Pogo et al., 1968; Allfrey, 1968). Similar observations have been reported for cortisol-treated rat livers, PHA-stimulated lymphocytes (Pogo et al., 1966), and estradiol-stimulated rat uterus (Libby, 1968). Furthermore, indirect evidence for the participation of histone acetylation in the increase of transcriptional activity has been obtained in avian erythrocytes and granular leukocytes. Mature avian erythrocytes synthesize little or no RNA (see Chapter 5). Histone acetylation does not occur in these cells (Allfrey, 1968). In addition, when polymorphonuclear leukocytes are treated with PHA, RNA synthesis is greatly reduced. During this period of suppressed RNA synthesis there is a parallel decrease in histone acetylation (Pogo et al., 1967). In conclusion, it has been suggested that the purpose of acetylation of the arginine-rich histones is to alter the state of chromatin from that of condensed nature to a more diffuse state. This in return would increase the rate of transcription of DNA (Allfrey, 1968). However, it should be cautioned that more information is needed to clarify fully the role of histone acetylation in gene regulation.

4. *Histones and RNA Synthesis*

Huang and Bonner (1962) first demonstrated that histones suppress DNA–dependent RNA synthesis. Since then, histones have been shown to inhibit DNA polymerase (Gurley et al., 1963), and a variety of other metabolic events, such as protein synthesis, amino acid transport, and oxidative phosphorylation (for review, Allfrey, 1966). Thus, if these various nonspecific inhibitory effects of histones on cellular metabolism are considered, then histones as specific repressors of transcription must be suspect. This is particularly true from the observations that have shown that histones from human, calf, and pea tissues are almost identical (MacGillivray, 1968; Stellwagen and Cole, 1969). This suggests that histones have conserved their basic structure and amino acid composition during evolution. The lack of evolution of these macromolecules may suggest that they are are adapted for a specific function, e.g., a structural protein. It should also be mentioned at this time that the histone composition of repressed heterochromatin is no different from that of euchromatin (Comings, 1967). Then, how is it that histones can continue to be implicated in the regulation of gene activity?

Recent interest has turned toward methylation, phosphorylation, acetylation, and cysteine disulfide linkages as possible mechanisms for increasing the heterogeneity of histones (for review, Allfrey, 1966, 1968; Langan, 1968; Stellwagen and Cole, 1969). It is generally felt, however, that methylation of histones is probably insufficient to cause much alteration in the polymeric structure of the proteins. In addition, in those cell systems investigated, histone methylation takes place long after gene activation has occurred, e.g., liver regeneration, PHA-stimulated lymphocytes. On the other hand, both phosphorylation and acetylation of histones occur very early in gene activation in these same cell systems. Thus, as pointed out by Allfrey (1968) and Langan (1968), these metabolic alterations of histones could possibly be important in the transition of heterochromatin (repressed) to euchromatin (open cistrons). In any event, acetylation may likely be one of the initial changes in a series of molecular interactions that begin to loosen up the condensed chromatin. The role of cysteine and disulfide linkages is even less clear. Cysteine is present in the arginine-rich histones (Jellum, 1966). Cysteine participates in intra- and interpolypeptide covalent linkages. Because of this, Fambrough and Bonner (1968) have suggested that cysteine may be responsible for the dimerization of histone III. Thus, cysteine may be involved in polymeric formations of arginine-rich histones making them biologically inactive. Only monomer and dimer forms of histone III may be biologically active. It is interesting to note that the proportion of thiol-disulfide in histones of sea urchin eggs changes from less than 20% in an unfertilized egg to 59% just before cleavage (Ord and Stocken, 1968, 1969).

Bonner et al. (1968) have reviewed the interaction of chromosomal RNA and nonhistone (acidic) proteins with histones as a possible mechanism for controlling gene expression. Chromosomal RNA is characterized by a chain length of 40 to 60 nucleotides and contains a relatively high content (5 to 25%) of dihydrouridylic acid (Bonner and Huang, 1966). It is suspected to be very heterogeneous because it hybridizes with 5% of the total nuclear DNA (Bonner and Widholm, 1967). In addition, chromosomal RNA has been shown to form covalent bonds with nonhistone chromosomal proteins. This RNA–protein complex is then capable of forming hydrogen bonds with histones (Bonner, 1967). Because of these properties, it has been suggested that the following mechanism may apply to gene regulation in eucaryote cells. The chromosomal RNA has sufficient heterogeneity to have base sequence recognition. The complex of RNA and nonhistone protein then binds to that portion of the DNA with a base sequence complementary to the RNA. The ionically bound histones lead, therefore, to further masking of cistrons in the immediate area of nucleotide sequence recognition.

Further support for the role of histone–nonhistone protein complexes in the control of RNA synthesis has come from *in vitro* experiments. Wang (1968) and Marushige *et al.*, (1968) have shown that histones and acidic proteins form insoluble complexes *in vitro*. When acidic proteins are added to histones, they restore histone-inhibited, DNA-dependent RNA synthesis. The greatest restoration occurs upon the complexing of f3 (arginine-rich) histones (Wang, 1968). Recently, Teng and Hamilton (1969) have confirmed these observations in the rat uterus that has been stimulated by estrogen to synthesize RNA. In conclusion, it appears that histones alone probably do not regulate transcription. If they do, it would only be at a rather crude level, i.e., euchromatin vs heterochromatin. For example, Sonnenbichler (1969) has demonstrated that residual complexes from calf thymus chromatin consist of DNA complexed with histone. Removal of the histone by increasing salt concentrations revealed that the complex actually consists of a rosette of DNA with a protein core. These he has termed chromomeres. Apparently, this unfolding of the DNA–histone chromomere is similar to the phenomena of chromosomal puffing and lamp-brush chromosomes. However, mounting evidence seems to point toward molecular alterations of histones (methylation, phosphorylation, acetylation, and cysteine disulfide linkages) as the major role of these proteins in regulation of transcription.

G. Acidic Nuclear Proteins

The acidic nuclear proteins are defined as that class of proteins that is soluble in 0.05 N NaOH. They are precipitated when the pH is lowered to 6. The acidic nuclear proteins constitute from 30 to 50% of the total nuclear proteins. They are found in chromatin, nucleolus, and nuclear sap. Because of their solubility characteristics and the inability to resolve them with normal separation procedures, they still remain somewhat of an enigma (for review, Busch, 1965; Murray, 1965; Stellwagen and Cole, 1969).

The acidic proteins of the nucleus deserve further investigation because of their biochemical and physical properties. It is known that they turn over much more rapidly than histones and cytoplasmic proteins in both the liver and Walker carcinosarcoma cells (Busch, 1965). As mentioned above, they have recently been shown to form insoluble complexes with histones and may be involved in gene regulation by interacting with histones, chromosomal RNA, and DNA. It is also possible that the cytonuclear proteins described earlier in this chapter may belong to this group of proteins. In addition, other evidence has suggested that they may be an integral part of the regulatory mechanisms of gene expression. Thus, they have been shown to be more abundant in heterochromatin than in euchromatin (Frenster, 1965). They also appear to reverse the inhibition of DNA-dependent RNA synthesis by histones (Wang, 1968; Marushige et al., 1968). Recently, Langan (1968) has reviewed the literature on the acidic phosphoproteins of the nucleus. These proteins rapidly incorporate and turn over inorganic phosphate. They are also involved in histone–phosphoprotein complexes. Thus, increasing experimental evidence tends to point toward the participation of these proteins in gene regulation.

Finally, Howk and Wang (1970) have shown that a least one of the nonhistone proteins of chromosomes is DNA polymerase. The enzyme is capable of producing DNA templates. The templates are small, heterogeneous fragments with a molecular weight of 2.5×10^6. It is possible that other nuclear enzymes will eventually be placed in the acidic nuclear protein group.

III. Turnover of Proteins in Cytoplasmic Systems

A. TURNOVER OF MITOCHONDRIAL PROTEINS

That mitochondria turn over has been well established. In Chapter 5 it was mentioned that the half-life of mitochondrial DNA (mit-DNA) is 6.7 days (heart), 9.4 days (liver), 10.4 days (kidney), and 31 days (brain). Estimates on the turnover of mitochondrial proteins have indicated that they are more rapidly synthesized and catabolized than mit-DNA. For example, von Hungen et al. (1968) have shown that total mitochondrial RNA and protein in the rat brain turn over with half-lives of 12 and 20 days, respectively. However, Fletcher and Sanadi (1961a) have demonstrated that the turnover of four mitochondrial components (insoluble and soluble proteins, lipids, and cytochrome c) of the rat liver approximates the value obtained for mit-DNA, i.e., 10.3 days. In addition, these times were not different when the turnover rates were compared between young and senescent rats (Fletcher and Sanadi, 1961b). More recently, Swick et al. (1968), using another labeled precursor, have shown that these components of the rat liver mitochondria turn over more rapidly than mit-DNA and at different rates. The half-lives range from 4 to 6 days for soluble enzymes, structural proteins, and cytochrome c, while inducible enzymes are renewed in a matter of hours (see below).

The dynamic state of the proteins of the inner and outer mitochondrial membranes has also been investigated (Beattie, 1969). The proteins of the outer membrane have a half-life of 7.0 days as compared to 8.4 days for the inner mitochondrial membrane. This difference in the turnover of the two membrane systems has been confirmed by DeBernard et al. (1969). In addition, the proteins of mitochondria that are soluble in water and KCl are renewed at similar rates, i.e., 7 to 8 days. In conclusion, mitochondria, the constituent proteins, and RNA of mitochondria are in a constant state of synthesis and degradation. However, the rate of renewal of mitochondrial components depends largely upon the choice of labeled precursors (Swick et al., 1968; Druyan et al., 1969).

The heterogeneity of the metabolism of various enzymes in mitochondria has been stressed by Druyan et al. (1969). Cytochromes b and c, which are present in the inner mitochondrial membrane, turn over every 5.5 and 6.1 days. Cytochrome b_5, an enzyme of the outer membrane, is renewed every 4.4 days. On the other hand, inducible enzymes are more rapidly synthesized and degraded. The enzymes alanine and ornithine transferase, catalase, and δ-aminolevulinic acid synthetase are renewed every 0.73, 1.03, 1½ to 3½, and 1 day, respectively (Tschudy et al., 1965; Swick et al., 1968; Pool et al., 1969).

As mentioned in Chapter 5, some of the mitochondrial enzymes and possibly proteins of the inner mitochondrial membrane are probably coded in mit-DNA. The subject has been adequately reviewed by Roodyn and Wilkie (1968). Therefore, only a few comments are in order. Roodyn and Wilkie (1968) have suggested that soluble outer membrane proteins as well as cytochrome c are synthesized on cytoplasmic ribosomes. The finished proteins are then transferred to the mitochondria where they become integral parts of the outer membrane.

The proteins that are coded in mit-DNA and synthesized on mitochrondrial RNA and ribosomes are just now being elucidated. Most of the evidence has been obtained from respiratory mutants of yeast and Neurospora. It is hoped that these observations will be extended to higher eucaryotes in the near future. At least three types of respiratory mutants are recognized in yeast: petite mutant, suppressive petite, and the rho-minus mutant. They lack cytochromes a and b, and the mutations are cytoplasmically inherited. In addition, some types of mutants have been shown to lack mitochondrial DNA (Moustacci and Williamson, 1966).

In Neurospora the cytoplasmic respiratory mutants also lack cytochromes a and b. Thus, it appears that cytochromes a and b are coded in mito-chondrial DNA. It has also been demonstrated in these same mutants that a mitochondrial structural protein (MSP) is altered in amino acid composition. In two strains of mutants the protein contains one less tryptophan residue. This amino acid substitution is sufficient to decrease the association of the MSP with NADH, ATP, and MDH. This in turn leads to a decrease in respiratory efficiency (Woodward and Munkres, 1966). In conclusion, it appears that cytochromes a and b as well as one structural protein of the inner mitochondrial membrane have their cistrons located in mit-DNA. It could be possible that the differences in the turnover rates of inner and outer mitochondrial membrane proteins may result from the different sites of synthesis, i.e., mitochondrial vs cytoplasmic polysomes.

B. RIBOSOMES

Ribosomes have received considerable attention in the past decade because of their central role in protein synthesis. As a result several recent reviews have been published on their physical and biochemical properties (Darnell, 1968; Osawa, 1968; Lengyel and Söl, 1969; Schlessinger, 1969). For the purpose of this chapter the subjects of the ribosome cycle and cellular sites of the origin of ribosomal proteins will be discussed.

1. The Ribosome Cycle

It is now recognized that ribosomes of the cell exist in four physical states: (1) polysomes, (2) individual free ribosomes, (3) ribosomal subunits, and (4) membrane-bound ribosomes (Darnell, 1968; Attardi et al., 1969).

The membrane-bound ribosomes are defined as those ribosomes that are fixed to or associated with the rough endoplasmic reticulum. The proportion of membrane-bound ribosomes to total cellular ribosomes varies from cell type to cell type. This variation depends upon the metabolic and secretory functions of the cell. Thus, the membrane-bound ribosomes are much higher in the zymogenic cells of the pancreas which secrete proteins (Redman et al., 1966) than in HeLa cells (Attardi et al., 1969) and undifferentiated hepatocytes (Dallner et al., 1966a,b). The obvious function of the membrane-bound ribosomes in zymogenic cells is the synthesis of proteins destined for secretion. However, in those cells such as differentiating hepatocytes and HeLa cells, in which membrane-bound ribosomes constitute only 10 to 20% of the total ribosomal pool, it has been suggested that they are responsible for the synthesis of the proteins (including enzymes) of the endoplasmic reticulum (see Section III, C).

Recently, Fridlender and Wettstein (1970) have shown that free and membrane-bound polysomes of chick embryos are different with respect to one protein. Membrane-bound polysomes have a protein that bands in poisition 1 on polyacrylamide gels, while this is replaced by a protein in position 2 in free polysomes. If these preliminary observations are accurate, then they demonstrate that free and bound polysomes are structurally different. The functional purpose of this difference may lie in the fact that the proteins may select for either membrane or nonmembrane specificity of free polysomes. Thus, the differences in protein composition may restrict different ribosomes to the translation of certain species of mRNA (Glick and Warren, 1969).

The intracellular events of the ribosomal cycle have been most extensively studied in HeLa cells. When cytoplasmic extracts of HeLa cells are centrifuged in a sucrose gradient, 75 to 90% of the ribosomes sediment as polysomes (100 S to 400 S values). These are capable of synthesizing protein *in vitro* (Warner *et al.*, 1963). The remaining ribosomes sediment as either free single ribosomes (75 S to 80 S values) or as subunits. The subunits consist of a large 60 S ribosomal subunit (RSU) which contains the 28 S, 5 S, and 7 S rRNA. The other RSU sediments at 40 S and contains the 18 S rRNA (see Chapter 5). As the finished RSU's leave the nucleolus and nucleoplasm with their respective rRNA molecules, they enter the cytoplasm and become part of the subunit pool. The RSU's produce 80 S ribosomes upon attachment to the mRNA. The mRNA generally has several 80 S ribosomes attached to it, forming polysomes. The now "active" ribosomes are stable once attached to the mRNA. At this time they resist dissociation in low concentrations of Mg^{++}. Once the read out is completed the active ribosomes dissociate and enter the RSU pool. The mechanism for ribosome dissociation is not fully understood. It has been suggested that low Mg^{++} concentrations may be responsible for the production of RSU upon completion of translation. However, in *E. coli* the dissociation appears to controlled by a protein factor (Subramanian *et al.*, 1969). Once the RSU's reenter the cytoplasmic pool they reassociate with newly synthesized RSU at random (Vaughan *et al.*, 1967; Schlessinger, 1969). The rate of turnover of the ribosomal cycle depends upon the half-life of the mRNA. As mentioned in Chapter 5, mRNA in mammalian cells can have half-lives ranging from 30 minutes (short-lived mRNA) to 80 hours (long-lived mRNA). The ribosomes and the rRNA, however, are renewed once every 5 to 9 days depending upon the tissue (see Chapter 5).

A slightly more complicated ribosome cycle has been suggested by Adamson *et al.* (1969) and Baglioni *et al.* (1969). The present data on this subject are insufficient to warrant a detailed description. However, a few points of interest should be elucidated at this time. The RSU's that are found in the cytoplasm constitute only 10% of the total cytoplasmic pool of ribosomes. These are derived from both newly synthesized RSU's as well as from the dissociation of 80 S ribosomes. They have a relatively slow rate of entry and exchange with 80 S ribosomes and polysomes. On the other hand, 80 S ribosomes are easily recruited into polysomes. The difference in the behavior of the RSU's when compared to the 80 S ribosomes is not understood. However, it could result from the existence or absence of a protein factor (Fridlender and Wettstein, 1970). Recently, Hunt and Laycock (1969) have suggested that ribosome association and activation may be determined by properties of the mRNA. The exact mechanism that controls the ribosome recycling will probably be elucidated in the near future.

2. Cellular Sites of Ribosomal Protein Synthesis and Packaging

The nucleolus as the site of synthesis of ribosomal RNA has been discussed in Chapter 5. Considerable evidence has now accumulated showing that ribosomal protein precursors exist in the nucleolus. In addition, rRNA becomes attached to ribosomal precursor protein in the nucleolus and the nucleoplasm (for review, Darnell, 1968). An attempt will be made to briefly review these events.

Ribonucleoprotein particles (RNP), which contain the precursors of rRNA, have recently been isolated from the nucleoli of L-cells (Liau and Perry, 1969). Three RNP particles exist that sediment at 62 S, 78 S, and 110 S in sucrose gradients. These fit into a maturation sequence of 110 S → 78 S → 62 S. At the present time it appears that the rRNA's of these particles are: 110 S (45 S, 41 S [?], 36 S, 32 S rRNA); 78 S (36 S [?], 32 S rRNA), and 62 S (32 S, 28 S rRNA). Thus, this sequence of maturation probably leads to the production of the 60 S RSU. The point of production of the RNP for the 40 S RSU is not known. It probably arises at the time that 41 S rRNA is cleaved to form the 20 S rRNA precursor of 18 S rRNA (see Chapter 5). It is interesting to note that the 110 S RNP has a high ratio of protein to rRNA (about 57%). As the maturation of the RNP continues the protein content decreases to 53% (78 S RNP), 44.2% (62 S RNP), and 43.4% (60 S RSU). Thus, protein as well as rRNA is lost during the maturation of RNP. The processing within the nucleolus from 110 S to 62 S RNP takes about 15 minutes. Finally, the proteins of the 62 S RNP appear to be almost identical to those of the 60 S RSU. The only exceptions are those proteins that become associated with the RSU in the cytoplasm (Warner and Soeiro, 1967).

At present there is little information on the number and properties of proteins in ribosomes of mammalian cells. The proteins of ribosomes come from three sources. The first class, ribosomal structural proteins, are derived from the nucleolus, probably as RNP. In addition to rRNA they make up the structural elements of the RSU. These constitute approximately 60% of the ribosomal proteins. The second class, which comprises about 20% of the total protein, is derived from a cytoplasmic pool. These have been referred to as cytoplasmic ribosomal proteins. The remaining 20% is a poorly defined class of proteins. They are not firmly bound to the ribosome and can be extracted in 0.2 M NaCl (Warner, 1966). It is possible that this group may be enzymes attached to the ribosomes (Wang and Wang, 1962). For example, Collier and Traugh (1969) and Gill *et al.* (1969) have shown that one of these enzymes, aminoacyl transferase II, which transfers amino acids from aminoacyl-tRNA to growing polypeptide chains, is inactivated by diphtheria toxin.

The ribosomal structural proteins derived from the nucleolus consist of a minimum of 10 to 12 discrete bands on polyacrylamide gels (Warner, 1966). These proteins appear to be sequentially added to the RNP during synthesis. In spite of this sequential addition of proteins, it takes from 30 to 120 minutes for the large RSU to enter the cytoplasm from the first moment of incorporation of labeled amino acids. This delay is longer than that observed for the 28 S rRNA and the RNP particles. Thus, there appears to be a large pool of structural ribosomal proteins that are added sequentially to the RNP (Warner, 1966; Darnell, 1968; Baglioni *et al.*, 1969). The small RSU, on the other hand, enters the cytoplasm by 15 minutes after the initial synthesis and addition of precursor proteins (Baglioni *et al.*, 1969). Once having entered the cytoplasm, the cytoplasmic ribosomal proteins are added to the subunits (Warner, 1966). The newly completed RSU then slowly enter the pool of 80 S ribosomes and polysomes.

Both the structural and cytoplasmic ribosomal proteins are derived from a pool of precursors. Whether this is a pool of either monomers or completed polymers is not known. However, several lines of evidence indicate that the pool is large. If protein synthesis is completely inhibited by cycloheximide, without affecting rRNA synthesis, RSU continue to appear in the cytoplasm for at least 3 hours following treatment (Warner *et al.*, 1966). Confirmation of these observations was obtained from the fact that analysis of proteins on polyacrylamide gels have no evidence of missing bands. Furthermore, during cycloheximide inhibition new ribosomal protein synthesis did not occur, as evidenced by the lack of incorporation of ^{14}C-leucine (Warner, 1966). Finally, in methionine-deficient cells, a condition that prevents methylation of rRNA precursors, ribosomal proteins are assembled into rRNA particles of the nucleolus. The assembly of a limited number of RNP's continues although rRNA maturation is blocked by lack of rRNA methylation. Thus, the addition of proteins from the pool to RNP does not require rRNA maturation (Maden and Vaughan, 1968).

C. SYNTHESIS AND TURNOVER OF MEMBRANE PROTEINS

Recent evidence has shown that the proteins of cellular membranes are heterogeneous. They probably consist of enzymes as well as structural proteins (Kiehn and Holland, 1968, 1970a,b). The cell membrane of erythrocytes contains up to 15 different proteins (Azen et al., 1965). Schnaitman (1969) has shown in liver cells that the inner mitochondrial membrane contains 23 proteins, 12 in the outer membrane, and 15 each in the membranes of the smooth and rough endoplasmic reticulum. The heterogeneity of membrane proteins results from the presence of both enzymes and structural proteins. Thus, it is now accepted, for example, that the outer mitochondrial and the microsomal membranes contain NADH–cytochrome c reductase and cytochrome b_5. However, other enzymes, such as monoamine oxidase and kynurenine hydroxylase, are only found in the outer mitochondrial membrane, while most of the enzymes of the glycolytic pathway are present in the microsomal membranes. Finally, the inner mitochondrial membrane contains almost all of the enzymes of the respiratory chain, particularly cytochromes a and b. Thus, the multitude of membrane functions—active transport, contact inhibition, cell recognition, and communication—results not only from structural proteins, but also from the array of enzymes that are present.

Recently, Kiehn and Holland (1970b) have demonstrated that membrane proteins from a variety of cell types are complex, heterogeneous, and have molecular weights that range from 45,000 to 85,000 daltons. Based upon gel electrophoresis, they were able to demonstrate only small differences in membrane proteins obtained from the plasma membrane, microsomes, and mitochondria from each of several cultured cell types. Presumably, the slight variation in protein composition among these membranes results from different enzyme content. Also, membrane proteins are essentially indistinguishable among cultured cells of different species, e.g., L-cells, HeLa, BHK–21 hamster kidney cells, chick embryo fibroblast. However, organ-specific differences in membrane proteins in mouse tissues (liver, heart, lung, kidney) were found. This probably reflects organ-specific functions.

The rates of incorporation of labeled amino acids into membrane proteins have also been reported (Kiehn and Holland, 1968, 1970a; Warren, 1969). The incorporation of amino acids and the subsequent labeling pattern of membranes from mitochondria, nucleus, microsomes, and plasma membrane are the same when cells are labeled for only a few minutes, several hours, or for days. Thus, membrane proteins are rapidly synthesized, are uniformly labeled, and immediately become an integral part of the various cell membranes. The rate of turnover of individual membrane proteins varies considerably. This fact alone suggests that the proteins of cellular membrane are heterogeneous because of differential turnover rates (Kiehn and Holland, 1968, 1970a). These differences in turnover have been confirmed by Warren (1969). However, measurements of the half-life of cellular membrane proteins have not been adequately made. The problems associated with such studies must consider membrane precursor pool, individual organelles, generation time, and organ-specific physiology.

Various data and observations that have been reported in the literature permit some speculation on the biogenesis of the membranes of the Golgi complex. Dallner *et al.* (1966a,b) have examined the structural and chemical differentiation of the rough and smooth endoplasmic reticulum of developing rat hepatocytes. Just before birth the endoplasmic reticulum is predominantly rough with fixed ribosomes. Following birth the endoplasmic reticulum increases in size, mainly from the biogenesis of the smooth membranes of the Golgi complex. Similar electron microscopic observations have been reported by Flickinger (1969b) during the cytodifferentiation of rat epididymal cells. Moreover, these cytological observations suggest that the Golgi complex may be synthesized and, thus, derived from the rough endoplasmic reticulum during cytodifferentiation.

Dallner *et al.* (1966a) have shown that ^{14}C-leucine and ^{14}C-glycerol are incorporated into the rough endoplasmic reticulum for the first few hours following injection. The labeled proteins and lipids are then slowly transferred to the membranes of the Golgi complex over the next 10 hours. Similarly, the enzymatic activities of constitutive enzymes, glucose-6-phosphatase, and NADH–cytochrome *c* reductase first appear in the rough endoplasmic reticulum and are eventually detectable in the Golgi complex.

Nuclear transplantation studies in *Amoeba proteus* have given additional information on the biogenesis of the Golgi complex. The membranes of the Golgi cannot be detected in the cytoplasm of amoebae 5 days after enucleation. When a nucleus is reintroduced at the end of the five days, the following events have been observed by electron microscopy. The Golgi complex is not observable at 15 minutes after renucleation. From 1 to 6 hours later, aggregations of Golgi complexes are present in the cytoplasm. The membranes of the Golgi complex increase in size, have continuous attachments to the membranes of the rough endoplasmic reticulum, and are completely regenerated by 5 days following renucleation (Flickinger, 1969a). Thus, in the amoeba the integrity and maintenance of the Golgi complex are dependent upon the nucleus and possibly the rough endoplasmic reticulum.

It is quite possible that both the rough and smooth endoplasmic reticulum are derived from the nuclear membrane in a conveyor belt system. This can be deduced from the fact that the fixed ribosomes are a product of the nucleolus. These leave the nucleus and become attached to the membrane of the rough endoplasmic reticulum upon entering the cytoplasm. Once complexed with the rough endoplasmic reticulum, they begin directing the synthesis of membrane proteins and lips of the Golgi complex, as mentioned above. Many of these proteins are destined for secretion, e.g., pancreatic acinar and goblet cells. In the zymogenic cells of the mammalian body the time of transport of these proteins, from the fixed ribosomes to the Golgi complex, into zymogenic granules and out of the cell takes 11 hours (parotid gland), 6 hours (Paneth cell), and 30 to 60 minutes (pancreas). Finally, Neutra and Leblond (1966a,b) have shown that the Golgi complex of goblet cells turns over within 20 to 40 minutes following the incorporation of labeled sugars into glycoproteins. Their estimates indicate that individual cisternae containing labeled glycoproteins are released every 2 to 4 minutes. In conclusion, the membranes, proteins, and contents of the endoplasmic reticulum (rough and smooth) turn over. The rate of turnover varies greatly from one cell type to the next and is probably influenced by intrinsic differences in the metabolism of cells, e.g., pancreas vs goblet cells (for more detail, see Section V, C and D).

D. The Soluble Phase of the Cell

The soluble phase of the cell is defined as the supernatant remaining after sedimentation of all particulate. It contains both cytoplasmic and nuclear components. In reality, it is poorly defined and consists of a myriad of moieties that interact with the particulates of the cell (e.g., ribosomes, chromatin, mitochondria). The components of the soluble phase consist of *micromolecules* (ions: Na^+, K^+, Mg^{++}, Ca^{++}, etc.), *meromolecules* (nucleotides, amino acids, sugars, metabolic intermediates, etc.), and *macromolecules* (soluble RNA, lipids, lipoproteins, and several enzymes). The subject has been adequately reviewed by Anderson and Green (1967). As a result of this review and for brevity further literature citation will be limited.

It should be obvious to the reader that the components of the soluble phase interact with the particulate material of the cell. Thus, ions are responsible not only for maintenance of membrane potentials, but are also cofactors in enzymatic reactions. The meromolecules are essentially the building blocks of proteins, lipids, and nucleic acids. In general, they have large intracellular pools that turn over rapidly (4 to 30 minutes) upon the introduction of labeled molecules. For example, it is well established that intracellular thymidylic acid turns over in 2 to 4 minutes, while its half-life in the plasma is about 20 minutes. Similar estimates for the turnover of other nucleotides and amino acids have been made (see Feinendegen, 1967).

The macromolecules, in addition to lipoproteins, consist of a large number of enzymes of intermediary metabolism. These include enzymes for amino acid activation, nucleic acid synthesis, nucleotide metabolism, fatty acid synthesis, glycolysis, pentose–phosphate oxidative cycle, and glycogen metabolism. It should be pointed out at this time that it is difficult to separate many of these enzymes from functioning in close relationship with the particulate of the cell. Although these proteins probably have limited life span and, thus, turnover, it is felt that to cover this subject would be too cumbersome. It is hoped as a result of this brief coverage that an appreciation of the possible interactions between the components of the soluble phase and the particulates of the cell has been obtained.

IV. Proteins and the Cell Cycle

A. Introduction

Considerable energy and effort have been put forth by many investigators to unlock the temporal events leading up to cell division (in other words, "trigger"). The basic fallacy of this approach lies in the fact that many individuals have considered mitosis to be the "active" event of cell, while those cells in interphase are "resting" cells. Although this point was mentioned in the introduction to this chapter, it is felt that it should be emphasized again at this time. Because, as unfortunate as it is, this concept of cell division and cytodifferentiation still exists in modern textbooks and is still presented to students of biology by many lecturers. I wish to point out at this time that most of the protein metabolism, with the exception of histones, that has been presented in this chapter takes place in interphase cells. Thus, it is reasonable to assume that the problem of cell division does not result from a trigger to division, but probably lies in the realm of differences or changes in both transcriptional and translational control mechanisms of the cell. This is particularly evident when one considers the differences between normal liver parenchyma and regenerating liver as well as the enzymatic and biochemical differences between a cryptal progenitor cell and its progeny—the surface absorbing cell.

The trigger hypotheses for cell division and differentiation were simplistic and very mechanistic. After all, they were put forth long before molecular biology became the vogue. Several hypotheses gained popularity. These include the critical mass, nuclear–cytoplasmic volume ratios, energy reservoirs (Prescott, 1956; Swann, 1957; Rustad and Rustad, 1960; Gelfant, 1960), and, finally, the induction of enzymes for thymidine metabolism and DNA synthesis (Maley and Maley, 1960; Greulich *et al.*, 1961; Hotta and Stern, 1963). In addition, efforts were also made to explain differentiation through the concept of differential mitosis, i.e., daughter cells were endowed at division with either different DNA complements or some other cellular constituent (Osgood, 1961; Talmage and Claman, 1964).

At present no one objects to the fact that cells double their cellular organelles, DNA, RNA, and protein during G_1, S, and G_2 of the cell cycle. However, to state that this duplication process attains a critical mass or nuclear–cytoplasmic ratios beyond which the cell cannot survive, is no longer acceptable. As a matter of fact, Prescott (1956) demonstrated that critical mass or volume ratios are not operative in the division of *Amoeba proteus*. He performed repeated cytoplasmic amputations on *Amoeba* in order to prevent the increase of mass or volumes. He showed that loss of cytoplasm by repeated amputations did not delay division in three out of five experiments. In the remaining two cases division eventually took place.

The concept of an energy reservoir for mitosis gained its support from the facts that cells in division have a decreased uptake of oxygen. In addition, inhibitors of oxidative phosphorylation were ineffective in preventing division, when introduced to cells just prior to mitosis (Swann, 1957). Recently, Robbins and Morrill (1969) have shown that oxygen uptake during the cell cycle of HeLa cells correlates with macromolecular synthesis. Oxygen uptake increases linearly during the first 2 hours of G_1. Oxygen consumption during early G_1 accounts for approximately 22% of the total uptake over the cycle. It is used for protein and RNA synthesis as well as intermediary metabolism. The period of DNA synthesis accounts for almost 55% of the total oxygen uptake, while the events of mitosis and probably G_2 consume the remaining 23%. It is of interest to point out that during the S phase the rates of RNA and protein synthesis double because of gene dosage effects. Also, histones are synthesized just prior to and during S. The macromolecular events of DNA, RNA, and protein synthesis require 80% of the total oxygen consumed during the S phase, while the remaining 20% is spent on ion transport, lipid metabolism, and intermediary metabolism. On the other hand, very little oxygen is consumed for macromolecular synthesis during cell division as a result of the absence of detectable RNA synthesis and reduced protein synthesis at this time. Thus, almost all of the oxygen taken up during mitosis (less than 10% of the total O_2 consumption of the cell cycle) is probably spent on the mechanism of division. In conclusion, almost all of the oxygen consumed during the cell cycle is spent on the synthesis of macromolecules. These synthetic activities are almost nonexistent during division because of chromatin condensation and polysome disaggregation. Because of this, the oxygen consumed during division is precluded for macromolecular events of the cell. It is spent, therefore, on division and intermediary metabolism. The total amount of oxygen consumed during division is sufficient to maintain the cell and obviates the requirement of energy stored in the form of trinucleotides.

With respect to the role of thymidine kinase and other enzymes responsible for metabolism of thymidylic acid and DNA, it can be said that these have now been defined as nothing more than biochemical events in the cell cycle (Baserga, 1968). It is more likely that the control mechanisms for cell division probably occur at the translational level just after division and at the transcriptional level just before division. This will be discussed in greater detail below.

To cover the arguments against the differential mitosis hypothesis is out of the scope of this particular chapter. For those individuals interested in the subject the following papers and reviews are recommended (Cairnie et al. (1965a,b); Leblond et al. (1966); Thrasher (1966, 1970); Gurdon and Woodland (1968).

B. Protein Synthesis over the Cell Cycle

Protein synthesis begins at the time of nuclear reconstruction in late telophase to early G_1. It commences without new RNA synthesis and appears to result from mRNA that is carried over from the previous cell cycle (Steward et al., 1968; Hodge et al., 1969). The incorporation of labeled amino acids into total cellular proteins continues at a linear rate through G_1. At or just before the beginning of the S phase, total protein synthesis increases two- to threefold (Klevecz and Ruddle, 1968; Bosmann and Winston, 1970). This sudden increase probably results from a gene dosage effect (see Chapter 5) as well as synthesis of histones and enzymes related to nucleic acid metabolism. The high rate of protein synthesis continues throughout S and G_2 and abruptly diminishes during mitosis (Prescott and Bender, 1962). The initiation of a new round of replication in a continuously proliferating cell in vitro results from the reassembly of polysomes with persistent mRNA mentioned above. However, the situation in vivo where on the average one half of the daughter cells differentiate is not understood (Baserga, 1968; see below).

Bosman and Winston (1970) have investigated the synthesis of glycoproteins, proteins, glycolipids, and lipids in the synchronized cell cycle of mouse lymphoma cells, L_{5178Y}. Glycoproteins and proteins are synthesized at a linear rate throughout G_1 and increase two- to threefold during the S phase. On the other hand, the synthesis of glycolipids and lipids occur almost exclusively in G_2 and mitosis. The temporal macromolecular events as described by these authors may suggest that the synthesis of glycolipids and lipids are dependent upon enzymes that are translated in S and G_2. It might be that lipids and glycolipids are the last macromolecules to be synthesized and incorporated into membranes in preparation for division.

The synthesis and appearance of enzymes in the cell cycle are periodic and in certain instances occur at precise times. For example, the enzymes lactic acid dehydrogenase (LDH) and glucose-6-phosphate dehydrogenase (G6PD) undergo periodic outburst of enzymatic activity and synthesis over the cell cycle of Chinese hamster cells. The enzymatic activities of these two enzymes have three peaks that occur at 3.5-hour intervals after mitosis. The activity and synthesis of these enzymes, however, are greatest during DNA synthesis at the time of peak protein synthesis. These cyclic fluctuations appear to result from changes in the amount of enzyme synthesis (Klevecz and Ruddle, 1968; Klevecz, 1969). Whether or not the control lies at either or both the transcriptional or translational levels has not been determined.

The other enzymes that have been extensively investigated are those responsible for the metabolism of deoxynucleotides, particularly thymidylic acid, and DNA synthesis (for reviews, Baserga, 1968; Mueller, 1969). These enzymes appear in a transitional period in late G_1 just before the cell enters DNA synthesis. Once DNA synthesis has been completed they are degraded and disappear. Apparently, this phenomenon is present in continuously proliferating cells *in vitro* as well as *in vivo* cell populations, e.g., regenerating liver. It is because of this sudden appearance and disappearance of these enzymes that considerable attention was paid to these macromolecular events of the cell cycle as a point of control of division. The enzymes investigated to date have been thymidine and thymidylic acid kinases, thymidylate synthetase, deoxycytidylic acid deaminase, and DNA polymerase. The time of appearance of these enzymes is delayed by early treatment of G_1 cells with metabolic inhibitors (actinomycin D, puromycin, etc.). However, once the block is removed the cells continue to synthesize these enzymes and eventually divide. These observations support the conclusions of Prescott (1964a), i.e., once the transition from G_1 to S has been made, DNA synthesis ensues and division occurs. The macromolecular events that preclude DNA synthesis must occur in early G_1.

The synthesis of microtubule proteins in HeLa cells has recently been reported by Robbins and Shelanski (1969). Advantage was taken of the fact that colchicine selectively binds with microtubule proteins. These proteins sediment at 6 S on sucrose gradients and appear to be homogeneous (Shelanski and Taylor, 1967). The amount of ^{3}H-colchicine that binds with newly synthesized microtubule protein is remarkably constant over the cell cycle. Thus, microtubule proteins are synthesized at relatively the same rate through the cycle. It may also be possible that cells tend to accumulate and conserve microtubule proteins from one cell cycle for utilization in the following mitosis (Robbins and Shelanski, 1969).

C. Control of Cell Division and Differentiation

Only a few comments will be made on this subject at this time. The mechanisms that may be operative in the control of cell division and differentiation have been the subject of several reviews (Prescott, 1964a; Baserga, 1968; Gurdon and Woodland, 1968; Mueller, 1969). Therefore, only a few words of caution are in order.

Continuously proliferating cells *in vitro* have a different karyotype than their *in vivo* predecessors. This phenomenon has been adequately demonstrated in investigations on changes in the simple karyotypes of the marsupial mouse (Moore and Uren, 1966) and the black-tailed wallaby (Moore and Uren, 1965; Moore and Radley, 1968) in tissue culture. The changes in the karyotypes occur in the state of ploidy ($2n \rightarrow 4n$), chromosome morphology (deletions and translocations), and in an increase in the number of late replicating units. Assuming that late replicating DNA (heterochromatin) is genetically inactive, then it appears that cells may shift gene activity and transcription toward adjustment to the new environment *in vitro*. This transformation of gene expression is away from precise *in vivo* control that, in general, regulates the generation time and the balance between cell birth and cell death in the adult animal, toward that of continuous proliferation. Perhaps this transformation may be reflected in the fact that cells *in vitro* have mRNA that persists through division and causes polysome reaggregation in the new cell cycle. These mRNA molecules are responsible for the translation of at least six polypeptides. Thus, attention toward control of cell division may have to be placed upon differences that exist in these early translational events between cells *in vitro* and *in vivo*. Tomkins *et al.* (1969) have recently made this point in their review on the expression of mammalian genes by repressors acting upon the translation of mRNA. Recently, Baltimore and Huang (1970) have demonstrated the existence of a group of heterogeneous neutral and acidic cytoplasmic proteins that bind with RNA in HeLa cells. These could possibly be translational repressors. However, more data are needed to confirm this speculation.

In renewing cell populations *in vivo* the problem of regulation of the cell cycle and cell differentiation is even more difficult to approach than *in vitro*. First of all, it is difficult to apply data and experimental methods from *in vitro* cell populations to cell proliferation *in vivo*. Especially when *in vivo* cell populations appear to have a feedback control mechanism that maintains the steady state. The other problems *in vivo* arise from the fact that renewing cell populations consist of several compartments. Each compartment must be individually analyzed with respect to macromolecular events. In most instances it has proved difficult to separate and obtain well-defined populations of cells in similar stages of differentiation. Recently, this has been attacked in the small intestine of rodents by two different methods. One involves separating villus cells from cryptal cells by continuous vibration of inverted sacs of the small intestine (Webster and Harrison, 1969). The other method entails the sequential planing of the mucosal surface with a micrometer-mounted razor blade. This latter technique permits the analysis of the enzyme composition of the following portions of the intestinal mucosa: villus, cryptovillus junction, upper crypt, and lower crypt (Imondi *et al.*, 1969). Both approaches have demonstrated changes in enzymes and other macromolecules during migration and differentiation of intestinal epithelial cells.

Webster and Harrison (1969) have shown that levels of cytochrome oxidase and G6PD remain constant in cells of the crypt and villus. On the other hand, the activities of the enzymes NADH–cytochrome c reductase, invertase, alkaline phosphatase, esterase, and leucine aminopeptidase increase during migration toward the villus tip. In addition, the RNA content is highest in the crypt, while the DNA/protein ratio is constant throughout all levels of the epithelium.

Imondi *et al.* (1969) have demonstrated differences in the activities of other enzymes. Thymidine kinase is exclusively restricted to the cryptal cells. An observation consistent with the role of this enzyme in the metabolism of thymidine in proliferating cells. In addition, thymidylate phosphatase and adenylate deaminase are uniformily distributed throughout the epithelium. The presence of these catabolic enzymes in the villus epithelium is significant from the fact that thymidine kinase is not demonstrable in the villus epithelium. Other enzymes that accompany the migration and differentiation of the mucosal cells are adenosine deaminase, nucleoside phosphorylases, and purine phosphoribosyl transferase.

Although these approaches have demonstrated specific differences in the enzymology of proliferating and differentiated cells of a renewing cell population, they still have not begun to answer the question of the control mechanisms involved. It is possible that the higher content of RNA in the cryptal cells could mean that these cells have transcribed RNA that is used for the synthesis of enzymes as cell migration and differentiation take place. This could be analogous to the persistent mRNA of cells *in vitro*. It should prove interesting in the near future to determine if differentiation in renewing cell populations results from preprograming by persistent mRNA, through interaction of the cell with the new environment of the villus epithelium or by translational repressors. It is hoped that some of these newer methodologies designed to microdissect renewing epithelia can be applied toward answering some of these questions.

V. Protein Metabolism in Special Cell Systems

A. PROTEIN SYNTHESIS IN THE IMMATURE AND ADULT LENS

The immature and adult lenses are excellent cell systems in which to investigate protein metabolism during the cytodifferentiation of a single epithelial cell type. During early postfetal growth of the lens, cell division occurs at the germinative zone near the equatorial regions. The newly formed lens fibers begin to elongate and form the cortical lens fibers. As the neonatal animal continues to grow and mature more lens fibers are produced by appositional addition of cells formed by divisions in the proliferative zone. The old lens fibers, which gradually become deeply embedded into the matrix of the lens, disintegrate and produce the nucleus or body of the lens. During this period of cytodifferentiation the water-soluble proteins that are synthesized in the proliferating cells and cortical lens fibers are transformed into the insoluble albuminoid proteins of the cortical and nuclear regions (see Fig. 10, Chapter 5) (Fulhorst and Young, 1966; Young and Fulhorst, 1966).

Autoradiographic and radiobiochemical studies of protein synthesis have been accomplished in the developing rat lens. The data are summarized in Table V. At 1 hour following injection of labeled amino acids almost all

TABLE V

DISTRIBUTION OF RADIOACTIVITY AMONG DIFFERENT LENS CONSTITUENTS AT DIFFERENT DAYS FOLLOWING INJECTION OF ^{35}S-L-METHIONINE

Lens fraction	Percent of radioactivity recovered after injection		
	1 day[a]	28 days[a]	49 days[b]
Cortex	92.4	71.6	60.5
Nucleus	5.4	22.9	60.5
Albuminoid	1.6	3.5	39.3
Lipid	<0.1	<0.1	—
Other	0.6	2.0	0.2

[a] Young and Fulhorst (1966).
[b] Fulhorst and Young (1966).

protein synthesis is restricted to the lens capsule, epithelium, and cortex (Hanna, 1965). One day after the injection over 90% of the radioactivity is recovered in the soluble proteins of the cortex. Continuous apposition of new lens fibers at the equator progressively buries the labeled proteins into the nucleus of the lens. This is evident by the fact that at 4 weeks after administration of labeled amino acids 22.9 and 3.5% of the total radio-activity are present in the soluble proteins and insoluble albuminoids of the nucleus, respectively (Young and Fulhorst, 1966). In another study, Fulhorst and Young (1966) have shown that by 7 weeks after injection of labeled amino acids the amount of radioactivity in the insoluble albumi-noids has increased to 39%. Thus, the lens proteins (α-, β-, γ- crystallins) are first synthesized in the cells of the equatorial region and the elongating lens fibers. As these cells are covered by appositional addition of new cells from the equatorial region, the crystallin proteins are slowly converted to insoluble albuminoids.

The conversion of the soluble crystallin proteins into insoluble albumi-noids occurs in normal as well as cataractous lenses. The composition of proteins of both normal and cataractous lenses have been investigated in a variety of animals. In the rat lens the small molecular weight β- and γ-crystallins appear to transform into insoluble albuminoids (Lerman et al., 1966). Recently, Harding (1969), while examining the nature and origin of insoluble proteins in the rat lens, has shown that they are divisible into either urea-soluble or insoluble fractions. Further characterization of these two fractions by amino acid analysis and starch gel electrophoresis has demonstrated that the urea-soluble albuminoids contain an α-crystallin major component, while the urea-insoluble proteins are similar to γ-crystallins. Both albuminoid fractions, however, appear to be produced from a mixture of all soluble crystallins. Thus, in the course of cytodiffer-entiation of the normal rat lens, all three crystallins are converted to in-soluble albuminoids.

In the aging and advanced cataractous human lenses, soluble crystallins decrease markedly, while the insoluble albuminoids increase (Malik et al., 1969; Francois et al., 1969; Clark et al., 1969). Changes in the concentration of lens crystallin in different types of cataracts are given in Table VI. No changes are observable in the concentration of the soluble lens crystallins in immature cataracts. However, in aged and advanced cataracts the β- and γ-crystallins decrease in concentration, while α-lens proteins increase. Concomitant to this is a rise in the concentration of insoluble albuminoids. In the human lens it appears that the albuminoids are mainly derived from the α-crystallins. The insolubilization of crystallins probably results from an increase in disulfide cross-links in the protein. The mechanism by which this occurs is poorly understood.

TABLE VI

CHANGES IN HUMAN LENS CRYSTALLIN PROTEINS DURING CATARACT FORMATION[a]

Lens type	Concentration (%) of crystallin proteins in various cataracts			Change in concentration during cataract development		
	α	β	γ	α	β	γ
Normal	42.60	41.60	15.72	—	—	—
Immature senile nuclear cataract	47.03	35.93	16.73	—	—	—
Immature senile cortical cuneiform cataract	47.85	43.72	16.85	—	—	—
Immature senile cortical cupuliform cataract	48.32	40.73	13.44	—	—	—
Nuclear black senile cataract	55.39	41.82	4.32	Rise	—	Fall
Mature senile cortical cataract	54.07	45.93	0	Rise	—	Fall
Hypermature senile cataract	61.94	33.90	4.18	Rise	Fall	Fall
Developmental cataract	61.60	33.24	9.02	Rise	Fall	—

[a] Modified from Malik et al. (1969).

B. RENEWAL OF OUTER SEGMENT IN RODS AND CONES

The photoreceptor cells of the adult vertebrate retina, rods and cones, are highly specialized cells. They are very sensitive to light and convert this sensitivity into nerve impulses that are transmitted to second-order neurons. The structural basis of these coordinated functions has been attributed to the polarity and compartmentalization in these cells (Hall et al., 1969; Young, 1969b; Cohen, 1969). Figure 1 schematically demonstrates this compartmentalization of rods and cones.

The cone differs from the rod in that its outer segment is shorter, cone-shaped, and contains fewer stacked discs (Young, 1969a). Outside of this, the rest of the structure of rods and cones is similar. The photoreceptor cells are divisible into an outer segment, inner segment, nuclear region, and synaptic body. The outer segment consists of a stack of saccules or discs. It is connected to the inner segment by a modified cilium that has a 9 + 0 fibrillar arrangement. The inner segment is divisible into an outer ellipsoid region containing mitochondria and an inner myoid region that contains most of the cellular RNA and ribosomes. The myoid is connected to the nuclear region by the fiber. RNA synthesis occurs in the nucleus, which continually supplies newly synthesized RNA to the myoid portion of the cell (Bok, 1966; Young, 1969b).

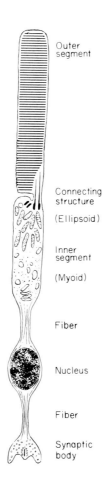

Outer segment

Connecting structure

(Ellipsoid)

Inner segment

(Myoid)

Fiber

Nucleus

Fiber

Synaptic body

FIG. 1. Schematic representation of a rod photoreceptor that demonstrates the compartmentalization of this cell. Protein synthesis takes place in the myoid portion. Newly synthesized protein then migrates through the ellipsoid and accumulates at the base of the outer segment in the connecting structure. The protein is then packaged into the membranous discs of the outer segment. The newly formed discs then slowly migrate (or are displaced) toward the pigment epithelium. (Courtesy of R. W. Young.)

The cellular site of protein synthesis in rods and cones has been demonstrated by electron microscope autoradiography in a variety of animals (for review, Young, 1969b). Within 10 minutes following administration of labeled amino acids silver grains are localized over the myoid region of free and membrane-bound ribosomes. A shift of labeled proteins to the Golgi complex occurs by 30 minutes and maximum labeling is reached by 1 to 2 hours after injection. The protein-bound radioactivity moves through the ellipsoid region and accumulates at the base of the connecting cilium. The labeled protein then moves through the cilium where it is incorporated into the membranous discs at the base of the outer segment (Droz, 1963; Young, 1967, 1968; Young and Droz, 1968; Young and Bok, 1969). At 2 hours and later following injection of labeled amino acids, a distinct difference in the labeling pattern of the outer segments of rods and cones has been observed (Young, 1969a).

In the cones of the frog retina the incorporation of labled protein into the discs is diffuse. Beginning between 2 and 4 hours after the injection a weak, diffuse labeling pattern in the membranous discs is present. After 8 hours little or no increase in the labeling of the cone outer segments occurs. It has been suggested that the diffuse incorporation of newly synthesized protein into the cone outer segment may be due to the differences in the fine structure of cones when compared to that of rods. The cones have a conical outer segment, fewer discs, wider spaces between the discs, and a larger connecting cilium (Young, 1969a). However, more information is needed to determine if the labeling pattern observed in cones reflects true biochemical and physiological differences between rods and cones.

In the rods the labeled protein is incorporated into newly formed discs at the base of the outer segment. The incorporated protein appears as a distinct band of membrane-bound protein. This band then moves toward the pigment epithelium with time after administration of labeled amino acids. In the frog retina these discs are formed at the rate of 36 per day in the red rods and 25 per day in the green rods at $22.5°C$ (Young and Droz, 1968). The time that it takes (renewal time) for the outer segment to turn over completely is 5 to 6 weeks (green rods) and 6 to 7 weeks (red rods). In the retina of rats and mice, the photoreceptor outer segments are renewed completely in about 9 days. In addition the rate of renewal of the outer segments in the frog retina doubles with each $10°C$ rise in temperature. Also, the rate of renewal appears to accelerate in animals maintained in visible light for several days, and is slower in animals kept in total darkness (Young, 1967).

The incorporation of inorganic ^{35}S into mucopolysaccharides (MPS) of rat photoreceptors is similar to the labeling pattern seen with amino acids (Hall et al., 1965; Ocumpaugh and Young, 1966). The sulfated MPS are synthesized in the myoid region of the inner segment. They are then displaced into the extracellular spaces between the outer segments of the rods. The labeled MPS reach maximum concentration as determined by grain counts in autoradiograms in the inner segment by 1 hour after injection. The outer segments are maximally labeled in a diffuse manner by 7 days after injection of ^{35}S. Labeled MPS are almost completely lost from both

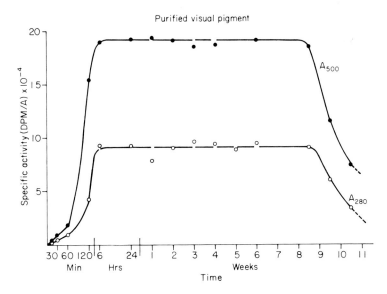

Fig. 2. Specific activity of outer segment visual pigments (rhodopsin, A_{500}; apo-protein, A_{280}) as a function of time after injection of labeled amino acids. See text for further details. (Courtesy of D. Bok; from Hall et al., 1969.)

inner and outer segments by 14 days following administration of the isotope. Possibly, the slower turnover in the discs of labeled MPS when compared to labeled protein could result from reutilization of the ^{35}S from the break-down of MPS.

Recently, Hall et al. (1969) have investigated the synthesis and turnover of the visual pigment, rhodopsin, in the inner and outer segments of the rods in the frog retina. Rhodopsin is currently considered to be a struc-tural protein of the membranes of the outer segment discs. Their results are summarized in Fig. 2. For the first hour after injection of tritiated leucine and phenlylalanine, the amino acids are incorporated into the pro-teins of the inner segment. Between 1 and 2 hours after injection the specific activity of rhodopsin rises sharply to 60 to 80% of the maximum. Maximum labeling of the visual pigment in the outer segment occurs by 6 hours after administration of the labeled amino acids. The specific activity of the visual pigment remains constant for a period lasting 8.5 weeks, after which it rapidly declines. In electron microscope autoradiograms the label associated with the visual pigment is present in the form of migrating bands of silver grains in the discs of the outer segment similar to that described by Young and Droz (1968). Thus, the visual pigment, rhodopsin, is synthesized in the inner segment of the photoreceptor cell. Rhodopsin (A_{500}) with its apoprotein (A_{280}) is then rapidly transported through the myoid portion of the rod where it accumulates in the modified cilium at the base of the outer segment. It is then incorporated into the membranes of the discs. The discs are slowly displaced toward the pigment epithelium over the next 9.5 weeks, by the addition of new discs containing visual pigment at the base of the outer segment.

It is now accepted that the discs as well as the visual pigment of the outer segment of the rod undergo a continuous process of formation and displacement. Until recently, however, the mechanism for removal of worn-out discs was not understood. The process of removal now appears to involve phagocytic activity of the pigment epithelium. Young and Bok (1969) and Hall et al. (1969) have demonstrated the presence of fragments of labeled discs in the cytoplasm of pigment epithelial cells. It appears, therefore, that as the labeled membranous discs reach the outermost portion of the outer segment of the rod they are detached from the outer segment and appear in the cytoplasm of pigment cells as labeled phagosomes.

Recent evidence from autoradiographic observations on the renewal of rod outer segments in normal and dystrophic rats have suggested that the phagocytic activity of the pigment cells is necessary in order to maintain the normal functional integrity of the photoreceptor cells (Herron et al., 1969). The dystrophic rats have a normal renewal rate of the outer segment until about the eighteenth day of life. After this age the normal rate of renewal of the outer segment gradually diminishes. The outer segment of the dystrophic rat retina then undergoes a retrograde degeneration with an ensuing blindness. This slower renewal rate and the retrograde degeneration are accompanied by a loss of phagocytic activity of the pigment epithelial cells. This results in a build-up of degenerated and disorganized labeled discs between the photoreceptor cells and the pigment epithelium. Thus, it seems reasonable to assume that the loss of phagocytic activity of the pigment epithelium in these retinal distrophic rats may be the cause of hereditary retinal degeneration.

C. Synthesis and Transport of Glycoproteins and Mucopolysaccharides

Proteins containing carbohydrates are widely distributed in animal tissues. Because of their ubiquity and importance in diseases (e.g. serum sickness, dermatomyositis, scleroderma, tumors, cystic fibrosis) they have been the subject of numerous reviews and symposia (Spiro, 1963; Gottschalk, 1966; Coutts and Smail, 1966; Rossi and Stoll, 1968; White et al., 1968). They are classified into two categories: the mucopolysaccharides complexed with proteins and the glycoproteins.

TABLE VII

MUCOPOLYSACCHARIDES[a]

Type	Sugar composition	Location
Nonsulfated		
Hyaluronic acid	Glucuronic acid, N-acetylglucosamine	Skin, umbilical cord, aqueous humor, synovial fluid, heart valves
Chondroitin	Glucuronic acid, N-acetylgalactosamine	Cornea, embryonic cartilage
Sulfated		
Chondroitin sulfate A	Glucuronic acid, N-acetylgalactosamine-4-sulfate	Tendon, embryonic cartilage, aorta, bone, cartilage, cornea
Chondroitin sulfate B	Iduronic acid, N-acetylgalactosamine-4-sulfate	Aorta, heart valves, ligaments
Chondroitin sulfate C	Glucuronic acid, N-acetylgalactosamine-6-sulfate	Cartilage, tendon, embryonic cartilage, umbilical cord
Keratosufate	Galactose, galactose-6-sulfate, N-acetylglucosamine-6-sulfate	Bone, cornea, nucleus pulposus, cartilage
Heparitin sulfate	Glucuronic acid-2-sulfate, glucosamine-6-sulfate, N-acetyl or N-sulfate	Aorta, liver, lung, mast cells

[a] From Coutts and Smail (1966); White et al. (1968).

The mucopolysaccharides are listed in Table VII. They are found as a major constituent of the ground matrix of connective tissues. They are acidic, and contain hexuronic acid or sulfate esters or both of this carbohydrate. The polysaccharide moiety consists of glucuronate, iduronate, or galactose as well as amino sugars, galactosamine and glucosamine. The polysaccharide molecule is associated with the protein complex by either ionic linkages or labile covalent bonds.

The glycoproteins (Tables VIII and IX) differ from the mucopolysaccharides in several ways. The carbohydrate moiety is firmly linked to the polypeptide by covalent bonds. They do not contain either hexuronic acid or sulfate esters. The carbohydrate constituents are the amino sugars, glucosamine and galactosamine; the neutral sugars, mannose, galactose, and fucose; and various derivatives of neuraminic acid (N-acetyl, N-glycol, N–O-diacetyl, and N-acetyl, O-diacetyl). The neuraminic acid compounds have been collectively referred to as sialic acids (Spiro, 1963).

TABLE VIII

DISTRIBUTION OF GLYCOPROTEINS IN THE MAMMALIAN BODY[a]

I. *Plasma glycoproteins:* Orosomucoid, fetuin, ceruloplasm, glycoproteins, hapto-
globulins, macroglobulins, transferrin, prothrombin, fibrinogen, 7 S globulins,
19 S globulins

II. *Glycoprotein hormones and related substances:* ICSH, FSH, human chorionic
gonadotropin, pregnant mare's serum gonadotropin, erythropoietin, TSH,
thyroglobulin

III. *Glycoproteins with blood-group activity:* Present in red blood cells, pseudomucinous
ovarian cysts, gastric mucosa, meconium, saliva, gastric juice, amniotic
fluid, urine

IV. *Glycoproteins of mucous secretions:* Submaxillary, sublingual, cervical, tracheo-
bronchial, gastric, biliary, epithelium of large and small intestines

V. *Glycoproteins from egg white:* Ovalbumin, ovomucoid, ovomucin, avidin

VI. *Glycoproteins of connective tissue:* Collagen, reticulin, basement membranes, lens
capsule, Descemet's membrane, soluble glycoproteins

---

[a] Adapted from Spiro (1963).

The incorporation of ^{35}S-sulfate into mucopolysaccharides has been
followed autoradiographically (Peterson and Leblond, 1964; Neutra and
Leblond, 1966a, b). Inorganic sulfate is incorporated in the Golgi complex
by 5 minutes after injection. The autoradiographic reactions are observable
in only a few types of cells. These are the goblet cells of the large and small
intestine, the surface mucous cells of the stomach, epithelial mucous cells,
and mucous glands of the trachea and chondrocytes (Table X). Apparently,
the sulfation of mucopolysaccharides takes place in the Golgi complex of
the cell. The sulfated mucopolysaccharides then slowly accumulate in the
extracellular matrix and secretory products over the next 4 hours following
injection of the isotope. The incorporated labeled sulfate represents acid
mucopolysaccharides because it is enzymatically removed by treatment of
histological sections with hyaluronidase and β-glucuronidase.

The cellular sites of the incorporation of labeled amino acids and sugars
(^{3}H-glucose, ^{3}H-galactose, and ^{3}H-mannose) have been investigated in a
variety of cell types that are known to synthesize and secrete both glycoproteins and mucopolysaccharides (Peterson and Leblond, 1964; Neutra
and Leblond, 1966a,b; Whur *et al.*, 1969). Neutra and Leblond (1966b)
compared the distribution of ^{3}H-galactose with that of ^{3}H-glucose and ^{35}S-
sulfate. Glucose was incorporated into all cell types secreting glycoproteins
and mucopolysaccharides, while ^{35}S- and ^{3}H-galactose were found in only
certain cell types (see Table X). The incorporation of glucose into the Golgi
complex of all mucous-secreting cells occurs mainly from the fact that this

TABLE IX

CARBOHYDRATE COMPOSITION OF A FEW REPRESENTATIVE GLYCOPROTEINS

Protein	Hexoses (%)	Galactose (%)	Mannose (%)	N-acetyl-glucosamine (%)	N-acetyl-galactos-amine (%)	Sialic acid (%)	Fucose (%)	Total (%)	Reference
Orosomucoid	—	6.5	4.8	15.2	—	10.8	1.0	38.3	Yamashina (1956)
Haptoglobulin	11.3	—	—	7.1	—	5.5	0.2	24.1	Schultze (1958)
Transferrin	2.4	—	—	2.0	—	1.4	0.1	5.6	Schultze et al. (1958)
FSH	2.1	—	—	3.5	0	1.9	0.5	8.0	Gröschel and Li (1960)
Thyroglobulin	—	1.3	3.5	4.2	0	1.1	0.5	10.6	Spiro and Spiro (1963)
Cervical mucin	—	27.5	—	18.9	14.1	13.8	5.1	79.4	Gibbons (1969)

TABLE X

INCORPORATION OF ^{3}H-GLUCOSE, ^{3}H-GALACTOSE AND ^{35}S-SULFATE INTO THE GOLGI
COMPLEX BETWEEN 5 AND 15 MINUTES AFTER INJECTION[a]

Cell type	^{3}H-glucose	^{3}H-galactose	^{35}S-sulfate
Small intestine			
Goblet	+++	—	+++
Columnar	+/−	++	—
Large intestine			
Goblet	++++	++	+++
Columnar	+/−	+	—
Brunner's gland			
Mucous	++++	+++	—
Stomach			
Surface mucous	++++	+/−	++
Mucous neck	+	—	—
Salivary glands			
Sublingual mucous	+++	++	—
Submaxillary mucous	+	—	—
Trachea			
Epithelial mucous	++	+	+
Mucous gland	+++	—	+++
Serous gland	+/−	—	—
Pancreas			
Acinar cells	+/−	+	—
Liver Parenchyma	—	+	—
Epididymis epithelium	+/−	++	—
Proximal tubule (kidney)	—	++	—
Chondrocytes			
Trachea	+	+	++
Knee joint	+++	+++	+++

[a] From Neutra and Leblond (1966b).

Key: +, relative grain concentration; +/−, grains observable only after high doses.

sugar is converted into other monosaccharides. These are then synthesized
into the polysaccharide moiety of glycoproteins and mucopolysaccharides
(Spiro, 1963; Dorfman, 1963). Galactose, on the other hand, was not taken
up by all mucous-secreting cells. This was particularly evident in the goblet
cells of the small intestine, the mucous cells of the stomach, submaxillary
mucous cells, and the mucous cells of the trachea. However, this does not
mean that the glycoproteins of these cells do not contain galactose. Rather,
it may suggest that all mucous-secreting cells do not have the enzymes

necessary for the incorporation of galactose. Another interesting point is that some of the mucous cells incorporate ^{35}S-sulfate in addition to the sugars. Therefore, at least some of these cells synthesize and secrete both glycoproteins and mucopolysaccharides, e.g., goblet cells of the small intestine, surface mucous cells of the stomach, etc. Finally, from these data it is possible to conclude that the addition of glucose, galactose, and sulfate to the peptide moiety appears to take place in the Golgi complex.

The time course of the incorporation of labeled sugars into glycoproteins has also been investigated (Neutra and Leblond, 1966a, Whur *et al.*, 1969). Neutra and Leblond (1966a,b) have shown that ^{3}H-glucose is rapidly incorporated into the Golgi complex of the rat colon. By 20 minutes after administration of the labeled sugars both the Golgi region and nearby mucigen granules are heavily labeled. The incorporated glucose by 40 minutes after administration is almost completely associated with cytoplasmic mucigen granules. The mucigen granules then migrate toward the apical portion of the cell over the next 3 hours. Once reaching the membrane of the apical region of the goblet cell, the mucigen granules are secreted with their membranes intact. According to their interpretation of the data, the Golgi complex is the site of synthesis of complex carbohydrates and the addition of these polysaccharides to the polypeptide of the glycoprotein. The Golgi saccules are then transformed into mucigen-containing granules with an intact Golgi membrane surrounding each granule. Granules are released from the Golgi complex at a rate of one every 2 to 4 minutes.

Whur *et al.* (1969) have investigated the time course of events of the incorporation of tritium-labeled galactose, mannose, and leucine into thyroglobulin of the rat thyroid. Autoradiographic observations have shown that the uptake of leucine and mannose by thyroid cells is diffuse at 5 minutes after injection. The diffuse autoradiographic images are associated with the rough endoplasmic reticulum. The uptake of both mannose and leucine is inhibited by puromycin, indicating that their incorporation is into newly synthesized protein. The silver grains from ^{3}H-leucine are concentrated over the vesicles of the apical portion of the cell by 1 hour and appear in the colloid material by 2 hours following administration of the amino acid. ^{3}H-mannose passes from the rough endoplasmic reticulum to the Golgi apparatus by 1–2 hours and appears in the apical vesicles by 3 hours after injection. ^{3}H-galactose, on the other hand, first appears over the Golgi zone at 5 minutes after injection. Its incorporation into glycoproteins is unaffected by puromycin. The label associated with galactose is then rapidly transferred to the apical vesicles during the first hour and appears in the colloidal material of the thyroid thereafter. Thus, the steps in the synthesis of thyroglobulin are the incorporation of ^{3}H-leucine and

³H-mannose in the rough endoplasmic reticulum. The carbohydrate–
polypeptide molecule is then transported to the Golgi complex during the
next hour. Once in the Golgi saccules ³H-galactose is added. The thyroglobulin then appears in the apical viscles over the next 2 hours and is
secreted thereafter into the colloid substance of the thyroid follicles.

D. SYNTHESIS AND TRANSPORT OF PROTEINS IN ZYMOGENIC CELLS

In general, cells containing zymogen granules are associated with the
gastrointestinal track. Their major metabolic function is the synthesis and
secretion of digestive enzymes (Table XI) in a liquid medium that also
contains ions, bicarbonate, and glycoproteins. The stimulus for the secretion of these enzymes comes from gastrointestinal hormones. These hormones in turn are released by such factors as protein, polypeptides, vagal
stimulation, intestinal chyme, and probably even distension of the intestinal lumen (for review, Davenport, 1966; Ganong, 1967). The end
result of such physiological responses to ingested food causes the secretion
of as much as 1500 ml of saliva and 2000 ml of pancreatic juices per day
in man.

The cytology of the zymogenic cells is neatly packaged to fit this metabolic demand. The cells are cone-shaped with the base of the cell adjacent to
the basement membrane. The apex borders on the lumen of the gland. The
apical cytoplasm contains large membrane-bound zymogenic granules. An
extensive Golgi complex lies in a supranuclear position, while the rough
endoplasmic reticulum is between the nucleus and the basement membrane.
The digestive enzymes are synthesized on the fixed ribosomes of the rough
endoplasmic reticulum and then rapidly transported to the Golgi region of

TABLE XI

ZYMOGENIC CELLS AND THEIR SECRETORY PRODUCTS

Organ	Cell	Digestive enzyme	Reference
Salivary glands	Serous	Ptyalin, amylase	—
Stomach	Chief	Pepsin	Grossman and Marks (1960)
Small intestine	Paneth	Unspecific acid phosphatase, E 600-resistant esterase, β-glucosaminidase, β-glucuronidase	Riecken and Pearse (1966)
Pancreas	Acinar	Chymotrypsin A and B, trypsin, carboxypeptidase, lipase, amylase, ribonuclease	Desnuelle and Rovery (1961)

the cell. The Golgi saccules release the membrane-bound zymogen granules, which are then secreted into the lumen of the gland at the apical portion of the cell. In the zymogen cells of the parotid gland, the membrane of the zymogen granule fuses with the cell membrane at the time of secretion. In this manner the membrane of the granule is probably reutilized. The secretory cycle from the time of synthesis to the release of the granules takes about 11 hours in the parotid gland (Amsterdam et al., 1969).

The chief cells of the gastric mucosa also undergo a similar secretory cycle following the injection of pilocarpine. Within 1 hour after the injection the zymogen granules in the apical portion of the cell are depleted. Only those granules near the base of the chief cell remain. At the end of 6 hours following the injection of pilocarpine signs of the replenishment of the granules are present. The pilocarpine-stimulated chief cell returns to its normal appearance by 16 hours after the injection (for review, Hirschowitz, 1957). However, Grossman and Marks (1960) have shown that pepsinogen is continuously secreted from the pyloric glands of both control and fed dogs. This secretion amounts to a total effluent volume of 2.0 to 2.5 ml per hour that contains approximately 20 to 25 units of pepsin activity per ml. Similar observations on human subjects have also been made (Go et al., 1970).

The Paneth cell still remains somewhat of an enigma. Its granules have been described as either zymogenic or lysosomal in character (for review, Lewin, 1969). However, Riecken and Pearse (1966) have shown by histochemical techniques that the granules of the Paneth cell contain lysosomal enzymes (Table XI). They have suggested that the Paneth cell is probably a digestive gland that empties its lysosomal granules directly into the lumen of the crypt in the small intestine. This concept has been supported by Trier et al. (1967) who examined the uptake and turnover of ^{3}H-leucine by Paneth cells. At 20 minutes after the injection of the labeled amino acid, silver grains in autoradiograms were demonstrable over the rough endoplasmic reticulum at the base of the cell. The newly labeled protein is transported to the Golgi region at 1 hour and to the apical cytoplasm in the granules at 6 hours after administration of labeled leucine. By 12 hours after the injection 92% of the Paneth cells are no longer labeled. The labeled proteins and granules are observable at this time in the contents of the lumen of the crypt. According to their results the Paneth cell continuously synthesizes and secretes proteins. The secretory activity of the cell is not affected by diet, but is accelerated by the injection of pilocarpine and is reduced after the administration of atropine. In conclusion, the Paneth cell probably contains lysosomes. The time between the initial synthesis of the lysosomal enzymes and their secretion into the cryptal lumen takes approximately 12 hours in both fed and starved mice.

The cellular sites of synthesis, transport, storage, and secretion of pancreatic enzymes have been investigated both by autoradiographic (Warshawsky *et al.*, 1963; Nadler, 1963; van Heyningen, 1964) methods and cellular fractionation (Siekevitz and Palade, 1960a,b; Jamieson and Palade, 1967a,b, 1968a,b) methods. In autoradiograms labeled amino acids are detectable over the fixed ribosomes of the rough endoplasmic reticulum from 1 to 5 minutes following injection. From there the newly synthesized proteins are transported to the Golgi complex where they accumulate during the following 10 to 30 minutes (Warshawsky *et al.*, 1963; van Heyninger, 1964). Calculations of the turnover times of the labeled proteins have indicated that two classes of proteins are synthesized in the pancreatic acinar cells. Some proteins of undetermined nature and function turn over very slowly in the rough endoplasmic reticulum. These have been termed sedentary proteins and turn over with a half-life of about 63 hours. On the other hand, the majority of pancreatic proteins, termed exportable proteins, turn over very rapidly. The exportable proteins spend about 5 minutes in the rough endoplasmic reticulum, and 12 minutes in the Golgi complex where they are packaged into zymogen granules. Thereafter, the labeled proteins spend 36 minutes in the zymogen granules of the apical cytoplasm before evidence of secretion. The average life span of a zymogen granule is about 48 minutes (Warshawsky *et al.*, 1963; Nadler, 1963). The sedentary proteins and those labeled proteins that remain in the acinar cells from 3.5 to 12 hours after injection of labeled amino acids appear to be structural proteins (van Heyningen, 1964). Siekevitz and Palade (1960a,b) have shown by cell fractionation techniques that amylase, RNase, trypsinogen, and chymotrypsin-activatible proteolytic activities are first demonstrable at the site of synthesis in the rough endoplasmic reticulum. These enzymes are then transported through the Golgi complex and accumulate in the zymogen granules. More recently, Jamieson and Palade (1968a,b) have shown that the intracellular transport of the secretory proteins from the site of synthesis to the zymogen granule continues when protein synthesis is inhibited by cycloheximide. In addition, the transport mechanism to the condensing vacuoles of the Golgi complex is insensitive to glycolytic inhibitors, but is blocked by inhibitors of respiratory enzymes and oxidative phosphorylation.

E. Synthesis and Turnover of Liver Proteins

1. *Introduction*

The functions of the liver in the mammalian body have been extensively investigated. The liver and its metabolic functions have, therefore, been the subject of several excellent reviews. For brevity these will be listed for those individuals who wish to do further reading on liver physiology: (1) metabolism of bilirubin and bile salts (Combes, 1964; Hargreaves, 1968); (2) vitamins (Wiss and Weber, 1964); (3) steroids (Cameron, 1964); (4) lipid metabolism (Favarger, 1963); (5) carbohydrate metabolism (Pesch and Topper, 1963); (6) metabolism of amino acids and plasma proteins Tarver, 1963; Schultze and Heremans, 1966). The discussion on liver proteins will be restricted for the most part to a description of the dynamic state of liver proteins. This will cover the functional unit of the lobule—the liver acinus, the synthesis and turnover of plasma proteins, the turnover of inducible enzymes, and the role of diurnal rhythms in liver protein metabolism.

2. The Liver Acinus and Protein Metabolism

A structural and functional unit of the liver has been devised by Rappaport (1963). It eliminates the classic liver lobule as the metabolic unit of the liver and presents, instead, the simple liver acinus. The liver acinus is diagrammatically represented in Fig. 3. The frame of reference is shifted from the central vein, hereafter termed the terminal hepatic venule, to the portal canal. The portal canal contains the hepatic arteriole, portal venule, bile duct, and lymphatics. Radiating from the portal canal are the terminal portal venule and hepatic arteriole. Blood from the portal vein

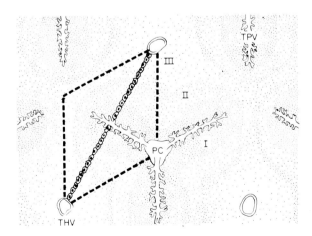

FIG. 3. Diagram of an area of rat liver showing a portal canal (PC), terminal portal venule (TPV), terminal hepatic venule (THV) and the metabolic zones (I, II, and III). A simple liver acinus is outlined by the dashed line. Within the acinus is a row of hepatic cells extending the length of the acinus. (From LeBouton, 1968.)

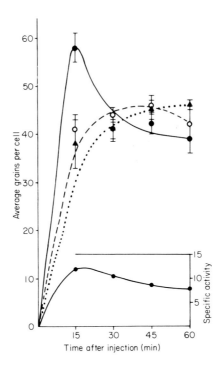

Fɪɢ. 4. Upper: This graph depicts the zonal radioactivity at various times after injection of ³H-leucine for each metabolic zone of the liver acinus diagramed in Fig. 3. Zone I (●—●), Zone II (○ - - - - ○) and Zone III (▲ · · · · · · ▲). A vertical line at each point represents the standard error of the mean. Lower: This graph shows the specific activity (cpm/μg protein) of soluble intracellular proteins at various times after injection of ³H-leucine. (From LeBouton, 1968.)

and hepatic artery trickles from the terminal vessels of the acinus through the sinusoids toward the terminal hepatic venule.

Although Rappaport's description of the liver acinus is based upon observations from pathophysiological material, cytochemical, histochemical, and autoradiographic data support his conclusions. For example, the cells immediately surrounding the portal canal contain more RNA than those hepatocytes near the terminal hepatic venule. On the other hand, some of the oxidative enzymes have an opposite pattern of distribution. Reduced nicotinamide adenine dinucleotide and alcohol dehyrogenase, for example, have distinctly higher histochemical reactions in liver cells near the terminal hepatic venule when compared to those surrounding the portal canal (Wachstein, 1963; Morrison and Brock, 1967).

The concepts of the liver acinus and metabolic gradients within the acinus have been confirmed and extended by LeBouton (1968, 1969). Protein metabolism in hepatocytes was investigated by autoradiography from 10 to 60 minutes following the injection of ^{3}H-leucine into rats. The results from grain counts over hepatocytes have shown that the cells of the liver acinus can be divided into three general zones according to the incorporation of the amino acid and the turnover of labeled proteins. Zone I is approximately eight cells in width and immediately surrounds the portal canal and the terminal portal venule and hepatic arteriole. The cells of Zone III are situated around the terminal portal venule. Zone II includes all liver cells in the intermediate parenchyma.

The cells in Zone I incorporate ^{3}H-leucine into proteins and turn over the labeled proteins at a faster rate than cells in Zones II and III. Radioactivity in cells of Zone I reaches peak values by 15 minutes after injection and then decreases rapidly by 30 minutes. On the other hand, the amount of the radioisotope incorporated into cells of Zones II and III does not reach its highest value until 45 to 60 minutes after injection of the labeled amino acid (see Fig. 4). Thus, the cells of Zone I incorporate labeled amino acids and lose their label protein much more rapidly than the hepatocytes of Zone II and III of the liver acinus. This should be expected on the basis that the cells of Zone I contain more RNA (Wachstein, 1963). As pointed out by LeBouton (1968, 1969), it is possible that the function of liver cells in Zone I is that of synthesis and secretion of plasma proteins. The remaining liver parenchyma may carry out the metabolic activities of the liver listed above. However, this concept of the division of labor with in the liver acinus needs further experimental support before it can be accepted.

3. Synthesis and Turnover of Plasma Proteins and Inducible Enzymes

Outside of the proteins associated with mitochondria, ribosomes, and nuclei (these have been covered earlier in the chapter), liver proteins can be placed into one of two general categories. One category comprises the plasma proteins synthesized and secreted by liver cells (Madden and Whipple, 1940). The second group of proteins includes the endogenous enzymes that may be either inducible or noninducible and undergo constant intracellular turnover (Rechcigl, 1968).

Table XII lists the plasma proteins that are synthesized by the liver. Values for the mean concentration in the plasma, half-life, and percentage of turnover are also given (for review, Schultze and Heremans, 1966). Albumin has been the most extensively studied plasma protein. It will be used here as an example of the synthesis and turnover of a typical plasma

TABLE XII
TURNOVER OF PLASMA PROTEINS IN HUMANS[a]

Protein	Concentration of plasma (gm/ml)	Half-life of plasma (days)	Percent of plasma pool degraded/day
Albumin[b]	4.2	19 [17–23][j]	10 [7–11]
Transferrin[c]	0.24	8.5 [7–10][j]	8–17
α_1-Acid glycoprotein[d]	0.1	5.2 [5–7][j]	11.5–14[k]
Haptoglobulin[e]	0.1	3.5–4.0	—
Fibrinogen[f]	0.3	4.0–5.5	12–16
α_1-Lipoprotein[g]	—	4.2–4.5	14–16
$S_{f3-9}(\beta)$ lipotroteins[h]	—	3.1–3.4	20–22
Prealbumin[i]	0.034	1.9	36.3[k]

[a] Adapted from Schultze and Heremans (1966).
[b] Lewallen et al. (1959); Cohen et al. (1961); Jarnum and Schwartze (1960); Takeda and Reeve (1963); Beeken et al. (1962).
[c] Awai and Brown (1961); Jarnum and Lassen (1961); Katz (1961).
[d] Scanu and Hughes (1962); Weissman et al. (1961).
[e] Morretti et al. (1963).
[f] McFarlane (1963); Madden and Gould (1952); Gitlin and Borges (1953); Hammond and Verel (1959).
[g] Gitlin et al. (1958).
[h] Gitlin et al. (1958).
[i] Oppenheimer et al. (1965).
[j] Range.
[k] Percent of body pool degraded per day.

protein. As pointed out in Chapter 5, albumin and probably most of the plasma proteins are synthesized on long-lived mRNA in fixed polysomes. This is in contrast to ferritin, an endogenous liver protein, which is synthesized on free polysomes with a short-lived mRNA. (Hicks et al., 1969). Intrahepatic albumin reaches maximum specific activity between 15 and 30 minutes following injection of ^{3}H-leucine. Its specific activity rapidly falls, thereafter, with a half-life value of 70 to 80 minutes (Peters, 1962a,b; LeBouton, 1968). Plasma albumin reaches its maximum specific activity between 80 and 120 minutes following administration of the labeled amino acid. The maximum labeling of intrahepatic albumin corresponds with the peak radioactivity that is found in Zone I cells of the acinus. Thus, it is possible, as already mentioned, that the metabolic function of Zone I cells is that of synthesizing and replacing plasma proteins.

The dynamic state of the turnover of plasma proteins can be appreciated from Table XII. The half-life of plasma proteins ranges from 1.9 to 19 days. It has been estimated, for example, that albumin is synthesized and degraded in amounts of 10 to 16 gm daily (Schultze and Heremans, 1966). Similar values for degradation and turnover have been obtained for the other plasma proteins. Thus, it should be obvious that the liver synthesizes and secretes large quantities of plasma proteins per day.

According to Rechcigl (1968) very little information is available on the turnover of noninducible enzymes of the liver. He has pointed out that only two enzymes have been extensively investigated. Arginase has a half-life of 4 to 5 days. Another noninducible enzyme, catalase, has also been studied (Rechcigl and Heston, 1967; Rechcigl and Price, 1967). Although half-life values have not been calculated, this enzyme is synthesized at a rate of 28 μg/hr/gm of liver. The amount of the enzyme present in liver cells is regulated by its rate of degradation. Thus, the rate of synthesis of catalase is fairly constant, while its rate of degradation varies according to the physiological state of the animal (e.g., starvation) as well as genetic mechanisms as a result of substrain differences.

The dynamic state of protein metabolism in the liver is also demonstrable in studies that have investigated the turnover of inducible enzymes. This adaptation phenomenon, i.e., the induction of enzymes by substrates, is best described by the following statement. Following the administration of a suitable substrate or inducer, there is a period of accelerated enzyme activity that results from the synthesis of the induced enzyme. The activity of the newly synthesized enzyme remains high for several hours to days after induction. Subsequently, the rate of synthesis decreases and the level of enzymatic activity then returns to basal levels. Measurements of the

TABLE XIII

HALF-LIFE VALUES FOR INDUCIBLE ENZYMES IN THE LIVER

Enzyme	Half-life	Reference
Tryptophan pyrrolase	2–4 hours	Feigelsen et al. (1959); Nemeth (1962); Schimke et al. (1965)
Tyrosine transaminase	2–4 hours	Goldstein et al. (1962); Kenney (1962)
Serine dehydrase	3 hours	Pitot and Peraino (1964)
δ-Aminolevulinc acid synthetase	67–72 min	Marver et al. (1966)
3–P–glycerate dehydrogenase	14.6 hours	Fallon et al. (1966)
Glutamic-pyruvic transaminase	3½ days	Segal and Kim (1963)
Malate dehydrogenase	4 days	Tarentino et al. (1966)
L-α-Glycerophosphate dehydrogenase	4 days	Tarentino et al. (1966)

rate of decay of the enzyme activity are taken as estimates of the half-life of the enzyme. Table XIII lists several inducible enzymes that have been investigated. It can be seen from the table that most of the enzymes turn over with half-life values of 1 to 4 hours. However, a few decay over a period of days. In either case, it can be speculated at this time that new mRNA synthesis probably precedes the appearance of the induced enzyme. It would be interesting to determine if the mRNA is short-lived or long-lived and also to determine if translational mechanisms act to regulate the induction of new enzymes in the adult liver.

4. *Diurnal Rhythms in Liver Metabolism*

Superimposed upon the synthesis, turnover, and secretion of proteins by the liver are circadian (or diurnal) rhythms in hepatocyte metabolism. These rhythms are observable in animals that have been adapted to light cycles consisting of 12 hours of light and 12 hours of dark. Glycogen content of rodent livers is at its peak concentration at the end of the dark period through the beginning of first part of the light period. This is reversed at the end of the light period through the beginning of darkness (Haus and Halberg, 1966). RNA synthesis as determined by the incorporation of ^{32}P is greatest between 8 to 10 P.M., that is, from 2 to 4 hours after the light is turned off. The increased RNA synthesis occurs 6 to 8 hours earlier than peak DNA synthesis and mitotic activity in the liver of young mice (Barnum *et al.*, 1958). Interestingly, the rate of general protein synthesis is almost doubled at 12:00 midnight, close to 2 hours after peak RNA synthesis (LeBouton and Handler, 1970). Two hours after the period of increased protein synthesis, maximum concentration of plasma albumin and other proteins are observable (Scheving *et al.*, 1968). In addition, inducible enzymes, such as tyrosine transaminase and tryptophan pyrrolase, have maximum specific activity at the same time that the increase in protein metabolism is seen (Fuller and Snoddy, 1968; Hardeland and Rensing, 1968; Cohn *et al.*, 1970, Fuller, 1970).

Several physiological factors appear to influence the daily rhythm of protein metabolism in the rodent liver. Tyrosine transaminase and tryptophan pyrrolase are induced within 5 hours following the injection of cortisol or the administration of their respective substrates. The induction of the enzymes by the substrate is abolished with adrenalectomy. On the other hand, several other enzymes (glucose-6-phosphatase, alanine transaminase, serine dehydrase, and urea cycle enzymes) respond over a period of days to treatment with cortisol (for review, Rosen and Nichol, 1964; Potter *et al.*, 1967). Recently, Cohn *et al.* (1970) have shown that adrenalectomy of rats does not abolish the dirunal rhythm of tyrosine transaminase activity. However, the amplitude of the 24-hour rhythm is diminished under these experimental conditions. The rhythmicity of liver protein metabolism is also influenced by light. Scheving *et al.* (1968) have shown that the circadian fluctuation in plasma proteins of the rat can be abolished under constant lighting conditions. In addition, reversal of the light schedule also leads to a reversal in the rhythms of tyrosine transaminase activity (Cohn *et al.*, 1970). Finally, changes in the diet can also produce variations in the pattern of peak enzymatic activity. Fuller (1970) has shown that switching food intake from an *ad libitum* regimen to a single early morning feeding shifts the peak activity of tryptophan pyrrolase. In *ad libitum*-fed rats on a 12–12 light cycle the maximum enzymatic activity of this enzyme occurs between 8 and 11 P.M. In rats fed a single daytime meal, the activity of tryptophan pyrrolase peaks at 11 A.M., only 3 hours after the feeding. In these experiments no differences in the rhythm of corticosterone or tryptophan amino acid cycles could be observed in the daytime-fed animals. Starvation of animals, on the other hand, causes only a slight shift in the time that liver protein metabolism is at its maximum synthetic rate. LeBouton and Handler (1970) have shown that withholding of food from rats during the dark period shifts the time of maximum protein synthesis from 12 midnight to 2 A.M. in the starved rats. In conclusion, it is safe to assume that a primary circadian rhythm in liver DNA, RNA, and protein synthesis occurs. Such treatments as adrenalectomy, injection of cortisol, administration of amino acid substrates, alteration in feeding, and light regimens modify this rhythm at secondary and tertiary levels.

REFERENCES

Adamson, S. D., Howard, G. A., and Herbert, E. (1969). The ribosome cycle in a reconstituted cell-free system from reticulocytes. *Cold Spring Harbor Symp. Quant. Biol.* **35**, 547.

Allfrey, V. G. (1963). Nuclear ribosomes, messenger-RNA and protein synthesis. *Exp. Cell Res., Suppl.* **9**, 183.

Allfrey, V. G. (1966). Control mechanisms in ribonucleic acid synthesis. *Cancer Res.* **26**, 2026.

Allfrey, V. G. (1968). Some observations on histone acetylation and its temporal relationship to gene activation. *In* "Regulatory Mechanisms for Protein Synthesis in Mammalian Cells" (A. San Pietro, M. R. Lamborg, and F. T. Kenney, eds.), p. 65. Academic Press, New York.

Allfrey, V. G., Faulkner, R., and Mirsky, A. E. (1964). Acetylation and methylation of histones and their possible role in the regulation of RNA synthesis. *Proc. Nat. Acad. Sci. U.S.* **51**, 786.

Allfrey, V. G., Littau, V. C., and Mirsky, A. E. (1963). On the role of histones in regulating ribonucleic acid synthesis in the cell nucleus. *Proc. Nat. Acad. Sci. U.S.* **49**, 414.

Allfrey, V. G., Pogo, B. G. T., Pogo, A. O., Kleinsmith, L. J., and Mirsky, A. E. (1966). The metabolic behaviour of chromatin. *In* "Histones" (A. V. S. deReuck and J. Knight, eds.), p. 42. Ciba Foundation Symp., Little, Brown, Boston, Massachusetts.

Amsterdam, A., Ohad, I., and Schramm, M. (1969). Dynamic changes in the ultrastructure of the acinar cell of the rat parotid gland during the secretory cycle. *J. Cell Biol.* **41**, 753.

Anderson, N. G., and Green, J. G. (1967). The soluble phase of the cell. *In* "Enzyme Cytology" (D. B. Roodyn, ed.), p. 475. Academic Press, New York.

Asao, T. (1969). Behavior of histones and cytoplasmic basic proteins during embryogenesis of the Japanese newt. *Triturus pyrrhogaster. Exp. Cell Res.* **58**, 243.

Attardi, B., Cravito, B., and Attardi, G. (1969). Membrane-bound ribosomes in HeLa cells. I. Their proportion to total cell ribosomes and their association with messenger RNA. *J. Mol. Biol.* **44**, 47.

Awai, M., and Brown, E. B. (1961). Studies of the metabolism of human transferrin. *J. Lab. Clin. Med.* **58**, 797.

Azen, E. A., Orr, S., and Smithies, O. (1965). Starch-gel electrophoresis of erythrocyte stroma. *J. Lab. Clin. Med.* **65**, 440.

Baglioni, C., Vesco, C., and Jacobs-Lorena, M. (1969). The role of ribosomal subunits in mammalian cells. *Cold Spring Harbor Symp. Quant. Biol.* **35**, 547.

Baltimore, D., and Huang, A. S. (1970). Interaction of HeLa proteins with RNA. *J. Mol. Biol.* **47**, 263.

Barnard, E. A. (1969). Ribonucleases. *Annu. Rev. Biochem.* **38**, 677.

Barnum, C. P., Jardetzky, C. D., and Halberg, F. (1958). Time relations among metabolic and morphologic 24-hour changes in mouse liver. *Amer. J. Physiol.* **195**, 301.

Barondes, S. H. (1969). Cellular dynamics of the neuron. *Symp. Int. Soc. Cell Biol.* **8**, 375.

Baserga, R. (1968). Biochemistry of the cell cycle: a review. *Cell Tissue Kinet.* **1**, 167.

Beattie, D. S. (1969). The turnover of the protein components of the inner and outer membrane fractions of rat liver mitochondria. *Biochem. Biophys. Res. Commun.* **35**, 721.

Beeken, W. L., Volwiler, W., Goldsworthy, P. D., Garby, L. E., Reynolds, W. E., Stogsdill, R., and Stemler, R. S. (1962). Studies of I^{131}-albumin catabolism and distribution in normal young male adults. *J. Clin. Invest.* **41**, 1312.

Birnstiel, M. L., and Flamm, W. G. (1964). Intranuclear site of histone synthesis. *Science* **145**, 1435.

Bloch, D. P. (1966). Cytochemistry of histones. *Protoplasmatologia* **5**, 3d.

Bok, D. (1966). RNA and DNA metabolism in rat photoreceptors. *Anat. Rec.* **154**, 320.

Bonner, J. (1967). The role of histones in the regulation of RNA synthesis. *In* "Regulation of Nucleic Acid and Protein Biosynthesis" (V. V. Koningsberger and L. Bosch, eds.), p. 211. Elsevier, Amsterdam.

Bonner, J., and Huang, R. C. (1966). Histones as specific repressors of chromosomal RNA synthesis. *In* "Histones" (A. V. S. deReuck and J. Knight, eds.), p. 18. Ciba Foundation Symp., Little, Brown, Boston, Massachusetts.

Bonner, J., and T'so, P., eds. (1964). "The Nucleohistones." Holden-Day, San Francisco, California.

Bonner, J., and Widholm, J. (1967). Molecular complementarity between nuclear DNA and organ-specific chromosomal RNA. *Proc. Nat. Acad. Sci. U.S.* **57**, 1379.

Bonner, J., Dahmus, M. E., Fambrough, D., Huang, R. C., Marushige, K., and Tuan, D. Y. H. (1968). The biology of isolated chromosomes. *Science* **159**, 47.

Borun, T. W., Scharff, M. D., and Robbins, E. (1967). Rapidly labeled polyribosome-associated RNA having the properties of histone messenger. *Proc. Nat. Acad. Sci. U.S.* **58**, 1977.

Bosmann, H. B., and Winston, R. A. (1970). Synthesis of glycoproteins, glycolipids, protein and lipid in synchronized L$_{5168}$Y cells. *J. Cell Biol.* **45**, 23.

Bouvier, C. A., and Maurice, P. A. (1964). Liver and blood coagulation. *In* "The Liver" (C. Rouiller, ed.), Vol. 2, p. 177, Academic Press, New York.

Busch, H. (1965). Histones and other Nuclear Proteins." Academic Press, New York.

Bustin, M., and Cole, R. D. (1968). Species and organ specificity in very lysine-rich histones. *J. Biol. Chem.* **243**, 4500.

Butler, J. A. V. (1966). Complexity and specificity of histones. *In* "Histones" (A. V. S. deReuck and J. Knight, eds.), p. 4. Ciba Foundation Symp., Little, Brown, Boston, Massachusetts.

Butler, J. A. V., Johns, E. W., and Phillips, D. M. P. (1968). Recent investigations on histones and their functions. *Progr. Biophys. Mol. Biol.* **18**, 209.

Byers, T. J., Platt, D. B., and Goldstein, L. (1936a). The cytonucleoproteins of amebae. I. Some chemical properties and intracellular distribution. *J. Cell Biol.* **19**, 453.

Byers, T. J., Platt, D. B., and Goldstein, L. (1963b) The cytonucleoproteins of amebae. II. Some aspects of cytonucleoprotein behavior and synthesis. *J. Cell Biol.* **19**, 467.

Byvoet, P. (1966). Metabolic integrity of deoxynucleohistones. *J. Mol. Biol.* **17**, 311.

Byvoet, P. (1968). Differences in turnover between histones and their acetyl N-terminal groups. *Biochim. Biophys. Acta.* **160**, 217.

Cairnie, A. B., Lamerton, L. F., and Steel, G. G. (1965a). Cell proliferation studies in the intestinal epithelium of the rat. I. Determination of the kinetic parameters. *Exp. Cell Res.* **39**, 528.

Cairnie, A. B., Lamerton, L. F., and Steel, G. G. (1965b). Cell proliferation studies in the intestinal epithelium of the rat. II. Theoretical aspects. *Exp. Cell Res.* **39**, 539.

Cameron, C. B. (1964). The liver and steroid metabolism. *In* "The Liver" (C. Rouiller, ed.), Vol. 2, p. 92. Academic Pres , New York.

Clark, R., Zigman, S., and Lerman, S. (1969). Studies on the structural proteins of the human lens. *Exp. Eye Res.* **8**, 172.

Cohen, A. I. (1969). Rods and cones and the problem of visual excitation. *In* "The Retina" (B. R. Straatsma, M. O. Hall, R. A. Allen, and F. Crescitelli, eds.), p. 31. Univ. California Press, Berkeley, California.

Cohen, S., Freeman, T. and McFarlane, A. S. (1961). Metabolism of ^{131}I-labelled human albumin. *Clin. Sci.* **20**, 161.

Cohn, C., Joseph, D., Lavin, F., Shoemaker, W. J., and Wurtman, R. J. (1970). Influence of feeding habits and adrenal cortex on diurnal rhythm of hepatic tyrosine transaminase activity. *Proc. Soc. Exp. Biol. Med.* **133**, 460.

Collier, R. J., and Traugh, J. A. (1969). Inactivation of aminoacyl transferase II by diphtheria toxin. *Cold Spring Harbor Symp. Quant. Biol.* **35**, 589.

Comb, D. G., Savkar N., and Pinzino, C. J. (1966). The methylation of lysine residues in protein. *J. Biol. Chem.* **241**, 1857.

Combes, B. (1964). Excretory function of the liver. *In* "The Liver" (C. H. Rouiller, ed.), Vol. 2, p. 1, Academic Press, New York.

Comings, D. E. (1967). Histones of genetically active and inactive chromatin. *J. Cell Biol.* **35**, 699.

Coutts, R. T., and Smail, G. A. (1966). "Polysaccharides, Peptides and Proteins." William Heineman, London.

Dallner, G., Siekevitz, P., and Palade, G. E. (1966a). Biogenesis of endoplasmic reticulum membranes. I. Structural and chemical differentiation in developing rat hepato-cytes. *J. Cell Biol.* **30,** 73.

Dallner, G., Siekevitz, P., and Palade, G. E. (1966b). Biogenesis of endoplasmic reticu-lum. II. Synthesis of constitutive enzymes in developing rat hepatocytes. *J. Cell Biol.* **30,** 97.

Darnell, J. E. (1968). Ribonucleic acids from animal cells. *Bacteriol. Rev.* **32,** 262.

Davenport, H. C. (1966). "Physiology of the Digestive Tract; an Introductory Text." Year Book Medical Publ., Chicago, Illinois.

DeBernard, B., Getz, G. S., and Rabinowitz, M. (1969). The turnover of the protein of inner and outer mitochondrial membrane of the rat liver. *Biochim. Biophys. Acta* **193,** 58.

DeLange, R. J., Fambrough, D. M., Smith, E. L., and Bonner, J. (1968a). Amino acid sequence of histone IV: presence of ϵ-N-acetyllysine. *Proc. Nat. Acad. Sci. U.S.* **61,** 1145.

DeLange, R. J., Fambrough, D. M., Smith, E. L., and Bonner, J. (1968b). Calf and pea histone IV. I. amino acid composition and the identical COOH-terminal 19-residue sequence. *J. Biol. Chem.* **243,** 5906.

deReuck, A. V. S., and Knight, J., eds. (1966). "Histones," p. 115. Ciba Foundation, Symp., Little, Brown, Boston, Massachusetts.

Desnuelle, P., and Rovery, M. (1961). The proteins of the exocrine pancreas. *Advan. Protein Chem.* **16,** 139.

Dorfman, A. (1963). Polysaccharides of connective tissue. *J. Histochem. Cytochem.* **11,** 2.

Dounce, A. L., Tishoff, G. H., Barnett, S. R., and Freer, R. M. (1950). Free amino acids and nucleic acid content of cell nuclei isolated by a modification of Behrens' tech-nique. *J. Gen. Physiol.* **33,** 629.

Droz, B. (1963). Dynamic condition of proteins in the visual cells of rats and mice as shown by radioautography with labeled amino acids. *Anat. Res.* **145,** 157.

Druyan, R., DeBarnard, B., and Rabinowitz, M. (1969). Turnover of cytochromes labeled with δ-aminolevulinic acid-^{3}H in rat liver. *J. Biol. Chem.* **244,** 5874.

Fallon, H. J., Hackney, E. J., and Byrne, W. L. (1966). Serine biosynthesis in rat liver. Regulation of enzyme concentration by dietary factors. *J. Biol. Chem.* **241,** 4157.

Fambrough, D. M., and Bonner, J. (1968). Sequence homology and role of cysteine in plant and animal arginine-rich histones. *J. Biol. Chem.* **243,** 4434.

Fambrough, D. M., Fujimara, F., and Bonner, J. (1968). Quantitative distribution of histone components in the pea plant. *Biochemistry* **7,** 575.

Favarger, P. (1963). The liver and lipid metabolism. *In* "The Liver" (C. H. Rouiller, ed.), Vol. 1, p. 549, Academic Press, New York.

Feigelson, P., Dashman, T., and Margolis, F. (1959). The half-lifetime of induced trypoto-phan peroxidase *in vivo*. *Arch. Biochem. Biophys.* **85,** 478.

Feindegen, L. E. (1967). "Tritium Labeled Molecules in Biology and Medicine." Aca-demic Press, New York.

Felix, K. (1960). Protamines. *Advan. Protein Chem.* **15,** 1.

Fletcher, M. J., and Sanadi, D. R. (1961a). Turnover of rat-liver mitochondria. *Biochim. Biophys. Acta* **51,** 356.

Fletcher, M. J., and Sanadi, D. R. (1961b). Turnover of liver mitochondrial components in adult and senescent rats. *J. Gerontol.* **16,** 255.

Flickinger, C. J. (1969a). The development of Golgi complexes and their dependence upon the nucleus in amebae. *J. Cell Biol.* **43,** 250.

Flickinger, C. J. (1969b). The pattern of growth of the Golgi complex during the fetal and postnatal development of the rat epididymis. *J. Ultrastruct. Res.* **27,** 344.

Francois, J., Rabaey, M., and Boyen-Rikkers, I. (1969). Distribution of protein molecular groups in the normal and cataractous lens. *Exp. Eye Res.* **8**, 157.

Freedman, M. L., Honig, G. R., and Rabinovitz, M. (1966). The role of newly synthesized RNA on nuclear histone synthesis by chicken immature erythrocytes. *Exp. Cell Res.* **44**, 263.

Frenster, J. H. (1965). Nuclear polyanions and de-repressors of synthesis of ribonucleic acid. *Nature (London)* **206**, 680.

Fridlender, B. R., and Wettstein, F. O. (1970). Differences in the ribosomal protein of free and membrane bound polysomes of chick embryos. *Biochem. Biophys. Res. Commun.* **39**, 247.

Fulhorst, H. W., and Young, R. W. (1966). Conversion of soluble lens protein to albuminoid. *Invest. Ophthalmol.* **5**, 298.

Fuller, R. W. (1970). Daily variation in liver tryptophan pyrrolase and tyrosine transaminase in rats fed *ad libitum* or single daily meals. *Proc. Soc. Exp. Biol. Med.* **133**, 620.

Fuller, R. W., and Snoddy, H. D. (1968). Feeding schedule alteration of daily rhythm in tyrosine alpha-keto-glutrate transaminase in rat liver. *Science* **159**, 738.

Ganong, W. F. (1967). "Review of Medical Physiology." Lange Medical Publ. Los Altos, California.

Gelfant, S. (1960). The energy requirements for mitosis. *Ann. N.Y. Acad. Sci.* **90**, 536.

Georgiev, G. P. (1967). The nucleus. *In* "Enzyme Cytology" (D. B. Roodyn, ed.), p. 27. Academic Press, New York.

Gershey, E. L., Vidali, G., and Allfrey, V. G. (1968). Chemical studies of histone acetylation. The occurrence of ϵ-N-acetyllysine in the f_{2a1} histone. *J. Biol Chem.* **243**, 5018.

Gibbons, R. A. (1969). Chemical properties of two mucoids from bovine cervical mucin. *Biochem. J.* **73**, 209.

Gill, D. M., Pappenheimer, A. M., Jr., and Baseman, J. B. (1969). Studies on transferase II using diphtheria toxin. *Cold Spring Harbor Symp. Quant. Biol.* **35**, 595.

Gitlin, D., and Borges, W. G. (1953). Studies on the metabolism of fibrinogen in two patients with congenital afibrinogenemia. *Blood* **8**, 679.

Gitlin, D., Cornwell, D. G., Nakasato, D., Oncley, J. L., Hughes, W. L., and Janeway, C. A. (1958). Studies on the metabolism of plasma proteins in nephrotic syndrome II. The lipoproteins. *J. Clin. Invest.* **37**, 172.

Glick, M. C., and Warren, L. (1969). Membrane of animal cells. III. Amino acid incorporation by isolated surface membranes. *Proc. Nat. Acad. Sci. U.S.* **63**, 563.

Go, V. L. W., Hofmann, A. F., and Summerskill, W. H. J. (1970). Simultaneous measurements of total pancreatic, bililary and gastric outputs in man using a perfusion technique. *Gastroenterology* **58**, 321.

Goldstein, L., and Prescott, D. M. (1967). Proteins in nucleocytoplasmic interactions. I. The fundamental characteristics of the rapidly migrating proteins and the slow turnover proteins of the *Amoeba proteus* nucleus. *J. Cell Biol.* **33**, 637.

Goldstein, L., and Prescott, D. M. (1968a). Proteins in nucleocytoplasmic interactions. II. Turnover and changes in nuclear protein distribution with time and growth. *J. Cell Biol.* **36**, 53.

Goldstein, L., and Prescott, D. M. (1968b). Proteins in nucleocytoplasmic interactions III. Redistributions of nuclear proteins during and following mitosis in *Amoeba proteus*. *J. Cell Biol.* **39**, 404.

Goldstein, L., and Ron, A. (1969). On the possibility of nuclear protein involvement in the control of DNA synthesis in *Amoeba proteus*. *Exp. Cell Res.* **55**, 144.

Goldstein, L., Stella, E. J., and Knox, W. E. (1962). The effect of hydrocortisone on tyrosine-α-ketoglutarate transaminase and tryptophan pyrrolase activities in the isolated perfursed rat liver. *J. Biol. Chem.* **237,** 1723.

Gottschalk, A., ed. (1966). "Glycoproteins. Their Composition, Structure and Function." Elsevier, Amsterdam.

Greulich, R. C., Cameron, I. L., and Thrasher, J. D. (1961). Stimulation of mitosis in adult mice by administration of thymidine. *Proc. Nat. Acad. Sci., U.S.* **47,** 743.

Gröschel, U., and Li, C. H. (1960). On carbohydrate moiety of ovin and human pituitary gonadotropins. *Biochim. Biophys. Acta* **73,** 375.

Grossman, D., and Lang, K. (1962). Anorganiscne Poly-und Metaphosphatasen sowie Polyphosphate in Tierischen Zellkern. *Biochim. Z.* **336,** 351.

Grossman, M. I., and Marks, J. N. (1960). Secretion of pepsinogen by the pyloric glands of the dog, with some observations on the histology of the gastric mucosa. *Gastroenterology* **38,** 342.

Gurdon, J. B., and Woodland, H. R. (1968). The cytoplasmic control of nuclear activity in animal development *Biol. Rev.* **43,** 233.

Gurley, L. R., and Hardin, J. M. (1968). The metabolism of histone fractions. I. Synthesis of histone fractions during the life cycle of mammalian cells. *Arch. Biochem. Biophys.* **128,** 285.

Gurley, L. R., and Hardin, J. M. (1970). The metabolism of histone fractions. III. Synthesis and turnover of histone fl. *Arch. Biochem. Biophys.* **136,** 392.

Gurley, L. R., Irvin, J. L., and Holbrook, D. J. (1963). Inhibition of DNA polymerase by histones. *Biochem. Biophys. Res. Commun.* **14,** 527.

Gurley, L. R., Hardin, J. M., and Langham, W. H. (1968). The turnover of histone fractions related to DNA and RNA synthesis *in vivo. Fed. Proc. Fed. Amer. Soc. Exp. Biol.* **27,** 797.

Hall, M. O., Ocumpaugh, D. E. and Young R. W. (1965). The utilization of ^{35}S-sulfate in the synthesis of mucopolysaccharides by the retina. *Invest. Ophthalmol.* **4,** 322.

Hall, M. O., Bok, D., and Bacharach, A. D. E. (1969). Biosynthesis and assembly of the rod outersegment membrane system. Formation and fate of visual pigment in the frog retina. *J. Mol. Biol.* **45,** 397.

Hammond, J. D. S., and Verel, D. (1959). Observations on the distribution and biological half-life of human fibrinogen. *Brit. J. Haematol.* **5,** 431.

Hanna, C. (1965). Changes in DNA, RNA and protein synthesis in the developing lens. *Invest. Ophthalmol.* **4,** 480.

Hardeland, R., and Rensing, L. (1968). Circadian oscillation in rat liver tryptophan pyrrolase and its analysis by substrate and hormone induction. *Nature (London)* **219,** 619.

Hardin, J. A., Einem, G. E., and Lindsay, D. T. (1967). Simultaneous synthesis of histone and DNA in synchronously dividing *Tetrahymena pyriformis. J. Cell Biol.* **32,** 709.

Harding, J. J. (1969). Nature and origin of the insoluble protein of rat lens. *Exp. Eye Res.* **8,** 147.

Hargreaves, T. (1968). "The Liver and Bile Metabolism." Appleton, New York.

Haus, E., and Halberg, F. (1966). Persisting circadian rhythm in hepatic glycogen during inanition and dehydration. *Experientia* **22,** 113.

Herron, W. L., Riegel, B. W., Myers, O. E., and Rubin, M. I. (1969). Retinal dystrophy in the rat–A pigment epithelial disease. *Invest. Ophthalmol.* **8,** 595.

Hicks, S. J., Drysdale, J. W., and Munro, H. N. (1969). Preferential synthesis of ferritin and albumin by different populations of liver polysomes. *Science* **164,** 584.

Hirschowitz, B. I. (1957). Pepsinogen, its origin, secretion and excretion. *Physiol. Rev.* **37,** 475.

Hnilica, L. S. (1966). Studies on Nuclear proteins. I. Observations on the tissue and species specificity of the moderately lysine-rich histone fraction 2b. *Biochim. Biophys. Acta* **117,** 163.

Hnilica, L. S. (1967). Proteins of the cell nucleus. *Progr. Nucl. Acid. Res. Mol. Biol.* **7,** 25.

Hnilica, L. S., Taylor, C. W., and Busch, H. (1963). Analysis of peptides of the moderately rich histone fraction, f2b, of the Walker tumor and other tissues. *Exp. Cell Res. Suppl.* **9,** 367.

Hnilica, L. S., Edwards, L. J., and Hey, A. E. (1966a). Studies on nuclear proteins. II. Quantitative distribution of histone fractions in various tissues. *Biochim. Biophys. Acta* **124,** 109.

Hnilica, L. S., Liau, M. C., and Hurlbert, R. B. (1966b). Biosynthesis and composition of histones in Novikoff hepatoma nuclei and nucleoli. *Science* **152,** 521.

Hodge, L. D., Robbins, E., and Scharff, M. D. (1969). Persistence of messenger RNA through mitosis in HeLa cells. *J. Cell Biol.* **40,** 497.

Hotta, Y., and Stern, H. (1963). Molecular facets of mitotic regulation. I. Synthesis of thymidine kinase. *Proc. Nat. Acad. Sci. U.S.* **49,** 648.

Howk, R., and Wang, T. Y. (1970). DNA polymerase from rat liver chromosomal proteins. II. Formation of an enzyme-template complex and association of product with template. *Arch. Biochem. Biophys.* **136,** 422.

Huang, R. C., and Bonner, J. (1962). Histone, a suppressor of chromosomal RNA synthesis. *Proc. Nat. Acad. Sci. U.S.* **48,** 1216.

Hunt, J. A., and Laycock, D. G. (1969). Characterization of messenger RNA for hemoglobin. *Cold Spring Harbor Symp. Quant. Biol.* **35,** 579.

Imondi, A. R., Balis, M. E., and Lipkin, M. (1969). Changes in enzyme levels accompanying differentiation of intestinal epithelial cells. *Exp. Cell Res.* **58,** 323

Ingles, C. J., and Dixon, G. H. (1967). Phosphorylation of protamine during spermatogenesis in trout testis. *Proc. Nat. Acad. Sci., U.S.* **58,** 1011.

Ingles, C. J., Trevithick, J. R., Smith, M., and Dixon, G. H. (1966). Biosynthesis of protamine during spermatogenesis in salminoid fish. *Biochem. Biophys. Res. Commun.* **22,** 627.

Jamieson, J. D., and Palade, G. E. (1967a). Intracellular transport of secretory proteins in the pancreatic exocrine cell. I. Role of the peripheral elements of the Golgi complex. *J. Cell. Biol.* **34,** 577.

Jamieson, J. D., and Palade, G. E. (1967b). Intracellular transport of secretory proteins in the pancreatic exocrine cell. II. Transport to condensing vacoules and zymgine granules. *J. Cell Biol.* **34,** 597.

Jamieson, J. D., and Palade, G. E. (1968a). Intracellular transport of secretory proteins in the pancreatic exocrine cell. III. Dissociation of intracellular transport from protein synthesis. *J. Cell Biol.* **39,** 580.

Jamieson, J. D., and Palade, G. E. (1968b). Intracellular transport of secretory proteins in the pancreatic exocrine cell. IV. Metabolic requirements *J. Cell Biol.* **39,** 589.

Jarnum, S., and Lassen, N. A. (1961). Albumin and transferrin metabolism in infectious and toxic diseases. *Scand. J. Clin. Lab. Invest.* **13,** 357.

Jarnum, S., and Schwartze M. (1960). Bestemmels af albuminomsaetningen med ^{131}I–maerkt albumin. *Nord. Med.* **63,** 708.

Jellum, E. (1966). Thiol content of calf thymus histone fractions. *Biochim. Biophys. Acta,* **115,** 95.

Katz, J. H. (1961). Iron and protein kinetics studied by means of doubly labeled human crystalline transferrin. *J. Clin. Invest.* **40,** 2143.

Keir, H. M. (1965). DNA polymerase from mammalian cells. *Progr. Nucl. Acid Res. Mol. Biol.* **4,** 81.

Kenney, F. T. (1962). Induction of tyrosine-α-ketoglutarate transaminase in rat liver. *J. Biol. Chem.* **237,** 3495.

Kiehn, E. D., and Holland, J. J. (1968). Multiple protein components of mammalian cell membranes. *Proc. Nat. Acad. Sci. U.S.* **61,** 1370.

Kiehn, E. D., and Holland, J. J. (1970a). Membrane and nonmembrane proteins of mammalian cells. Synthesis, turnover and size distribution. *Biochemistry* **9,** 1716.

Kiehn, E. D., and Holland, J. J. (1970b). Membrane and nonmembrane proteins of mammalian cells. Organ, species and tumor specificities. *Biochemistry* **9,** 1729.

Kim, S., and Paik, W. K. (1965). Studies on the origin of ε-N-methyl-L-lysine in protein. *J. Biol. Chem.* **240,** 4629.

Kinkade, J. M., and Cole, R. D. (1966). A structural comparison of different lysine-rich histones. *J. Biol. Chem.* **241, 5798**.

Kischer, C. W., Gurley, L. R., and Sheperd, G. R. (1966). Nuclear histones and early embryogenesis of the chick. *Nature (London)* **212,** 304.

Kleinsmith, L. J., Allfrey, V. G., and Mirsky, A. E. (1966). Phosphoprotein metabolism in isolated lymphocyte nuclei. *Proc. Nat. Acad. Sci. U.S.* **55,** 1182.

Klevecz, R. R. (1969). Temporal order in mammalian cells. I. The periodic synthesis of lactate dehydrogenase in the cell cycle. *J. Cell Biol.* **43,** 207.

Klevecz, R. R., and Ruddle, F. H. (1968). Cyclic changes in enzyme activity in synchronized mammalian cell cultures. *Science* **159,** 634.

Krakow, J. S., Kammen, H. O., and Canellakis, E. S. (1961). The incorporation of ribonucleotides into terminal positions of deoxyribonucleic acid. *Biochim. Biophys. Acta* **53,** 52.

Langan, T. A. (1968). Phosphorylation of proteins of the cell nucleus. *In* "Regulatory Mechanisms for Protein Synthesis in Mammalian Cells" (A. San Pietro, M. R. Lamborg, and F. T. Kenney, eds.), p. 101. Academic Press, New York.

Langan, T. A. (1969). Phosphorylation of liver histone following the administration of glucagon and insulin. *Proc. Nat. Acad. Sci. U.S.* **64,** 1276.

Laskowski, M. (1967). DNases and their use in studies of primary structure of nucleic acids. *Advan. Enzymol.* **29,** 165.

Leblond, C. P., Clermont, Y., and Nadler, N. J. (1966). The pattern of stem cell renewal in three epithelia (esophagus, intestine and testis). *Can. Cancer Conf.* **7,** 3.

LeBouton, A. V. (1968). Heterogeneity of protein metabolism between liver cells as studied by radioautography. *Curr. Mod. Biol.* **2, 111.**

LeBouton, A. V. (1969). Relationship and extent of the zone of intensified protein metabolism in the liver acinus. *Curr. Mod. Biol.* **3, 4.**

LeBouton, A. V., and Handler, S. D. (1970). Diurnal incorporation of ³H-leucine into liver protein. *Fed. Eur. Biochem. Soc. Lett.* **10,** 78.

Lengyel, P., and Söll, D. (1969). Mechanism of protein biosynthesis. *Bacteriol. Rev.* **33,** 264.

Lerman, S., Zigman, S., and Forbes, W. F. (1966). Properties of cryoprotein in the ocular lens. *Biochem. Biophys. Res. Commun.* **22,** 57.

Lewallen, C. G., Berman, M., and Rall, J. E. (1959). Studies on iodoalbumin metabolism. *J. Clin. Invest.* **38,** 66.

Lewin, K. (1969). The Paneth cell in health and disease. *Ann. Roy. Coll. Surg. Engl.* **44,** 23.

Liau, M. C., and Perry, R. P. (1969). Ribosome precursor particles in nucleoli. *J. Cell Biol.* **42**, 272.

Liau, M. C., Hnilica, L. S., and Hurlbert, R. B. (1965). Regulation of RNA synthesis in isolated nucleoli by histones and nucleolar proteins. *Proc. Nat. Acad. Sci. U.S.* **53**, 626.

Libby, P. R. (1968). Histone acetylation by cell-free preparations from rat uterus: *in vitro* stimulation by estradiol–17β. *Biochem. Biophys. Res. Commun.* **31**, 59.

Lindahl, T., and Edelman, G. M. (1968). Polynucleotide ligase from myeloid and lymphoid tissues. *Proc. Nat. Acad. Sci. U.S.* **61**, 680.

McEwen, B. S., Allfrey, V. G., and Mirsky, A. E. (1963). Studies on energy-yielding reactions in thymus nuclei. III. participation of glycolysis and the citric acid cycle in nuclear adenosine triphosphate synthesis. *J. Biol. Chem.* **238**, 2579.

McFarlane, A. S. (1963). *In vivo* behavior of I[131]-fibrinogen. *J. Clin. Invest.* **42**, 346.

MacGillivray, A. J. (1968). The histones of some human tissues. *Biochem. J.* **110**, 181.

Madden, R. E., and Gould, R. G. (1952). Turnover of fibrinogen in the dog. *J. Biol. Chem.* **196**, 641.

Madden, S. C., and Whipple, G. (1940). Plasma proteins: their source, production and utilization. *Physiol. Rev.* **20**, 194.

Maden, B. E. H., and Vaughan, M. H. (1968). Synthesis of ribosomal proteins in the absence of ribosome maturation in methionine deficient HeLa cells. *J. Mol. Biol.* **38**, 431.

Maley, F., and Maley, G. F. (1960). Nucleotide interconversions. II. Elevation of deoxycytidylate deaminase and thymidylate synthetase in regenerating rat liver. *J. Biol. Chem.* **235**, 2968.

Malik, S. R. K., Gupta, A. K., Chatterji, S., and Agarwal, P. S. (1969). Soluble proteins in normal and cataractous human lenses. *Exp. Eye Res.* **8**: 93.

Marushige, K., Brutlag, D., and Bonner, J. (1968). Properties of chromosomal non-histone protein of rat liver. *Biochemistry* **7**, 3149.

Marver, H. S., Collins, A., Tschudy, D. P., and Rechcigl, M., Jr. (1966). δ-aminolevulinic acid synthetase. II. Induction in rat liver. *J. Biol. Chem.* **241**, 4323.

Mazia, D. (1961). Mitosis and the physiology of cell division. *In* "The Cell" (J. Brachet and A. E. Mirsky, eds.), Vol. 3, p. 77. Academic Press, New York.

Moore, R., and Radley, J. M. (1968). The nature of aneuploid change in JU56 cells and and its relationship to continued proliferation. *Exp. Cell Res.* **49**: 638.

Moore, R., and Uren, J. (1965). The pattern of DNA synthesis in short-term cultures of *Protemnodon bicolor* ♂. *Exp. Cell Res.* **38**, 341.

Moore, R., and Uren, J. (1966). Permanent cell lines of the marsupial mouse, *Antechinus swainsonii*. *Exp. Cell Res.* **44**, 273.

Moretti, J., Borel, J., Dubryszycka, W., and Jaćjle, M. F. (1963). Détermination de la demi-vie de L'haptoglobine plasmatique humane. *Biochim. Biophys. Acta* **69**, 205.

Morrison, G. R., and Brock, F. E. (1967). Quantitative measurement of alcohol dehydrogenase in the lobule of normal livers. *J. Lab. Clin. Med.* **70**, 116.

Moustacchi, E., and Williamson, D. H. (1966). Physiological variations in satellite components of yeast DNA detected by density gradient centrifugation. *Biochem. Biophys. Res. Commun.* **23**, 56.

Mueller, G. C. (1969). Biochemical events of the animal cell cycle. *Fed. Proc. Fed. Amer. Soc. Exp. Biol.* **28**, 1780.

Murray, K. (1965). The basic proteins of cell nuclei. *Annu. Rev. Biochem.* **34**, 209.

Nadler, N. J. (1963). Calculations of the turnover times of proteins in each region of the acinar cells of the pancreas. *J. Cell Biol.* **16**, 24.

Nemeth, A. M. (1962). The effect of 5-fluorouracil on the developmental and adaptive formatin of tryptophan pyrrolase. *J. Biol. Chem.* **237**, 3703.

Neutra, M., and Leblond, C. P. (1966a). Synthesis of the carbohydrate of mucus in the Golgi complex as shown by electron microscope radioautorgraphy of goblet cells from rats injected with glucose-H^3. *J. Cell Biol.* **30**, 119.

Neutra, M., and Leblond, C. P. (1966b). Radioautographic comparison of the uptake of galactose-H^3 and glucose-H^3 in the Golgi region of various cells secreting glycoproteins and mucopolysaccharides. *J. Cell Biol.* **30**, 137.

Novogrodsky, A., Tal, M., Traub, A., and Hurwitz, J. (1966). Phosphorylation of ribonucelic acid and deoxyribonucleic acid. II. Further properties of the 5'-hydroxylpolynucleotide kinase. *J. Biol. Chem.* **241**, 2933.

Ocumpaugh, D. E., and Young, R. W. (1966). Distribution of sulfated mucopolysaccharides in the retina of the rat. *Invest. Ophthalmol.* **5**, 196.

Oppenheimer, J. H., Surks, M. I., Bernstein, G., and Smith, J. L. (1965). Metabolism of iodine-131-labeled thyroxine binding prealbumin. *Science* **149**, 748.

Ord, M. G., and Stocken, L. A. (1968). Variations in the phosphate content and thiol/disulphide ratio of histones during the cell cycle. *Biochem. J.* **107**, 403.

Ord, M. G., and Stocken, L. A. (1969). Further studies on the phosphorylation and the thiol/disulphide ratio of histones in growth and development. *Biochem. J.* **112**, 81.

Orlova, L. V., and Rodionov, V. M. (1970). The time of histone synthesis in regenerating rat liver. *Exp. Cell Res.* **59**, 329.

Osawa, S. (1968). Ribosome formation and structure. *Annu. Rev. Biochem.* **37**, 109.

Osgood, E. E. (1961). Radiobiological observations on human hemic cells *in vivo* and *in vitro*. *Ann. N.Y. Acad. Sci.* **95**, 828.

Penman, S. (1966). RNA metabolism in the HeLa cell nucleus. *J. Mol. Biol.* **17**, 117.

Pesch, L. A., and Topper, Y. J. (1963). The liver and carbohydrate metabolism. *In* "The Liver" (C. Rouiller, ed.), Vol. 1, p. 606. Academic Press, New York.

Peters, T., Jr. (1962a). The biosynthesis of rat serum albumin. I. Properties of rat albumin and its occurrence in liver cell fractions. *J. Biol. Chem.* **237**, 1181.

Peters, T., Jr. (1962b). The biosynthesis of rat serum albumin. II. Intracellular phenomena in the secretion of newly formed albumin. *J. Biol. Chem.* **237**, 1186.

Peterson, M., and Leblond, C. P. (1964). Synthesis of complex carbohydrates in the Golgi region as shown by radioautography after injection of labeled glucose. *J. Cell Biol.* **21**, 143.

Piha, R. S., Cuenod, M., and Waelsch, H. (1966). Metabolism of histones of brain and liver. *J. Biol. Chem.* **241**, 2397.

Pitot, H. C., and Peraino, C. (1964). Studies on the induction and repression of enzymes in rat liver. I. Induction of threonine dehydrase and ornithine-δ-transaminase by oral intubation of casein hydrolysate. *J. Biol. Chem.* **239**, 1783.

Pogo, B. G. T., Allfrey, V. G., and Mirsky, A. E. (1966). RNA synthesis and histone acetylation during the course of gene activation in lymphocytes. *Proc. Nat. Acad. Sci. U.S.* **55**, 805.

Pogo, B. G. T., Allfrey, V. G., and Mirsky, A. E. (1967). The effect of phytohemagglutinin on ribonucleic acid synthesis and histone acetylation in equine leukocytes. *J. Cell Biol.* **35**, 477.

Pogo, B. G. T., Pogo, A. O., Allfrey, V. G., and Mirsky, A. E. (1968). Changing patterns of histone acetylation and RNA synthesis in regeneration of the liver. *Proc. Nat. Acad Sci. U.S.* **59**, 1337.

Pool, B., Leighton, F., and DeDuve, C. (1969). The synthesis and turnover of rat liver peroxisomes. II. Turnover of peroxisome proteins. *J. Cell Biol.* **41**, 536.

Potter, V. R., Watanabe, M., Becker, J. E., and Pitot, H. C. (1967). Hormonal effects on enzyme activities in tissue culture and in whole animals. *Advan. Enzyme Reg.* **5,** 303.

Prescott, D. M. (1956). Relations between cell growth and cell division. III. *Exp. Cell Res.* **11,** 86.

Prescott, D. M. (1964a). Comments on the cell life cycle. *Nat. Cancer Inst. Monogr.* **14,** 57.

Prescott, D. M. (1964b). Turnover of chromosomal proteins. *In* "The Nucleohistones" (J. Bonner and P. T'so, eds.), p. 193. Holden–Day, San Francisco, Calfiornia.

Prescott, D. M. (1966). The synthesis of total macronuclear protein, histone and DNA during the cell cycle in *Euplotes. J. Cell Biol.* **31,** 1.

Prescott, D. M., and Bender, M. A. (1962). Synthesis of RNA and protein during mitosis in mammalian tissue culture cells. *Exp. Cell Res.* **26,** 260.

Prescott, D. M., and Bender, M. A. (1963). Synthesis and behavior of nuclear proteins during the cell life cycle. *J. Cell. Comp. Physiol.* **62,** 175.

Quincey, R. V., and Wilson, S. H. (1969). The utilization of genes for ribosomal RNA, 5S RNA and transfer RNA in liver cells of adult rats. *Proc. Nat. Acad. Sci. U.S.* **64,** 981.

Rappaport, A. M. (1963). Acinar units and the pathophysiology of the liver. *In* "The Liver" (C. Rouiller, ed.), Vol. 1, p. 266. Academic Press, New York.

Rasmussen, P., Murray, K., and Luck, J. (1962). On the complexity of calf thymus histone. *Biochemistry* **1,** 79.

Rechcigl, M., Jr. (1968). Intracellular and molecular turnover of proteins. *Texas Rep. Biol. Med.* **26,** 147.

Rechcigl, M., Jr., and Heston, W. E. (1967). Genetic regulation of enzyme activity in mammalian system by the alteration of the rates of enzyme degradation. *Biochem. Biophys. Res. Commun.* **27,** 119.

Rechcigl, M., Jr., and Price, V. E. (1967). Studies on the turnover of catalase *in vivo. Progr. Exp. Tumor Res.* **10,** 112.

Redman, C. M., Siekevitz, P., and Palade, G. E. (1966). Synthesis and transfer of amylase in pigeon pancreatic microsomes. *J. Biol. Chem.* **241,** 1150.

Reid, B. R., and Cole, R. D. (1964). Biosynthesis of a lysine-rich histone in isolated calf thymus nuclei. *Proc. Nat. Acad. Sci. U.S.* **51,** 1044.

Reid, E., El–Aser, A. B. A., Turner, M. K., and Siebert, G. (1964). Enzymes of ribonucleic acid and ribonucleotide metabolism in rat liver nuclei. *Hoppe–Seyler's Z. Physiol. Chem.* **339,** 135.

Reid, B. R., Stellwagen, R. H., and Cole, R. D. (1968). Further studies on the biosynthesis of very lysine-rich histones in isolated nuclei. *Biochim. Biophys. Acta* **155,** 593.

Richardson, C. C. (1969). Enzymes in DNA metabolism. *Annu. Rev. Biochem.* **38,** 795.

Riecken, E. O., and Pearse, A. G. E. (1966). Histochemical study on the Paneth cell in the rat. *Gut* **7,** 86.

Robbins, E., and Borun, T. W. (1967). The cytoplasmic synthesis of histones in HeLa cells and its temporal relationship to DNA replication. *Proc. Nat. Acad. Sci. U.S.* **57,** 409.

Robbins, E. R., and Morrill, G. A. (1969). Oxygen uptake during the HeLa cell life cycle and its correlation with macromolecular synthesis. *J. Cell Biol.* **43,** 629.

Robbins, E., and Shelanski, M. (1969). Synthesis of colchicine-binding protein during the HeLa cell life cycle. *J. Cell Biol.* **43,** 371.

Roeder, R. G., and Rutter, W. J. (1969). Multiple forms of DNA-dependent RNA polymerase in eukaryotic cells. *Nature (London)* **224, 234**.

Roeder, R. G., and Rutter, W. J. (1970). Specific nucleolar and nucleoplasmic RNA polymerases. *Proc. Nat. Acad. Sci. U.S.* **65**, 675.

Roodyn, D. B., and Wilkie, D. (1968). "The Biogenesis of Mitochondria." Methuen, London.

Rosen, F., and Nichol, C. A. (1964). Studies on the nature and specificity of the induction of several adaptive enzymes responsive to cortisol. *Advan. Enzyme Reg.* **2**, 115.

Rossi, E., and Stoll, E. eds. (1968). "Biochemistry of Glycoproteins and Related Substances." Karger, Basel.

Rustad, R. C., and Rustad, L. C. (1960). Nuclear-cytoplasmic relations in the mitosis of sea urchin eggs. *Ann. N.Y. Acad. Sci.* **90**, 531.

Scanu, A., and Hughes, W. L. (1962). Further characterization of human serum D 1.063–1.21, α_1-lipoprotein. *J. Clin. Invest.* **41**, 1681.

Scheving, L. E., Pauly, J. E., and Tsai, T. H. (1968). Circadian fluctuation in plasma proteins of the rat. *Amer. J. Physiol.* **215**, 1096.

Schimke, R. T., Sweeeney, E. W., and Berlin, C. M. (1965). The roles of synthesis and degradation in the control of rat liver tryptophan pyrollase. *J. Biol. Chem.* **240**, 322.

Schlessinger, D. (1969). Ribosomes: Development of some current ideas. *Bacteriol. Rev.* **33,**445.

Schnaitman, C. A. (1969). Comparison of rat liver mitochondrial and microsomal membrane proteins. *Proc. Nat. Acad. Sci. U.S.* **63**, 412.

Schultze, H. E. (1958). Über glykoproteine. *Deut. Med. Wochenschr.* **83**, 1742.

Schultze, H. E., and Heremans, J. F. (1966). "Molecular Biology of Human Proteins," Vol. 1. Elsevier, Amsterdam.

Schultze, H. E., Schmidtberger, R., and Haupt, H. (1958). Untersuchungen über die gebundenen Kohlenhydrate in isolierten Plasmaproteiden. *Biochem. Z.* **329**, 490.

Segal, H. L., and Kim, Y. S. (1963). Glucocorticoid stimulation of the biosynthesis of glutamic-alanine transaminase. *Proc. Nat. Acad. Sci. U.S.* **50**, 912.

Sekeris, C. E., Sekeris, K. E., and Gallwitz, D. Z. (1967). Methylation of the histones of ral liver nuclei *in vitro*. *Hoppe-Seyler's Z. Physiol. Chem.* **348**, 1660.

Shelanski, M., and Taylor, E. (1967). Isolation of a protein subunit from microtubules. *J. Cell Biol.* **34**, 549.

Siebert, G. (1961). Nuclear function and nuclear enzymes. *Fifth Int. Congr. Biochem. Symp.* **2**, 93.

Siekevitz, P., and Palade, G. E. (1960a). A cytochemical study on the pancreas of the guinea pig. V *in vivo* incorporation of leucine-C^{14} into the chymotrypsinogen of various cell fractions. *J. Biophys. Biochem. Cytol.* **7**, 619.

Siekevitz, P., and Palade, G. E. (1960b). A cytochemical study on the pancreas of the guinea pig. VI. Release of enzymes and ribonucleic acid from ribonucleoprotein particles. *J. Biophys. Biochem. Cytol.* **7**, 631.

Sims, R. T. (1965). The synthesis and migration of nuclear proteins during mitosis and differentiation of cells in rats. *Quart. J. Microscop. Sci.* **106**, 229.

Sonnenbichler, J. (1969). Nucleoprotein complexes: Possible subunits of chromosomes. *Hoppe-Seyler's Z. Physiol. Chem.* **350**, 761.

Spalding, J., Kajiwara, K., and Mueller, G. C. (1966). The metabolism of basic proteins in HeLa cell nuclei. *Proc. Nat. Acad. Sci. U.S.* **56**, 1535.

Spiro, R. G. (1963). Glycoproteins: structure and metabolism. *N. Engl. J. Med.* **269**, 56.

Spiro, R. G., and Spiro, M. J. (1963). Carbohydrate of thyroglobulin. *Fed Proc. Fed. Amer. Soc Exp. Biol.* **22**, 538.

Starbuck, W. C., Mauritzen, C. M., Taylor, C. W., Saroja, I. S., and Busch, H. (1968). A large scale procedure for isolation of the glycine-rich, arginine-rich histone and the arginine-rich, lysine-rich histone in a highly purified form. *J. Biol. Chem.* **243**, 2038.

Stedman, Edgar, and Stedman, Ellen (1950). The cell specificity of histones. *Nature (London)* **166**, 780.

Stellwagen, R. H., and Cole, R. D. (1969). Chromosomal proteins. *Annu. Rev. Biochem.* **38**, 951.

Stevely, W. S., and Stocken, L. A. (1968). Variations in the phosphate content of histone fl in normal and irradiated tissues. *Biochem. J.* **110**, 187.

Steward, D. L., Schaeffer J. R., and Humphrey, R. M. (1968). Breakdown and assembly of polyribosomes in synchronized Chinese hamster cells *Science* **161**, 791.

Stocken, L. A., and Ord, M. G. (1969). Histone changes and cell division. *Biochem. J.* **114**, 51P.

Subramanian, A. R., Davis, B. D., and Beller, J. (1969). The ribosome dissociation factor and the ribosome polysome cycle. *Cold Spring Harbor Symp. Quant. Biol.* **35**, 223.

Suzuki, K., and Ando, T. (1969). Inhibition of RNA synthesis by clupeine and basic homopolypeptides. *J. Biochem.* **65**, 831.

Swann, M. M. (1957). The control of cell division: A review. I. General mechanisms. *Cancer Res.* **17**, 727.

Swick, R. A. (1958). Measurement of protein turnover in rat liver. *J. Biol. Chem.* **231**, 751.

Swick, R. W., Rexroth, A. K., and Strange, J. L. (1968). The metabolism of mitochondrial proteins. III. The dynamic state of rat liver mitochondria. *J. Biol. Chem.* **243**, 3581.

Takeda, Y., and Reeve, E. B. (1963). Studies of the metabolism and distribution of albumin with autologous I^{131}-albumin in healthy men. *J. Lab. Clin. Med.* **61**, 183.

Talmage, D. W., and Claman, H. N. (1964). Cell potential: Its mutation and selection. *In* "The Thymus in Immunobiology" (R. A. Good and A. E Gabrielsen, eds.), p. 49. Harper and Row, New York.

Tarentino, A. L., Richert, D. A., and Westerfield, W. W. (1966). The concurrent induction of hepatic α-glycerophosphate dehydrogenase and malate dehydrogenase by thyroid hormone. *Biochim. Biophys. Acta* **124**, 295.

Tarver, H. (1963). Metabolism of amino acids and proteins. *In* "The Liver" (C. Rouiller, ed.), Vol. 1, p. 450. Academic Press, New York.

Teng, C. S., and Hamilton, T. H. (1969). Role of chromatin in estrogen action in the uterus. II Hormone-induced synthesis of nonhistone acidic proteins which restore histone-inhibited DNA-dependent RNA synthesis. *Proc. Nat. Acad. Sci. U. S.* **63**, 465.

Thaler, M. M., Cox, M. C. L., and Villee, C. A. (1970). Histones in early embryogenesis. Developmental aspects of composition and synthesis. *J. Biol. Chem.* **245**, 1479.

Thrasher, J. D. (1966). Analysis of renewing epithelial cell populations. *Methods Cell Physiol.* **2**, 323.

Thrasher, J. D. (1970). The relationship between cell division and cell specialization in the mouse intestinal epithelium. *Experientia* **26**, 74.

Tidwell, T., Allfrey, V. G., and Mirsky, A. E. (1968). The methylation of histones during regeneration of the liver. *J. Biol. Chem.* **243**, 707.

Tomkins, G. M., Gelehrter, T. D., Granner, D., Martin, D., Jr., Samuels, H. H., and

Thompson, E. B. (1969). Control of specific gene expression in higher organism *Science* **166,** 1474.

Tonino, G. J. M. and Rozijin, T. H. (1966). On the occurrence of histones in yeast. *Biochim. Biophys. Acta* **124,** 427.

Trier, J. S., Lorenzsonn, V., and Groehler, K. (1967). Pattern of secretion of Paneth cells of the small intestine of mice. *Gastroenterology* **53,** 240.

Tschudy, D. P., Marver, H. S., and Collier, A. (1965). A model for calculating RNA-half-life: short lived messenger RNA in the induction of mammalian aminolevulinic acid synthetase. *Biochem. Biophys. Res. Commun.* **21,** 480.

van Heyningen, H. E. (1964). Secretion of protein by the acinar cells of the rat pancreas, as studied by electron microscopic radioautography. *Anat. Rec.* **148,** 485.

Vaughan, M. H., Warner, J. R., and Darnell, J. E. (1967). Ribosomal precursor particles in the HeLa cell nucleus. *J. Mol. Biol.* **25,** 235.

Vidali, G., and Neelin, J. M. (1968). The stability of acid-soluble chromosomal proteins from avian erythrocytes. *Can. J. Biochem.* **46,** 781.

von Hungen, K., Mahler, H. R., and Moore, W. J. (1968). Turnover of protein and ribonucleic acid in synaptic subcellular fractions of rat brain. *J. Biol. Chem.* **243,** 1415.

Wachstein, M. (1963). Cyto- and histochemistry of the liver. *In* "The Liver" (C. Rouiller, ed.), Vol. 1, p. 137. Academic Press, New York.

Wang, T. Y. (1966). Solubilization and characterization of the residual proteins of the cell nucleus. *J. Biol. Chem.* **241,** 2913.

Wang, T. Y. (1968). Restoration of histone-inhibited DNA-dependent RNA synthesis by acidic chromatin proteins. *Exp. Cell Res.* **53,** 288.

Wang, T. Y., and Wang, K. M. (1962). Enzymes associated with nuclear ribosomes. *Biochim. Biophys. Acta* **55,** 392.

Warner, J. R. (1966). The assembly of ribosomes in HeLa cells. *J. Mol. Biol.* **19,** 383.

Warner, J. R., and Soeiro, R. (1967). Nascent ribosomes from HeLa cells. *Proc. Nat. Acad. Sci. U.S.* **57,** 1984.

Warner, J. R., Knopf, P., and Rich, A. (1963). A multiple ribosomal structure in protein synthesis. *Proc. Nat. Acad. Sci. U.S.* **49,** 122.

Warner, J. R., Girard, M., Latham, H., and Darnell, J. E. (1966). Ribosome formation in HeLa cells in the absence of protein synthesis. *J. Mol. Biol.* **19,** 373.

Warren, L. (1969). The biological significance of turnover of the surface membrane of animal cells. *Curr. Topics Develop. Biol.* **4,** 197.

Warshawsky, H., Leblond, C. P., and Droz, B. (1963). Synthesis and migration of proteins in the cells of the exocrine pancreas as revealed by specific activity determinations from radioautographs. *J. Cell Biol.* **16,** 1.

Webster, H. L., and Harrison, D. D. (1969). Enzymic activities during the transformation of crypt to columnar intestinal cells. *Exp. Cell Res.* **56,** 245.

Weissman, S., Goldsmith, B., Winzler, R., and Lepper, M. H. (1961). Turnover of plasma orosomucoid in man. *J. Lab. Clin. Med.* **57,** 7.

White, A., Hander, P., and Smith, E. L. (1968). "Principles of Biochemistry" McGraw-Hill, New York.

Whur, P., Herscovies, A., and Leblond, C. P. (1969). Radioautographic visualization of the incorporation of galactose-^{3}H and mannose-^{3}H by rat thyroids *in vitro* in relation to the stages of thyroglobulin synthesis. *J. Cell Biol.* **43,** 289.

Wiss, O., and Weber, F. (1964). The liver and vitamins. *In* "The Liver" (C. Rouiller, ed.), Vol. 2, p. 135. Academic Press, New York.

Woodward, D. O., and Munkres, K. D. (1966). Alterations of a maternally inherited mitochondrial structural protein in respiratory-deficient strains of *Neurospora.* *Proc. Nat. Acad. Sci. U.S.* **55,** 872.

Yamashina, I. (1956). On carbohydrate components of α_1-acid glycoprotein of human plasma. *Acta Chem. Scand.* **10,** 1666.

Young, R. W. (1967). The renewal of photoreceptor cell outer segments. *J. Cell Biol.* **33,** 61.

Young, R. W. (1968). Passage of newly formed protein through the connecting cilium of retinal rods in the frog. *J. Ultrastruct. Res.* **23,** 462.

Young, R. W. (1969a). A difference between rods and cones in the renewal of outer segment protein. *Invest. Ophthalmol.* **8,** 222.

Young, R. W. (1969b). The organization of vertebrate photoreceptor cells. *In* "The Retina" (B. R. Straatsma, M. O. Hall, R. A. Allen, and F. Crescitelli, eds.), p. 177. Univ. California Press, Berkeley, California.

Young, R. W., and Bok, D. (1969). Participation of the retinal pigment epithelium in the rod outer segment renewal process. *J. Cell Biol.* **42,** 392.

Young, R. W., and Droz, B. (1968). The renewal of protein in retinal rods and cones. *J. Cell Biol.* **39,** 169.

Young, R. W., and Fulhorst, H. W. (1966). Regional differences in protein synthesis within the lens of the rat. *Invest. Ophthalmol.* **5,** 288.

CHAPTER 7

The Dynamics of Extracellular and Cell Surface Protein Interactions

Harold C. Slavkin

I.	Introduction	221
II.	Epigenetic Controls Regulating Differentiation: The Problem	223
	A. Contact Guidance	225
	B. Cell Adhesion	226
	C. Contact Inhibition	226
III.	Outer Cell Surface Properties and Their Role in the Formation of Metazoan Systems	228
	A. Introduction	228
	B. Specific Cell Ligands	228
	C. Electrophoretic and Chemical Characterization of the Charged Groups at the Outer Surface of Mammalian Cells	230
	D. Metabolic Turnover of the Outer Cell Surface	232
	E. Architecture of Cell Membranes	233
	F. Limitations of Unit Membrane Concepts	237
IV.	Epithelial–Mesenchymal Interactions	239
	A. Morphogenetic Aspects during Embryogenesis	240
	B. The Basal Lamina	244
	C. Extracellular Microfibrils	245
	D. Morphogenetic Aspects of Collagen	246
V.	The Extracellular Matrix Influences upon Cellular Differentiation	248
	A. Glycosaminoglycans and Cell Differentiation	249
	B. The Extracellular Matrix: An Inductive Substratum	254
	C. Observations of the Collagen and Noncollagenous Protein Complexes: Cornea	259
	D. Tropocollagen, Fibrils, and Fibers	260
	E. Problems in Extracellular Matrix Protein Patterning: Self-Assembly	264
	References	267

I. Introduction

Morphogenesis during embryonic development and subsequent maturation involves an enormous succession of interactions between component parts of the mammalian organism. In attempting to analyze the myriad of such interactions one can select interactions between the organism and the physical–social environment, an organ system relating to the intact organism, a tissue component of a functioning organ, the cells within a tissue or in juxtaposition to a dissimilar tissue, the molecules at the cell surfaces interacting with adjacent cell surface materials, fluctuations of materials within the microenvironment, or interactions between solvents, solutes, and macromolecules. One of the most challenging problems in contemporary biology is the identification and function of sources of specificity in developmental patterns. How does one translate genetic specificity into epigenetic consequences? The physical and chemical attributes of outer cell surface materials and extracellular fibrous protein matrix constituents are, themselves, rich sources of biological specificity. Is there a process by which molecular specificity within ground substance and cell surfaces can impose specificity upon cell associations which, in turn, can be translated into specific tissue order and subsequent patterns of organization at the organismic level? During the organization of this chapter, I have attempted, in progressive steps, to evolve from the level of cellular interactions to the level of molecular structure. I shall attempt to argue that quantitative molecular differences are capable of translation into many of the structural specificities of cellular matrix tissue and organ architecture. In principle, the regulation of rates of synthesis, adsorption, absorption, and turnover should be extremely critical to an understanding of morphogenesis.

The observer of the many exquisite patterns of cellular interactions during embryogenesis and the various patterns imposed upon extracellular fibrous proteins often senses frustration in designing critical experiments. How might one isolate and characterize the outer cell surface materials recently resolved by electron microscopic methodology? If material is transferred between dissimilar cells during development, how might one obtain direct data for such phenomena? Can extracellular proteins be isolated and characterized from organic matrices and shed light upon their *in situ* organization? The following sections of this chapter are designed to state many of the *in situ* observations, attempts which have tried to elucidate many of these problems *in vitro*, and the opportunities currently available for molecular studies and their implications toward specificity. The reversible *in vitro* precipitation of structural proteins from solution, for example, collagen, and the formation of familiar-looking membranes from solutions of proteins and lipids are appealing indicators of contemporary advances in understanding basic mechanisms of *in vivo* organization. During growth and development, from embryo to senescence, the mammalian organism undergoes remodeling, often rapid renewal and turnover of many constituents. Differential gene action in determining protein structure and function is far better understood than the process of cellular orientation and the organization of structural fibrous proteins. My strategy is to focus upon the spatial and functional interactions between outer cell surfaces and extracellular matrices involved in rapid development using relevant cytological and biochemical criteria to disclose possible mechanisms controlling organization.

For purposes of experimental investigation or theoretical consideration the subject of this chapter can conveniently be divided into subtopics, relevant to the theme of this discussion. I propose to examine this topic utilizing information from the literature, and to a much lesser extent from the observations of some experiments of my own. No attempt will be made to exhaustively review the pertinent literature. References have, for the most part, been limited to studies which emphasize the biochemical and morphological basis of cell–cell interactions. The biosynthesis of many constituents of the outer cell surface and extracellular organic matrices have been the subject of recent separate monographs and, therefore, will not be included in this chapter. Emphasis will be placed on cellular and extracellular modifications, in molecular terms wherever possible, which are thought to effect or affect developmental patterns.

II. Epigenetic Controls Regulating Differentiation: The Problem

It is now axiomatic that all somatic cells contain the same complement of deoxyribonucleic acid (DNA). Often studies of genetic control of cell differentiation have excluded the environment in which cells operate. Differentiation within the organism must depend to a large extent upon epigenetic (extrinsic) factors which impinge upon the cell. Numerous studies have shown that the differentiation of a given cell type requires the action of an effector or inducer molecule (see reviews by Toivonen, 1967; Tiedemann, 1967, 1968; and T. Yamada, 1967), presumably transferred from one cell type to another cell type (Ambrose, 1967). Evidence continues to accumulate suggesting that differentiating cells influence one another by exchanging small molecules (Loewenstein, 1967) and direct gene products (RNA) (Ambrose, 1967). Other reviewers have pointed out the lack of critical experiments to verify such assumptions (Holtzer, 1963, 1968; Ebert, 1965; S. Cohen, 1965). Is RNA transferred from cell to cell thereby influencing subsequent cell differentiation, or might RNA complex with extracellular macromolecules to effect specific steric configurations? Appreciable numbers of investigators have found RNA in cell membranes

(Warren and Glick, 1968), in the outer cell periphery (reviewed by L. Weiss, 1968; Beierle, 1968), and in extracellular organic matrices (Slavkin *et al.*, 1969a).

The course of cell differentiation can be influenced by effectors acting at the cell surface. It now appears that collagen, or materials associated with it, play a major role in regulating many diverse differentiative events (Koningsberg and Hauschka, 1965; Grobstein and Cohen, 1965; J. Gross *et al.*, 1963; Wessels and Evans, 1968). The mechanism by which the availability of such a molecule during embryonic induction can influence differentiation is completely obscure. The data imply that an essential contribution of mesoderm to epithelial differentiation during morphogenesis is collagen (Wessels and Cohen, 1968). Grobstein (1967) has given special attention to the observation that in several inductive systems a "morphogenetic event" preceded the first recognizable cytological changes within the cells. P. R. Gross (1968) has presented a review of the biochemistry of differentiation in which differentiation is defined with emphasis upon the molecular events preceding those consequences of induction resolved in cytomorphological studies using light and electron microscopy. Given two distinctly different reproducing cell populations in an organism, do the propagated differences depend upon the influence of their mutual surroundings (epigenetic factors) or are they intrinsic? This question has been tested by placing each cell type into a common environment as an isolated cell suspension free of heterotypic cells and observing behavior as homotypic cell isolates and as disimiliar cell recombinants. Epithelial–mesenchymal embryonic systems are extremely suitable for such studies (see Symposia edited by Fleischmajer and Billingham, 1968). Common to such experiments is that each primary cell culture will lose a degree of its phenotype (dedifferentiation); however, each cell population in isolation will remain different from the other cell type (there is something intrinsic within a cell that is not lost when homotypic cells are placed into a common environment). The environment, the presence of heterotypic cells, intercellular substance, outer cell surface macromolecules, the nature of the surrounding medium—these factors profoundly influence the development of a cell's phenotype: cellular differentiation.

The principle that animal cells have mechanisms for regulating replication and subsequent biosynthetic activities depends upon information coming from the environment. The cell surface has the role of a "sensor" which receives information from the environment and presumably transmits this to a suitable regulatory site (Dulbecco, 1965). How do modifications in outer cell surfaces influence genetic and regulatory mechanisms is a problem of extreme importance.

A. CONTACT GUIDANCE

In 1914, Harrison noted that tissue cells do not swim in a medium as do spermatozoa but appear to require a "solid" substratum upon which to move. P. Weiss (1934, 1945) put forth his contact guidance theory in which his observations suggested that the nature of the substratum upon which he cultured various animal cells imposed its orientation upon the cells moving over it and their subsequent patterns of movement. He observed that fibroblasts orient preferentially in tissue culture with respect to glass, plastic fibers, in grooves scored in a glass substratum, and along lines of stress in a plasma clot (P. Weiss and Garber, 1952; P. Weiss, 1961). Such observations concluded that the substratum has a profound influence upon the patterns and nature of cell movements. Further, the morphogenetic significance of these observations provided a means whereby simple physicochemical changes within the extracellular environment could orient cells and influence the nature of their adherence to the substratum. In developing the concept of contact guidance, Weiss drew attention to the manner in which the structural organization of the substratum can directly influence the movement of cells. The observation is of obvious significance; for example, the longitudinal orientation that fibroblasts early adopt between the severed ends of a nerve or tendon. Several additional examples of the substratum influences upon cells *in vivo* should be considered: pigment cells and nerve axons orient along blood vessels, regenerating nerve axons grow out along a path determined by the degenerating cut axon and along myotome boundaries, and heart-forming mesodermal cell groups orient along oriented endoderm over which they are moving (DeHaan, 1963). Neural crest cells move down the sides of the neural tube regardless of the orientation of the tube in the embryo (Weston, 1963; Johnston, 1965). Melanocytes extend long dendritic processes along oriented rows of barbule cells. It is not clear, however, how cells orient along a substratum! Weiss suggested that cells secrete specific macromolecular materials which coat the substratum and form a "ground matrix" in the interface between cell and substratum that serves as the information for subsequent cell migrations (P. Weiss, 1961). Rosenberg (1962) found that cells in culture do release macromolecular materials which coat the substratum. It remains as yet evasive whether the secretions are under genetic or epigenetic control, whether the cells extrude cytoplasm as they migrate, and whether the remnant materials observed after cell migration (footprints) have a biological control in selectively directing cell movements. One possibility is that increased substratum surface area, due to grooves in glass or the deposition of biological material on glass, enhances the opportunities for cell adhesion to the substratum on the basis of complementarity between charge groups. It has been shown that cells do adhere preferentially to one substratum over another (Rosenberg, 1968). The cells seem to be guided by differential contact with properties of the substratum, however, not by the more obvious orientations of the substratum (see discussion by Carter, 1965). Concrete evidence for cells actually being oriented by macromolecular materials *in vivo* is lacking; this exciting area appears to be open for a variety of investigative research efforts.

B. Cell Adhesion

The differential adhesion hypothesis of Steinberg (1964) proposed that cells segregate and assume characteristic positions in mixed cell aggregates as a direct result of random mobility and innate quantitative differences in their general outer surface adhesiveness. However, the possibility of chemotaxis must not yet be discarded. It is notable that trypsin, EDTA, and other dissociating agents apparently do not have significant long-term effects on adhesiveness and mobile properties of metazoan cells. Given adequate time, treated cells recover from the effects of the cell-dissociating agents and function in terms of their inherent or acquired surface properties. Such properties are epigenetic, it must be argued, and perhaps best describe the cell's adaptation to its environment. Cells in monolayer may well possess different surface properties from cells in spinner culture, or indeed, cells *in vivo*. Studies on the nature of the cell surface and of the forces holding cells together have increased with a growing realization of the paramount importance of the outer cell surface in cell movement, contact, cell differentiation, and carcinogenesis (Abercrombie and Amrose, 1962; Curtis, 1966; Pethica, 1961; Humphreys, 1963, L. Weiss, 1967b; Steinberg, 1964; Grobstein, 1961; 1967; Moscona, 1968; Lilien, 1968; Beierle, 1968; Gustafson and Wolpert, 1963; Slavkin, 1970).

C. Contact Inhibition

The little known about regulation of growth and development in animal cells suggests that the outer cell surface macromolecules play a central role. Both direction and extent of cell movement appear to be controlled at the cell surface and are responsive to the nature of the substratum contacted by the cells. Abercrombie and Heaysman (1954) have analyzed the phenomenon of "contact inhibition" between fibroblasts in culture. Time-lapse cinemicrophotography has shown that fibroblasts *in vitro* move (as do many cell types) by means of a ruffled cell membrane developed at the leading margin. If contact is made with another cell, the plasma membrane ceases its movements, and a firm intercellular adhesion is formed. In time a new ruffled plasma membrane develops in a new location, presumably by a renewal of specific membrane properties, and the temporarily immobile fibroblast moves off in a new direction. When the fibroblast in question is surrounded by other fibroblasts, it is effectively immobilized. This hypothesis has been drawn upon to describe the cessation of many embryonic cell migrations (neural crest) and the behavior of fibroblasts in repairing wounds (James, 1969).

Contact inhibition is not an invariable occurrence (Curtis, 1961). The incidence of contact inhibition is dependent on the composition of the medium bathing the cells and on modification of the substratum upon which the cells move. Carter (1965) showed that inhibition is diminished in fibroblasts grown upon cellulose acetate coated with a very thin layer of palladium. If the palladium coat is thickened, the fibroblasts form monolayers to the expected extent. Carter concluded that the loss of contact inhibition involved a decrease in the adhesiveness of cell to substratum, so that encountering fibroblasts moved over one another's cell surfaces.

In this connection, preliminary results from studies with the scanning electron microscope are extremely pertinent (James, 1969). Earlier studies (Curtis, 1964) using an interference technique, showed that parts of fibroblasts cultured on glass surfaces approached to within 100 Å of the glass substratum. These regions of adhesion were confined to the peripheral cell margins and the cellular cytoplasmic extensions (filopodia). If fibroblasts are cultured in a medium containing a small concentration (0.05 M) of urea, they demonstrate a marked diminution of contact inhibition (J.A. Weston, personal communication). James (1969) utilized this observation and studied the behavior of fibroblasts in tissue culture by scanning electron microscopy and found that this technique would clearly distinguish between cell overlap and actual fibroblast migrations over or under neighboring cells. Numerous stereopaired scanning electron micrographs of migrating urea-treated fibroblasts showed that the ruffled membrane of the advancing cell retained contact with the substratum. Contact inhibition did not, under these special conditions, fail as a consequence of loss of cell-to-substratum adhesion on the part of the ruffled membrane as Carter's hypothesis would suggest (1965). Rather, it appears that the advancing ruffled membrane must insinuate itself between the substratum and the margin of the cell it encounters, implying that the latter is less adherent than the former (James, 1969).

III. Outer Cell Surface Properties and Their Role in the Formation of Metazoan Systems

A. INTRODUCTION

The ontogeny of multicellular organisms depends upon selective adhesion of cells. The rationale for this aspect of metazoan phylogeny may seem apparent, for it is at the outer cell surface that cells interact with their immediate environment (Davis and Warren, 1967). A multiplicity of outer cell surface structures (often referred to as specific cell ligands) have evolved in response to specific functional stresses elicited by the environment (epigenetic) for subsequent survival and reproduction. Assuming that cell aggregation is a critical aspect of metazoan development, the surface adhesional alterations profoundly affect development. Either changes in cell adhesion properties or modifications of the extracellular matrix (substratum) will enhance or inhibit aggregation. A further assumption required for such an argument is that the molecular composition of the outer cell surface, in a real sense, reflects the phenotype of eucaryotic cells. Therefore, cellular organization should be considered with respect to properties of the cell surfaces; their physicochemical affinities for the specific intercellular milieu (L. Weiss, 1967a). The theoretical analysis of cell interactions by Heinmets (1968) is an excellent review of the argument briefly presented.

B. SPECIFIC CELL LIGANDS

Despite the apparent importance of the outer cell surfaces and their adjacent extracellular matrices, little evidence relating molecular composition with specific cell functions in mammalian systems has been elucidated. In contrast, it has been shown that histogenetic attachment and aggregation of dissociated *Microciona prolifera* and *Haliclona occulata* (sponge cells) are controlled by specific macromolecular products localized at the outer cell surface, and between cells. These cells' ligands function as a specific adhesive (Humphreys, 1963; Moscona, 1963; Margoliash *et al.*, 1965; Galanti and Gasic, 1967). The surface and intercellular material is easily separated from the cells by washing the cells in cold seawater free of divalent cations. Upon addition of the removed material the cells will reaggregate into multicellular masses.

Using two species of sponges it was observed that the aggregation-enhancing solution was species specific (Moscona, 1968). *Microciona* cells in suspension with *Haliclona* cells can only aggregate with their own species; the isolated materials are also species specific. Moscona (1968) and Humphreys (1967) have presented conclusive evidence for the existence of specific factors which function in the histogenetic attachment and aggregation of sponge cells. These factors have been isolated from living systems and were shown to retain the essential functional properties that characterized the original ligand site on the outer cell surface. These cell ligands participate structurally in linking sponge cells into multicellular systems. Since biological and biochemical properties of sponge cell ligands have been determined (Moscona, 1968; Humphreys, 1967), I include a brief account of this information to serve as guidelines for future, detailed analysis of the origin, composition, structure, biosynthesis, and mode of function of comparable cell ligands in mammalian cell systems (see discussion by Slavkin, 1970).

It has been shown that the cell ligand's biological activity is present in a particulate fraction that contains unit particles with diameters of 20–25 Å that were sedimented by high-speed centrifugation (Margoliash et al., 1965; Galanti and Gasic, 1967). From analyses of amino acid and carbohydrate composition, the molecular weight of the unit particles was estimated to be 15,000; each particle may represent one ligand unit. The carbohydrate and protein moieties do not separate when the aggregation-enhancing factor is passed through Sephadex gel columns. After 80% of the protein is removed by proteolytic enzymes, the carbohydrate remains attached to a peptide residue (Moscona, 1968). If carbohydrate monomers are linked into a chain and then attached to a peptide residue, this configuration could have a structural polarity important to cell aggregation. The definitive nature of the carbohydrate species is not as yet known.

Of extreme biological importance is the fact that exogenously supplied ligands bind with greater efficiency to unwashed cells (cells with ligands) than to calcium–magnesium-free, seawater-washed, trypsin-treated, or Pronase-treated cells. Aggregation-enhancing materials bind to sites provided by either residual ligands remaining on the surface of dissociated cells, or by specific receptors on the outer cell surface (or by both).

It is of interest, at this point, to digress and point out that whereas cell aggregation in heterotypic sponge cells is species specific, aggregation of embryonic vertebrate cells is preferentially tissue specific (Moscona, 1962; Steinberg, 1964). Specific outer cell surface constituents with functional properties fundamentally analagous to those isolated from the sponge cells may also be involved in intercellular attachments in higher organisms. This is supported by the isolation from embryonic chick cells of materials with cell type-specific, aggregation-enhancing activity (Kuroda, 1968; Lilien and Moscona, 1967). The interesting work of Lilien (1968) on the isolation, specificity, antigenicity, uptake, and utilization of an aggregation-enhancing factor from embryonic chick retina cells has provided fresh insights into this complex problem. Several recent studies have employed outer cell surface probes such as EDTA or trypsin in order to selectively isolate different species of cell periphery material (Benedetti and Emmelot, 1967; L. Weiss, 1967a,b). The isolation and characterization of extracellular components from Wilm's tumor (nephroblastoma) (Allerton et al., 1970) and the preliminary characterization of the outer cell surface material from normal and polyoma virus-transformed fibroblasts (Beierle, 1968) are noteworthy examples employing this experimental approach. Various aspects of aggregation enhancement and methodology are to be found in recent reviews (Davis and Warren, 1967; Peachey, 1968; Manson, 1968; L. Weiss, 1967a; Lilien, 1969; Steinberg, 1970).

C. Electrophoretic and Chemical Characterization of the Charged Groups at the Outer Surface of Mammalian Cells

The technique of microelectrophoresis enables the measurement of the zeta potential at the surface of mammalian cells (Heard and Seaman, 1960). The electrophoretic mobility of cells has been shown to be dependent upon pH, ionic strength, and counterion concentration in the culture medium. Such information has implied the presence of specific ionic groupings at the outer cell surface (Cook et al., 1962). The advent of neuraminidase has complemented such studies by providing a well-defined enzyme reaction for the modification of cell surface components (as an α-glycosidase the enzyme functions to cleave terminal sialic acid residues from sialoproteins).

It has been repeatedly shown (see review by L. Weiss, 1967a) that all mammalian cells have a net negative surface charge which gives an anodic mobility. This mobility has been found to be the algebraic sum of both cationic and anionic contributions. Diazomethane has been used as a reagent to esterify surface carboxyl groups. For example, Ward and Ambrose (1969) using CL_3 ascites cells demonstrated that all the anionic groups on the outer cell surface over a wide pH range were carboxyl groups.

The use of neuraminidase clearly showed that sialic acid is a primary surface-charge determinant (i.e., reduces the electrophoretic mobility of cells after neuraminidase treatment). Other reagents have been used to show that after sialic acid removal by enzyme digestion, an increased concentration in cell surface amino groups is apparent. The removal of sialic acid appears to be followed by a reorientation of surface proteins determined by the large increase in contributions of amino and carboxyl groups. This reorientation is explained if one assumes that sialic acid functions as the primary determinant of membrane configuration. Removal of the acidic carboxyl groups of sialic acid ($pK_a = 2.6$) by neuraminidase may necessitate the reformation of the tertiary structure of the residual surface proteins so as to present a more hydrophilic outer cell surface to the adjacent external microenvironment. This would account for the observed increased surface charge density (L. Weiss, 1967a,b; Ward and Ambrose, 1969). It is conceivable that sialic acid *in vivo* produces subtle changes in pH at the interface between outer cell surfaces and environment. This could result in the membrane configuration alterations often observed at the cell membrane. The biological ubiquity of this surface-bound molecule (sialic acid) further suggests this basic function.

Sialic acid is the source of many carboxyl groups found at the outer cell surface. In addition, other carboxyl groups can be found in various parts of surface proteins (C terminal chain ends of proteins; glutamic or aspartic acids within protein chains). Without amino acid analysis of purified membrane fragments, differentiation between the various sources of surface carboxyl groups is not possible and numerous alternatives must be considered.

Trypsin has also been used to isolate a sialomucopeptide from the surface of human erythrocytes; this enzyme does not change the electrophoretic mobility of the ascites cells (Ward and Ambrose, 1969). Lack of reactivity of ascites cells with trypsin was interpreted as implying that outer cell surface proteins lack an appreciable amount of such basic amino acids as lysine and arginine (necessary for the specificity of trypsin activity). The lack of trypsin reactions suggests that the preponderance of *N*-acylated amino sugars are attached to outer surface proteins at the N-terminal chain ends. Pronase treatment of cells removes sialic acid and surface proteins, thereby exposing surface phosphate groups as a dominant ionic species (Ward and Ambrose, 1969) and significantly altering the electrophoretic mobility.

Dissociated invertebrate and vertebrate cells are increasingly being used in examinations of the outer cell surface and studies inquiring into the reaggregation and tissue reconstruction of embryonic organs. After enzymatic, mechanical treatment, or treatment of cells with cation-chelating methods (ethylenediaminetetraacetate, EDTA), many of the salient characteristics of the *in vivo* physicochemical properties may be drastically altered. Caution must be exercised when interpreting evidence from such studies in that outer cell surface properties of cells freshly isolated from embryonic tissues by standard techniques (i.e., mild trypsinization), have been shown to demonstrate artifactual changes (Barnard *et al.*, 1969). Studies into the effects of trypsinization, EDTA washings, neuraminidase, Pronase, and other mechanical, enzymatic, or cation-chelating methods for cell dissociation appear to be essential in order to further our understanding of the outer cell surfaces and subsequent cell aggregation phenomena.

D. Metabolic Turnover of the Outer Cell Surface

From the literature on metabolic turnover *in vivo* and *in vitro* has emerged the concept that there is very little turnover in growing cell populations, but that there is considerable turnover or renewal of components in corresponding nongrowing cell populations (Mandelstam, 1960). In this section, I wish to discuss briefly outer cell surface material turnover in mammalian cells. Studies of the behavior of the surface membrane of L cells demonstrated that the size and number of cells and surface membranes do not change; therefore, the data could be explained by a relatively large turnover of the membrane (Warren and Glick, 1968). Eagle and his colleagues (1957; 1959) reported that various growing and nongrowing cells in tissue culture had essentially the same rate of turnover of protein (0.7–1.1% per hour). The fact that the surface membrane of nongrowing cells turns over while that of growing cells presumably does not may provide a basis for a qualitative difference between the membranes in these various states, differences in membrane permeability, antigenicity, and receptivity to cell interactions. It is a curious observation, however, that at high concentrations cell suspensions do not grow. Why these cells do not grow is not known. With this in mind, it is surprising that cells in tissue culture maintain a fairly constant rate of synthesis whether or not the cell is dividing. It is assumed that normal cells and contact-inhibited cells demonstrate a depressed state of synthesis and turnover (Levine *et al.*, 1965).

Recently, experiments designed to study the dynamics whereby component macromolecules of the outer cell surface gain access to the external surface of the plasma membrane, following their intracellular synthesis, have been reported (Marcus and Schwartz, 1968; Kraemer, 1966). Methods have been employed to monitor the reappearance of sialic acid (N-acetylneuraminic acid or NANA) on the outer cell surface of HeLa cells after neuraminidase treatment and subsequent removal of the enzyme from the growth medium (Marcus and Schwartz, 1968). These studies demonstrated that the shortest half-life of the return of sialic acid-terminating outer cell surface receptors in HeLa cells can be measured chemically ($T_{1/2} = 4$ hours). This methodology enables one to detect logically the reappearance of any outer cell surface molecule accessible to neuraminidase treatment. Comparable studies are possible using trypsin or EDTA. During epithelial–mesenchymal interactions *in vitro*, recombined cell suspensions (obtained by mild trypsinization) repeatedly have been observed to show a lag period of 24–48 hours before reaggregation occurs (see review by Grobstein, 1967). This has been repeatedly observed during odontogenic cell interactions (Slavkin *et al.*, 1968b; Kollar and Baird, 1969; Koch, 1967). Does this lag period represent the renewal of the outer cell surface materials implicated in cell aggregation, or does cell recognition require, independent of the outer cell surface materials, 24–48 hours? What is the consequence of trypsin or EDTA dissociation of embryonic cells and what effects might the nature of the tissue culture medium have upon subsequent outer cell surface metabolism? I encourage the reader to evaluate several recent studies dealing specifically with effects of the dissociation of mammalian cells (Barnard *et al.*, 1969; Kemp *et al.*, 1967; Moscona and Moscona, 1966).

E. ARCHITECTURE OF CELL MEMBRANES

With the application of electron microscopy to investigations of the basic macromolecular architecture of cell membranes (see symposia edited by Locke, 1964; Peachey, 1968; Dalton and Haguenau, 1968), a variety of information has been brought forth illustrating that several architectural patterns for cell membranes can and indeed do exist. Much difficulty has been introduced by preparative techniques required to view thin sections (ca. 400–700 Å). How valid is interpretation from such sections seen in the electron microscope? How much of the molecular architecture of the living cell membrane is modified by cell isolation and interactions between the membrane and the fixatives used for preparation? Even the thinnest sections used in electron microscopy (100–200 Å) are thicker than the subunits seen in cell membranes by such techniques as negative staining with phosphotungstic acid (PTA).

Until rather recently, electron microscopists were unable to observe materials outside of the trilaminar unit membrane complex. Advances in preparation methods (reviewed by Revel and Ito, 1967; Dalton and Haguenau, 1968) have greatly facilitated the visualization of outer cell surface moieties and immediately adjacent extracellular matrix materials. The introduction of histochemical methods applicable to electron microscopy further permitted studies of the distribution of a variety of protein and polysaccharide materials (Sjostrand, 1967; Pease, 1966) (Ramburg and Leblond, 1967a, 1967b). Perhaps the most common type of surface coating consists of fine microfilaments extending from the plasma membrane of a variety of cell types (Figs. 1 and 2). Such surface specialization has been cited in tooth development (Slavkin *et al.*, 1969b), renal glomerulous (E. Yamada, 1955), and a variety of other systems (Pease, 1966; Fawcett, 1962). Further surface specializations should be made visible in the near future as histochemical, enzyme cytochemical, immunological, and freeze-etching become more available for electron microscopic applications.

The surface coat of the intestinal epithelium has been extremely useful in that it contains an abundant surface coat (Ito, 1965), presumably sialo-

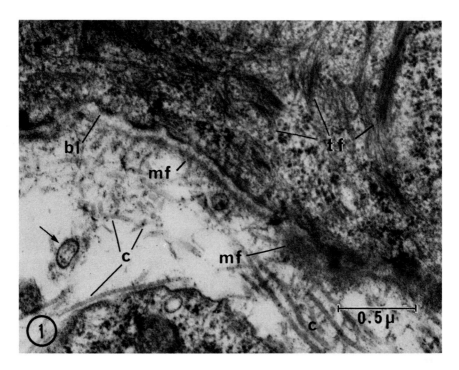

Fig. 1. Embryonic epidermal organ systems, in this case illustrated by embryonic mouse dorsal skin, demonstrates the dynamics of extracellular matrix formation (e. g., basement membrane) and specificity of the outer cell surfaces of each tissue component. Abbreviations: tf, tonofilaments; mf, microfilaments; c, collagen; bl, basal lamina. The arrow is pointing to a cell process of mesenchymal origin. Section is stained with lead citrate and uranyl acetate. 43,200 ×.

mucoprotein. The outer leaflet of the trilaminar membrane has a very low electron density and bears a branching mat of fine microfilaments arranged somewhat perpendicular to the outer cell surface (Revel and Ito, 1967). In the light microscope the outer edge of the striated border (area of the microvilli) stains PAS-positive and is metachromatic after staining with Toluidine Blue and with Alcian Blue. The use of colloidal thorium stain (Revel, 1964) on thin sections allows clear identification of the filaments as the site of polysaccharides detected in the histological sections. Failure to remove the microfilaments by various enzyme treatments (Pronase, neuraminidase, trypsin, hyaluronidase) suggests that this aspect of the extraneous coat of outer cell surfaces is membrane bound and not merely an adsorbed mucous material. Autoradiography in this system at the electron microscopic level (Revel and Ito, 1967) has provided very interesting information. After *in vitro* exposure of the intestinal mucosa to tritated glucose, galactose, and acetate, and even $^{35}SO_4$, there is initially an intense labeling of the epithelial cells. Chase experiments show that the grain density accumulates in the outer cell surface microfilaments within several hours. Eventually, the outer cell surface loses its label, implying that there is a rapid renewal of the outer cell surfaces; in addition, the distances between microfilaments suggest that the microfilaments provide negative charge, thereby preventing substances bearing a negative charge from approaching the outer cell surface. The radiochemical studies of Warren and Glick (1968) complement the high-resolution autoradiographic studies cited here.

Many mammalian cells appear to have filamentous outer cell surface material which is not visually continuous with the internal aspects of the plasma membrane (Figs. 1 and 2). The discontinuous surface materials are characterized by the presence of short filaments or a mat of amorphous

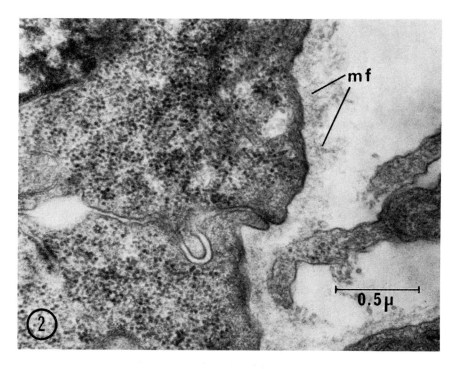

FIG. 2. A filamentous outer cell surface-bound material (microfilament, mf) is associated with many mammalian cell types. In this electron micrograph, the embryonic salivary gland is selected to show another example of this material. Section is stained with lead citrate and uranyl acetate. 46,000 ×.

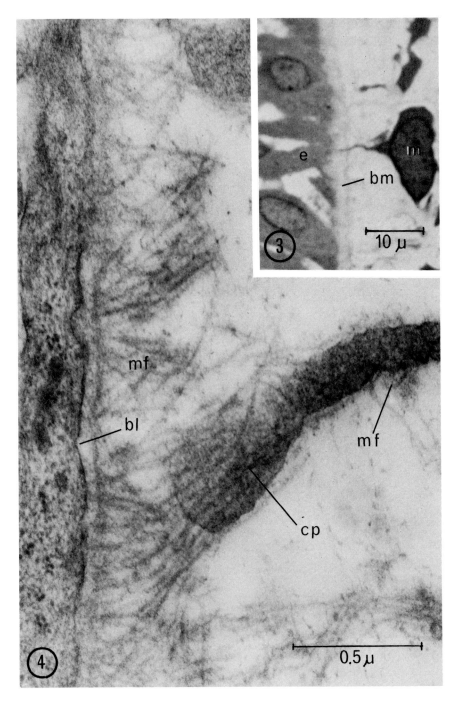

material facing the extracellular environment. The histochemical methods using light and electron microscopy have implicated acid mucopolysaccharides and sialomucoproteins as components of the outer cell surface materials. The implication lacks specificity. Polysaccharides have been shown in association with the outer surfaces of numerous animal cells (Pease, 1966; Fawcett, 1962); this may be a phylogenetic trait common to many procaryotic and eucaryotic cell types (Slavkin, 1970). At the base of the epithelium is a polysaccharide-rich complex referred to as the basement membrane (basal lamina) (Figs. 3 and 4). Muscle cells are invested in a PAS-positive coat, whereas connective tissue cells commonly are associated with mucopolysaccharide–protein complexes (e.g., epithelial–mesenchymal interactions). Enhanced resolution by electron microscopy and improved histochemical techniques, which can complement high-resolution ultrastructural studies, could distinguish between the unit plasma membrane and the outer cell surface materials intimately associated with cells of many types. It is difficult at present to ascertain what truly is the periphery of a cell, and what truly is the "sphere of influence" of a cell.

F. Limitations of Unit Membrane Concepts

It would seem appropriate that, for biological studies of cell interactions, the common view of the plasma membrane (the static sandwich-like structure), seen as the trilaminar membrane in the electron microscope and designated as the unit membrane (Robertson, 1964), be extended to include the outer cell surface, thereby conceptually extending the anticipated influence of one cell upon another and upon itself with respect to the environment (epigenetic). The exhaustive work done on the cell membranes of erythrocytes clearly has shown the complexity of the molecular ecology of the outer cell surfaces (enzymes, glycolipids, glycoproteins, blood group substances, etc.) (see Dalton and Haguenau, 1968 for a comprehensive review).

Fig. 3. The insert represents a light photomicrograph of epithelial–mesenchymal interactions associated with embryonic odontogenesis. Abbreviations: e, epithelia; m, mesenchyme; and bm, basement membrane which stains PAS-positive. 1600 ×.

Fig. 4. Higher resolution of the interface between extended mesenchymal cell process (cp) and proximal basal lamina (bl) which is coated with microfilaments (mf) on its undersurface. Microfilaments are also associated with the mesenchymal cell process. Although static, one observes what appears to be a transfer of material from cell to cell. The microfilamentous material presumably contains glycosaminoglycans. Section is stained with lead citrate and uranyl acetate. 70,000 ×.

Rubin (1966) has put forth a macromolecular membrane theory in which he proposed that the macromolecular units of the plasma membrane and outer cell surfaces are in flux with their immediate microenvironment, constantly being released from and replaced into the membrane. He assumed that the membrane units are held in association with one another by weak bonds easily broken by thermal energy. His evidence for such a phenomenon was obtained from large cell cultures in a medium and assaying the medium with respect to time. The medium, therefore, could be used to evaluate the surface molecules and their respective activities by isolating cell surface materials by various differential fractionation procedures (column chromatography, sucrose linear gradient, polyacrylamide gel electrophoresis, etc.)and evaluating the behavior of isolated material by reintroducing such materials back into culture. Cell surface materials from viral-transformed cells could be tested in control normal cultures and vice versa (for examples, see Beierle, 1968; Defendi and Gasic, 1963).

There is some evidence among multicellular organisms that membrane structure influences the fate of cells, although no such evidence exists that membrane structure in metazoan cells predetermines a patterned organization among progeny cells. Presumably, pre-existing patterns of structures in which surface macromolecules occur determine the pattern of these structures in subsequent cell generations. Paul Weiss (1962) suggested that certain macromolecules with hydrophilic groups at one end, and hydrophobic groups at the other, could be arranged at an oil–water interface with each group buried in the medium appropriate to it. The cellular metabolism would be adjusted to provide surface macromolecules in sufficient concentrations to obligate the position of the cell to be what might be considered most favorable to the functioning of the cell. The internal and external environments associated with a cell would directly affect what was synthesized and exported to the outer cell surface and, in turn, the function of that moiety, whether it be to adsorb, absorb, participate in secretions, or form a junction with another cell type from the same or a dissimilar cell population (Fig. 5). The surface arrangements of the macromolecules presumably determine the selective permeability properties of the cell and the distribution of other cell molecules progressing concentrically from the interior of the cell. By analogy, the distribution of molecules in complex mixtures was described by Weiss using the crystallization of hydroxyapatite on collagen fibrils as a model. A specific steric arrangement of collagen (640 Å periodicity) must be obtained before a particular higher order of complexity (mineralization) can be developed.

Most germane are the observations that the physical thickness and bulk properties of a specific substratum influences its interaction with cells (Rosenberg, 1962). Varying numbers of fatty acid monolayers were de-

Extracellular matrix formation

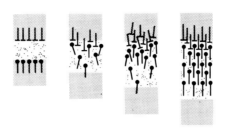

Fig. 5. Diagrammatic representation of the formation of an extracellular matrix (e. g., the interface during epithelial–mesenchymal interaction). Both heterotypic tissues contribute tissue-specific macromolecules to the molecular ecology of the matrix. This simple diagram illustrates tropocollagen migration toward the glycosaminoglycans presumed to be located on the undersurface of the basal lamina associated with epithelia. Differentiation of the extracellular matrix requires the selective localization of specific molecular populations (e. g., dentine, cartilage, bone, cornea). The physical and chemical processes which are translated into an orderly physical structure remain obscure.

posited at constant surface pressure on solid bases of different compositions. It was found that the time required for cell attachment to the substratum and the spreading of cells varied with the number of fatty acid monolayers and with the type of materials used to make the base substratum. It remains to be seen, however, whether comparable influences, such as in the distribution of molecules as new surface materials, can account for the intimate cell–cell interactions observed in the induction of cellular differentiation *in vivo*.

The finding of perpetuated membrane alterations in cells and propogated cell monolayer effects *in vitro* lends credibility, according to Rubin (1966), to the idea that developmental and malignant transformations arise from a heritable disruption in the distribution and configuration of cell surface macromolecules. This hypothesis requires critical experimentation.

IV. Epithelial–Mesenchymal Interactions

Within this decade there has been an appreciable influx of molecular techniques and new ideas into the field of developmental biology. Experimentation ranging from descriptions of the appearance of nascent enzymes or specific products to studies in which primitive tissues are tested for their ability to develop under a variety of conditions. The data accumulated are too often interpreted and discussed in terms of unproved assumptions using models of differential gene activity during organogenesis, wound healing, or neoplasia, to mention but a few.

Embryonic induction, described as an instructive biological event, is an appropriate concept to probe the dynamic interactions between dissimilar cells and between cells and adjacent extracellular matrices. Classically, this conceptual problem has been posed in terms implying the transmission of informational molecules from one cell to another cell (see reviews by Tiedemann, 1967; Grobstein, 1967; Holtzer, 1968). The mechanism of induction generally requires two assumptions: (1) An inducing cell or tissue releases a unique macromolecule which (2) instructs an undifferentiated, competent cell capable of responding (differentiating) into a more specialized cell. The inducing factor represses some genes in the responding cell and concurrently derepresses others (Lash, 1968). Embryonic induction, therefore, includes restriction of cell proliferation, specific morphological expressions, and the specific production of proteins and other macromolecules. These processes are both temporally protracted and biologically complex. The molecular and cellular requirements for inductive competence range from nonspecific to highly specific. I would like to briefly question these assumptions as related to epithelial–mesenchymal interactions, properties of outer cell surfaces, and relationships with the extracellular matrices. In this section I wish to include recent information suggesting that the molecular constituents of the extracellular organic matrices profoundly influence cellular differentiation.

A. MORPHOGENETIC ASPECTS DURING EMBRYOGENESIS

It is now axiomatic that epithelial–mesenchymal interactions are extremely important in development. Numerous examples of such interactions have been investigated and shown to have comparable properties (see review by Grobstein, 1967 and a recent symposium on this topic edited by Fleischmajer and Billingham, 1968). Two experimental approaches have elicited most of the information available: (1) Embryonic organ rudiments are enzymatically treated to isolate epithelial and mesenchymal tissue fragments which are reassembled in juxtaposition to a Millipore filter *in vitro* (transfilter experiments, Grobstein, 1956); and (2) tissue fragments are further dissociated into cell suspensions which can be reaggregated *in vitro* by rotation in flask cultures (Moscona, 1961), grafted to the chorioallantoic membrane (CAM) of chick embryos (Moscona and Moscona, 1965; P. Weiss and Taylor, 1960; Garber and Moscona, 1964; Slavkin *et al.*, 1968b), or cultured in the anterior chamber of the eye (Levak-Svajger and Moscona, 1964).

Interactions between epithelium and mesenchyme during organogenesis (e.g., thyroid gland, salivary gland, feather, hair follicle, pancreas, skin, lung, thymus gland, tooth formation, etc.) reflect the embryonic inductive process (Grobstein, 1967; 1969). Intimate association between the heterotypic tissues is essential to support histogenesis (the advanced differentiation of the cellular components within each tissue) and organogenesis. Homotypic cells or tissues will not develop unless placed in juxtaposition with an appropriate heterotypic cell population or tissue. The period of induction is that sequence in which both tissue types must be in association in order to interact. Developmental progression reflects the interdependency between epithelium and mesenchyme. Further, at given moments in time there is an oscillation in developmental significance between these tissues. Epithelium may become an inducer and the mesenchyme responds or the reciprocal relationship may dominate.

It has been repeatedly suggested through interpretations of various epithelial–mesenchymal interacting systems that several factors are involved in this type of induction. Drs. Kallman and Grobstein found that during pancreatic and salvary gland epithelial–mesenchymal interactions across a Millipore filter *in vitro*, collagen fibrils were observed in close association with the epithelial tissue (Kallman and Grobstein, 1965). Were these fibers secreted by the epithelium, a phenomenon recently shown in embryonic chick corneal epithelium (Hay and Revel, 1969), or were the collagen fibrils a product of the mesenchyme which had traversed the Millipore filter (80 μ) and polymerized at the epithelial basal lamina? To test such possibilities, Kallman and Grobstein (1966) had incubated one of the two tissues with labeled proline (tritiated) and the other tissue was left unlabeled. The mesenchyme, when labeled, transferred intracellular grain density to the extracellular interface (presumably the proline was incorporated in tropocollagen), whereas prelabeled epithelial tissue experiments showed grain density not in association with the extracellular matrix collagen. The grain density associated with collagen was removed by collagenase digestion but not by hyaluronidase treatment. Further studies (Bernfield, 1970) employed biochemical assays of hydroxyproline and proline-containing materials accumulated in Millipore filters during epithelial–mesenchymal interactions. These studies demonstrated that hydroxyproline is not synthesized by epithelium; this epithelium, however, regulates the synthesis of tropocollagen in mammalian mesenchyme during organogenesis. Autoradiographic data (Kallman and Grobstein, 1966) and biochemical data suggested that collagen, which deposits at the basal surface of the epithelium, has its developmental origin in mesenchyme. Does this material have a morphogenetic function during epithelial–mesenchymal interactions?

Enzyme digestion of collagen by collagenase during interactions suggests the collagen does have a biological activity during critical development (Grobstein and Cohen, 1965). Collagenase treatment of the mesenchyme, but not the epithelium, inhibits development by suppressing the morphogenetic expression of adenomer formation. Why does the collagen accumulate at the basal lamina? Perhaps this is, in part, a specific example of collagen fibrillogenesis; the fibrillogenesis due to polymerizing effects exerted by glycoproteins and mucopolysaccharides (MPS) produced by epithelium. Tritiated glucosamine labeling of the epithelium illustrated a concentration of grain density in association with the basal lamina. This was interpreted (Kallman and Grobstein, 1966) as indicating that the MPS-specific topographical locations participated in the observed collagen fibrillogenesis occurring in these regions. Labeling studies with tritiated

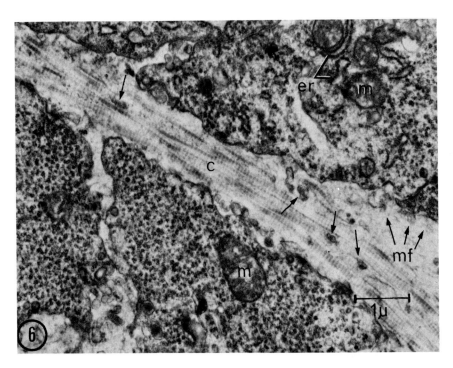

Fig. 6. Fibrillogenesis (c, collagen fibers) is commonly observed adjacent to meso-dermally derived preodontoblast cells during extracellular matrix formation. Within the intercellular spaces, membrane-bound cytoplasmic inclusions were observed (arrows) which could represent a merocrine-type secretion by these cells. Microfibrils (mf), either noncollagenous proteins or collagen precursors, were seen associated with the outer cell surfaces. Abbreviation: m, mitochondria; er, rough endoplasmic reticulum. Sections were stained with lead citrate and uranyl acetate. 15,000 ×.

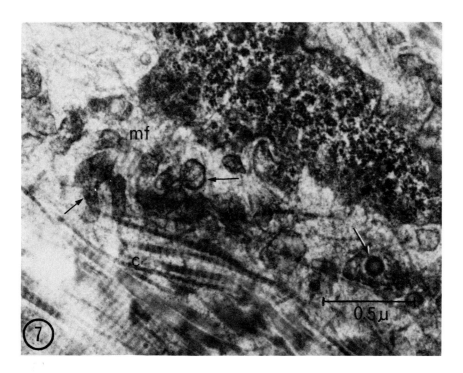

FIG. 7. Merocrine-like secretory mechanisms are observed with tropocollagen secretions from preodontoblasts [arrows refer reader to cell processes included within the intercellular collagen fiber formations (c)]. Numerous microfilaments (mf) are found within and adjacent to the fiber-forming regions. This section is stained with lead citrate and uranyl acetate. 50,500 ×.

proline were interpreted, on the basis of proline/hydroxyproline ratios, to show that the presence of epithelium increased the amount of collagen synthesized by mesenchyme per unit time; mesenchyme in the absence of epithelium, incubated with labeled precursors for collagen, showed a decrease in collagen biosynthesis (Bernfield, 1970). Hydroxylation of collagen appeared to occur in the mesenchyme with increased efficiency when epithelium was in juxtaposition. Perhaps the tropocollagen synthesized in the mesenchyme was assembled into fibrils at the surface of the mesenchyme and not in association with the epithelium? This is the case *in vivo* during epithelial–mesenchymal interactions during odontogenesis (Slavkin *et al.*, 1969b) (see Figs. 6 and 7). Grobstein's interpretation must be carefully considered for several reasons: (1) The pore size of the Millipore filter used in transfilter studies (0.4 μ) is ample for mesenchymal cell extensions to grow into; (2) collagen fibrils have been commonly noted in close association with mesenchymal cells as far as 6–10 μ from epithelium (indeed in epidermal-like organ systems such as skin, thyroid gland, salivary gland, etc.); (3) some tropocollagen may be extruded from mesenchymal cells and seen in association with the basal lamina of epithelium; however, these units may not show periodicity (either they are microfilamentous proteins other than collagen or collagen fibril precursors); and (4) tight cell junctions between dissimilar tissues are rarely observed. It appears that much additional research is essential in order to complement Grobstein's exciting interpretations or to establish somewhat different investigative paths to follow.

B. The Basal Lamina

The basal lamina is an interesting example of extracellular formation of a highly ordered molecular system. A brief discussion of its origin, composition, and suggested function is relevant to the theme of this chapter. It should be made clear, however, that much confusion yet remains in many of these aspects of the basal lamina.

The basal lamina has been considered to develop from the amorphous intercellular "ground substance" underlying the epidermal cells, but it is not certain whether this structure arises from ectoderm, mesoderm, or both (Revel and Hay, 1963). Other electron microscopic studies of the basal lamina suggested, after EDTA treatment, that the lamina has a definite contribution from the mesoderm (Goel and Jurand, 1968). Rambourg and Leblond (1967a,b) investigated the nature of the metachromatic basement membrane observed by light microscopy (see Fig. 3) with specific reference to the PAS-positive (periodic acid-Schiff) reaction at the ultrastructural level. Three distinct layers were found to compose the interface between epithelia and mesenchyme (see Fig. 4). The outer cell coat of the epithelia, the basal lamina, and the extracellular collagen fibrils are all stained by PAS and PAS–silver. Since only the epithelial cell coat and basal lamina are continuous, these investigators concluded that the PAS-positive interface, seen with the light microscope, represented this continuous layer. It was assumed that the PAS-positive reactions demonstrated glycoproteins as constituents of the basal lamina or as depositions on the undersurface of the lamina.

The exact chemical nature of the basement membranes has not been determined and, as one might suspect, numerous conflicting observations have been reported. Pierce (1966) reported that the basement membrane of the mammal is synthesized by epithelia; collagen need not be considered an integral part of the basement membrane of embryonic epithelia because this membrane is formed in the absence of collagen. Other workers observed that carbohydrate moieties in the basement membrane differ from those associated with collagen (Murkerjee *et al.*, 1965). In contrast, Revel and Hay (1963) considered epithelia to synthesize the collagenous material incorporated in amphibian adepidermal membranes. Lazarow and Speidel (1964) concluded that collagen is the major protein in glomerular basement membrane, and other studies formed comparable conclusions for the lens capsule (Dische, 1964).

P. Weiss and Ferris (1956) proposed that the basement membrane functions as a catalyst for polymerization of tropocollagen into fibrils. Kallman and Grobstein (1965, 1966) postulated from *in vitro* studies that tropocollagen units polymerize into collagen fibrils at the undersurface of the epithelial basal lamina. The precise role of epithelium or the basal lamina in collagen fibrilogenesis, however, is as yet unknown.

A variety of evidence has led to the interpretation that epithelial cells exhibit a pattern of differential adhesiveness of their basement lamina reflecting the glycosaminoglycans composition (Okazaki *et al.*, 1962; Kallman and Grobstein, 1966; Slavkin and Bavetta, 1968a). The mesenchymal cells with their extended cell processes "wander" over the substratum until selectively "trapped" by an area of high specific adhesiveness (see Fig. 4). It is suggested that the surface properties of the basement lamina, or extracellular matrix materials interposed between interacting dissimilar cell populations, may act as a template for the positioning and differentiation of cells (Dan, 1960; Gustafson and Wolpert, 1963).

C. EXTRACELLULAR MICROFIBRILS

Extracellular microfibrils appear to occupy a key role in the initial formation of the extracellular matrix during embryonic odontogenesis as well as in numerous other embryonic systems (Kallman and Grobstein, 1966; Kallman *et al.*, 1967; Low, 1968). That these fibrous protein–polysaccharide complexes originate solely in either heterotypic cell type is not known; morphological evidence is available to support either hypothesis (see Figs. 1, 2, 3, and 4). Other ultrastructural studies observed protein–polysaccharide filaments associated with the basal lamina of numerous types of epithelia (Fawcett, 1962; Pease, 1966; Kallman and Grobstein, 1966). The microfibrils appear to be involved in polymerization of collagen (Kallman and Grobstein, 1966) and the formation of elastin and reticulin (Greenlee *et al.*, 1966). These filaments could serve as "informational molecules" capable of supporting cell–cell communication. In this sense, communication represents the selective adhesive qualities of the undersurface of the basal lamina which could orient mesenchymal filopodia to specific sites by the nature of the polarity within a specific glycosamino-glycans complex (Slavkin and Bavetta, 1968a). It is significant that aggregations of microfibrils are attached to the basal lamina most frequently. Polymerized collagen units demonstrating an axial periodicity of 640 Å are repeatedly observed in association with the lamina. Collagen is repeatedly observed in locations peripheral to mesenchymal cells (Figs. 6 and 7); however, these fibrous macromolecules are an appreciable distance from the undersurface of the basal lamina during early stages of cell differentiation.

D. Morphogenetic Aspects of Collagen

The observed deposition of collagen at the interface during epithelial–mesenchymal interactions suggests a role for collagen in morphogenesis. It is much too simplistic to infer that collagen biosynthesis and secretion into the epithelial–mesenchymal interface is the function of the mesenchymal effect upon epithelium. The role of extracellular matrix collagen in secondary embryonic induction has been sought recently by J. Gross et al. (1963), Grobstein and Cohen (1965), Koningsberg and Hauschka (1965), Wessels and Cohen (1968), and Grillo et al., (1969).

Koningsberg studied the differentiation of clones of embryonic chick hindlimb muscle cells isolated by mild trypsinization. When muscle cells were grown on glass covered by a thin film of rat tendon collagen the muscle cells were able to continue to differentiate. When the muscle cells were grown in media conditioned with fibroblasts, they did not dedifferentiate but continued to develop. Kongingsberg concluded that the muscle cells were unable to differentiate in vitro unless the medium or substratum was conditioned by fibroblasts or collagen. It is significant to recall that embryonic inductions have often been studied using Millipore filters to separate heterotypic cell types involved in a given system. The pore size of the filters employed in these studies (see review by Grobstein, 1967) can easily accommodate the passage of collagen across the filter (Koningsberg and Hauschka, 1965). Kallman and Grobstein (1965) demonstrated that labeled proline material appears to traverse the filter from the mesenchymal tissue to the epithelial tissue (salivary gland and pancreas). Dodson (1967) had shown that epidermis does not differentiate in vitro; when grown upon a collagen substratum, in contrast, the epidermis differentiated. Such studies suggested, but were unable to demonstrate with direct data, that extracellular materials play critical roles in tissue interactions by determining the metabolic pattern that will occur in the induced tissues, enabling cells to retain metabolic products that they might otherwise deplete (Grobstein, 1967; Wessels and Cohen, 1968).

In vitro extracellular materials appear to influence tissue interactions or cellular differentiation. Is this the case *in vivo*? This is an extremely difficult question because methodology can create curious artifacts. *In vitro* systems use trypsinized cells, the result being the removal of the PAS-positive basal lamina associated with epithelium and other intercellular materials. Embryonic mammalian salivary gland epithelium does not incorporate labeled proline unless first trypsinized (Kallman and Grobstein, 1965). The incorporation of tritiated proline *in vitro* may merely be measuring the response of a "wounded" tissue synthesizing nascent tropocollagen in order to restore its plasma membrane and participate in the formation of the basal lamina.

Grobstein and Cohen (1965) showed that salivary epithelium, cultured for 48 hours in juxtaposition to salivary mesenchyme, develops to a certain stage. If this transfilter culture system is disassembled, and the epithelium treated with collagenase and thoroughly washed to remove the enzyme, the reassembled culture of collagenase-treated epithelium and untreated mesenchyme will not support the characteristic epithelial branching pattern seen in salivary gland morphogenesis. If the culture continues as the collagenase is metabolically depleted within the epithelium, a recovery of morphological contour is observed. If collagenase is maintained in the nutrient medium no advanced development is observed. These investigators implicated the loss of collagen by collagenase treatment in the retardation of epithelial–mesenchymal interactions during salivary gland morphogenesis.

More recently, analogous studies of cultured epithelia from embryonic lungs, ureteric buds, and pancreas pretreated with collagenase were reported (Wessels and Cohen, 1968). Lung morphogenesis stopped and ureteric buds lost their characteristic shape. If the mesoderm was recombined in cultures after collagenase treatment, lung development eventually continued and ureteric buds often showed the resumption of their shape. Pancreatic epithelia was unaffected by collagenase treatment and formed exocrine acini and differentiated cells in its presence. The results were interpreted by Wessels and Cohen (1968) to imply that collagen is an essential component of mesoderm which is transferred to epithelium in developmental systems in which epithelial branching occurs, but is not essential where acini are forming. Epithelial branching is correlated with a high mesodermal specificity which might stabilize epithelial morphology. There is no direct evidence to implicate collagen as an inducer in any epithelial–mesenchymal system.

The site of collagenase activity in an epithelial–mesenchymal interaction is the basal lamina. Collagenase is an excellent tool to separate epithelia from adjacent mesenchyme (for example, epidermis from dermis). Using the electron microscope, Kahl and Pearson (1967) studied the effects of injecting collagenase beneath epidermis. It is obvious that collagenase affects all collagenous constituents within the basal lamina and the collagen fibrils and fibers within the interface or extracellular matrix (see Kahl and Pearson, 1967 for a comprehensive discussion).

Grobstein and Cohen (1965) reported that lipase, elastase, EDTA ,and hyaluronidase failed to duplicate the morphogenetic effects of collagenase in transfilter studies of salivary gland. Is the stability of the basal lamina maintained by collagen, and, further, might this stability be crucial to subsequent heterotypic interactions? During transfilter experiments in which the homotypic tissue rudiments are first isolated by mild trypsinization, how long does it take for a new basal lamina to form? Or, if a new basal lamina does not form, does the interposed Millipore filter acquire the basic properties of the basal lamina and extracellular matrix (PAS-positive, microfilament, collagen, etc)? These questions are stated to promote experimental designs to further scrutinize the morphological interpretations so far presented. It should be recalled that it required 24–48 hours for trypsin-dissociated cells to reaggregate *in vitro*. In investigations studying reaggregation of epithelial–mesenchymal systems, reaggregation requires approximately 48 hours (see review by Grobstein, 1967). Reaggregation is well documented by the reappearance of the PAS-positive interface (see discussion of the significance of the PAS-positive interface by Slavkin and Bavetta, 1968a). In addition to searching for cell recognition factors or aggregation-enhancing factors, I urge that the effects of EDTA, collagenase, and trypsin be critically examined. It would appear extremely significant if the enzymes or chelating agents used in experimental embryological investigations were solely responsible for the reaggregation lag time, as opposed to the lag-reflecting properties intrinsic to development. Direct data are extremely difficult to obtain (see discussions by Kemp *et al.*, 1967; Barnard *et al.*, 1969).

V. The Extracellular Matrix Influences upon Cellular Differentiation

There are several important reasons for including considerations of the extracellular matrix and its influences upon cell differentiation. (1) During the history of experimental embryology, numerous significant roles have been associated with extracellular matrices during embryogenesis. (2) Recent investigations of such matrices in mammalian embryonic systems have ellicited new and exciting information quite relevant for the evaluation of contemporary molecular and developmental biologists as well as clinicians. Although the importance of "ground substance" in embryonic differentiation was described over 45 years ago (Baitsell, 1925), and although many embryologists accept the concepts of P. Weiss (1934; 1945; 1961) concerning the role of extracellular matrices and morphogenesis, little is known about the ecology of these matrices and which, if any individually, affects adjacent cellular development and organ formation.

Grobstein (1955) outlined an hypothesis for the function of extracellular matrices during embryonic induction. More recently Slavkin and Bavetta (1968a) discussed the relationships between tropocollagen and glycosaminoglycans in dentine collagen fibrillogenesis during embryonic tooth formation. P. Weiss (1945), Holtfreter (1948), Moscona (1968), Humphreys (1967), Rubin (1966), Urist (1969), Slavkin, (1970), Steinberg (1970), and many other investigators have all discussed the possible significance of outer cell surface materials and extracellular materials in the selective adhesion or contact inhibition between various embryonic cells. What do we know about extracellular matrices which might explain their roles in development? Further, what examples have been brought forth to illustrate direct influences of matrices upon cell differentiation? To answer such questions, it is not possible to cite all the pertinent investigations. My intention is to select examples which may prove highly instructive to illustrate aspects of the basic biological phenomena. In this discussion, ground substance designates the optically homogeneous viscous material which permeates the spaces between the various cells of the organism. Extracellular matrix includes the ground substance and, in addition, the fibrous proteins such as collagen and noncollagenous protein–mucopolysaccharide complexes.

A. Glycosaminoglycans and Cell Differentiation

The interface between epithelium and mesenchyme, the basement membrane in the light microscope, is formed by the confluence of materials derived from both epithelial and mesenchymal tissue components (Edds and Sweeny, 1960; Pierce et al., 1964; Pierce, 1966; Hay and Revel, 1963). Although not well characterized, the secretions of epithelium and mesenchyme, which comprise the extracellular interface (matrix), are composed of collagen, glycoproteins, and mucopolysaccharides. It is teleological to argue that all these constituents contribute to cell behavior. One aspect of cell differentiation, cell division, has been critically studied by Lippman (1968). Previously, reports have found that connective tissue extracts have both stimulatory (Takeuchi, 1966) and inhibitory (Parshley, 1965) effects on mitotic division. Lippman (1968) tested the influence of various molecules (hyaluronic acid, chondroitin-4-sulfate, chondroitin-6-sulfate, dermatan sulfate, heparatin sulfate, heparin and keratan sulfate) on mammalian cells and suggested, on the basis of her results, that cell differentiation may be controlled by the mesenchymal products of epithelial–mesenchymal interactions. She suggested that the metachromatic outer periphery around chondrocytes (free chondroitin sulfate) and the basement membrane to which both epithelium and mesenchyme contribute are critical sites where such control mechanisms may operate. Cell division could be inhibited or controlled at the G_2 level by the presence of glycosaminogycans acting as cation traps at the outer cell surface (Lippman, 1965). The implication that specific cell products, glycoproteins of epithelial secretions and polysaccharides and collagen of mesenchymal cells, may serve as feedback controls for cell division cycles is of extreme significance.

Before amplifying this hypothesis, I wish to digress to include the increasing literature on the presence of ribonucleic acid (RNA) and nucleotide intermediates (nucleotide sugars) as constituents of outer cell surface materials and extracellular matrices. RNA has been detected as a component of the outer cell surface of many mammalian cells (L. Weiss and Mayhew, 1966; 1967; Beierle, 1968; and see comments on cell periphery RNA by L. Weiss, 1968). These studies are compatible with direct analysis of isolated mammalian plasma membranes which also contain RNA (Warren and Glick, 1968). RNA has been isolated and partially characterized from the embryonic extracellular organic matrix interposed between rabbit epithelium and mesenchyme associated with tooth formation (Slavkin, et al., 1969a). It is not known whether the outer cell surface or extracellular matrix RNA is a unique species of RNA or whether it represents a degradative reflection of an intracellular species (e.g., chromosomal RNA, mRNA, rRNA, or tRNA). Neither is exclusive and both suggest that RNA could be transferred from one cell to another, mediated by the outer cell surface and extracellular matrix. An EDTA-extracted material from mammalian cells in tissue culture (normal baby hamster kidney cells and polyoma virus-transformed BHK cells) has been found to contain carbohydrate-rich materials in addition to a low molecular weight RNA (Allerton and Beierle, personal communication) at their outer surfaces. The phenol-extracted odontogenic extracellular matrix contains nucleotide sugars in addition to methylated RNA (Slavkin et al., 1970). Recently, a liporibonucleoprotein complex has been described as an integral component of mammalian cell plasma membranes; sucrose gradient ultracentrifugation indicates that 80% of the RNA corresponds to 10–12 S and 3.0–3.5 S RNA's (Davidova and Shapot, 1970). Studies in our laboratory indicate that embryonic tooth primordia synthesize in organ culture four discrete methylated RNA species (7 S, 5 S, 4 S, and 2 S) isolated from the extracellular matrix interposed between epithelia and mesenchyme (Slavkin, et al., 1970). The functional significance of these outer cell surface and extracellular matrix RNA molecules is that RNA could be exported and transferred by direct passage from cell to cell, analogous to the introduction of RNA-virus transformations in tissue culture cells. Numerous investigators have shown that exogenous RNA does enter mammalian cells and induces the subsequent synthesis of nascent protein molecules which reflect the phenotype of the exogenous RNA (Niu, 1963; Niu et al., 1961; Niu et al., 1968; Amos and Kearns, 1962; Amos and Moore, 1963; Amos, 1961; Ambrose, 1967; Michelazzi et al., 1965; and Thorp and Dray, 1968). It therefore seems most feasible to propose that if the outer cell surface RNA and extracellular matrix RNA described is informational, its transfer from one cell to another as a direct consequence of active cell migrations could result in its ingestion by the recipient cell with employment of its informational content in concert with the known steps of protein synthesis (see Fig. 8). Direct cell-to-cell transfer of information during development or neoplasia would be more economical in informational content than humoral transfer and would be deposited with great precision (Ambrose, 1967; Loewenstein, 1967).

Before returning to the hypothesis implicating glycosaminoglycans as critical controls of cell differentiation, it should be carefully noted that glucose is the most abundant and ubiquitous sugar found in nature, yet the distribution of glucose in mammalian cells is quite curious. With very rare exceptions, the hexose is not found in mammalian glycoproteins or mucopolysaccharides. It does occur, however, in glycolipids as the glycosyl residue closest to the lipid moiety, but does not occur in the distal parts of the heterosaccharide chains which extend into the aqueous environment.

Intercellular communication

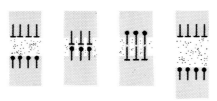

Fig. 8. Diagrammatic representation of intercellular communication between epithelia and mesenchyme during embryonic induction. Tight intercellular junctions at the cellular level or the exchange of microfibrils at the molecular level could easily mediate the transfer of developmental information between cells.

Presumably all mammalian cells have a carbohydrate-rich outer cell surface as demonstrated by the PAS staining reaction, the colloidal iron staining technique (Rambourg *et al.*, 1966), the Hale stain reaction (as exemplified in studies with ascites tumor cells by Gasic and Gasic, 1962), as well as by phosphotungstic acid (PTA) staining (Pease, 1966). Further, it has become axiomatic that trypsinization of mammalian cells removes the PAS-positive staining reaction and removes the basal lamina in association with epithelia. Carbohydrate material is released by trypsin, suggesting that the carbohydrate-bound material is in association with protein, and obviously accessible to the enzyme by being at the outer cell surface. At this point, one must caution in evaluation of the carboyhdrate released by mild trypsinization, for the liberation of sugars by this procedure is probably incomplete. It is interesting to note here that in studies of polysaccharide synthesis in various embryonic tissues, the polysaccharides will not migrate unless first digested with Pronase, indicating that the polysaccharide(s) were complexed with protein (see review by Lash, 1968). The function of carbohydrates or polymers of carbohydrates on the outer cell surface is not known. One attractive hypothesis (Shen and Ginsburg, 1968) is that they function as recognition cites for cellular interactions by forming highly specific structures recognized by complementary sites on other cells or macromolecules. A comparable suggestion was made to explain odontogenic cell-to-cell interactions (Slavkin and Bavetta, 1968a) and to explain collagen fibrillogenesis at the basal lamina (Kallman and Grobstein, 1966). The carbohydrates have significant informational value in that four different monosaccharides forming heterosaccharides can be arranged in many more combinations than can twenty amino acids in a polypeptide of comparable size (Shen and Ginsburg, 1968). Diversity and specificity can further be explained for carbohydrate material if one takes into account that monosaccharides can be linked to one another through any one of several hydroxyl groups by α- or β-glycosidic bonds and, in addition, that extensive branching is possible and commonly observed. The peculiar absence of glucose in mammalian outer cell surfaces is a finding compatible with the proposal that the glycosaminoglycans at the surface serve as recognition sites for cell interactions (Slavkin, 1970). If the polysaccharides are recognition sites at the cell surface, free glucose of the body fluids would inhibit the "recognition" of specific structures composed of glycosyl residues analogous to haptenes interfering with antigen–antibody interactions (Shen and Ginsburg, 1968; Gesner and Ginsburg, 1964).

Acknowledging the potential information in carbohydrate molecules serving as constituents of the outer cell surface and extracellular matrices, it is pertinent to examine briefly the metabolic pathways for glycoproteins, glycosaminoglycans, and nucleic acids. All three require nucleotide components in their respective biosynthesis. Aspects of the feedback inhibition have been presented for several systems (Kornfeld *et al.*, 1964; see review by Blakley and Vitols, 1968). In all cases in which the first step in biosynthesis is inhibited by the final product, a temporary accumulation of nucleotide sugars is to be expected (Ginsburg, 1964; Lippman, 1968). If this type of accumulation occurs, we must expect a shift in the utilization of the nucleotide sugar which could easily divert the pathways of polysaccharides to form intermediate RNA precursors, DNA precursors, or glycoproteins. These need not be considered totally exclusive of one another, and certain common pathways could profoundly affect two dissimilar end products. The importance of the regulation of the nucleotide pool's growth and utilization has been discussed (Mandel, 1964; Blakley and Vitols, 1968). Bucher and Swaffield (1966) have shown that 50% of the labeled uridine phosphates are located in the nucleotide sugars 16 minutes following the injection of ^{14}C-labeled orotic acid in early regenerating rat liver. Such experiments suggest that the nucleotide sugars draw substantially upon the UTP, UDP, and UMP.

It has been hypothesized by Lippman (1968) that when the synthesis of polysaccharides reaches a critical level, polysaccharide synthesis is inhibited and the nucleotide sugar pool increases signals to utilize the excess in different metabolic pathways; perhaps DNA. During the S period new polysaccharides are not produced to an appreciable extent. The hypothesis put forth by Lippman (1968) considers the G_2 phase of mitosis as the period required for the catabolism of existing outer cell surface glycosaminoglycans which would activate a permeability shift and calcium influx associated with the initiation of prophase. As a result of mitosis both the glycosaminoglycans and nucleic acids are again reduced and the cycle begins at G_1 anew. As long as nucleotide intermediates are being utilized in RNA and carbohydrate synthesis; for example, during rapid protein synthesis associated with extracellular organic matrix formation (cartilage, dentine, bone, corenea, wound healing), the availability of these nucleotide sugar pools for DNA synthesis is limited or inhibited. Those cells involved in chondrogenesis, dentinogenesis, osteogenesis, and wound healing (chondroblasts, odontoblasts, osteoblasts, and fibroblasts) do not demonstrate rapid cell division. In rapidly dividing, less specialized cell populations one should expect that normal feedback inhibition or allosteric inhibition turns off synthesis of carbohydrate polymers and turns on DNA synthesis. Experimentation on specific nucleotide intermediates should be pursued to characterize several basic conditions for cell differentiation in mammalian cells.

B. THE EXTRACELLULAR MATRIX: AN INDUCTIVE SUBSTRATUM

A unique capacity of several mammalian tissues, extracellular matrices such as bone and dentine, is to interact with "competent" cells for growth, remodeling, and repair. By competence it is meant that a cell possesses an intrinsic ability to interact with its environment and subsequently differentiate or modulate to another level of activity. The ability of a cell population to renew intracellular components and alter its synthetic activities for transfer or export is often considered to be an embryonic propensity for cellular interactions and cellular differentiation. It has repeatedly been shown that even embryonic cells in tissue culture as homotypic cell suspensions or monolayers fail to develop; they dedifferentiate. In epidermal-like organogenesis (epithelial–mesenchymal interactions), both cell or tissue types are essential for development. In this section a curious aspect of development is to be briefly outlined. Succinctly, it is possible for a homotypic cell population to differentiate in the presence of an inductive substratum. An inductive substratum is an extracellular organic matrix, presumably free of included cells, which can provide those "factors" essential for inducing a cell population to differentiate into specialized cells. Several examples of such phenomena are in the literature (see a comprehensive review of inductive substratum by Urist, 1969). Neither the character of these inductive substrata nor the time of transmission of the inductive activity is understood.

An additional observation of induction by an extracellular organic matrix is briefly described because it is the resultant of epithelial–mesenchymal interactions, represents a basement membrane which has developed, and has been shown to influence odontogenic epithelial and mesenchymal cells, as well as dermal fibroblasts, to differentiate as homotypic cell suspensions grafted to the chick CAM (Slavkin et al., 1969b).

Recently, Koch (1967) demonstrated that embryonic rodent incisor development could be studied by enzymatic separation of epithelial and mesenchymal tissues and placement of tissue isolates in juxtaposition on a Millipore filter. As in other epidermal organ developments, heterotypic tissues in juxtaposition developed; homotypic tissues in recombination did not differentiate. Our laboratory recently illustrated similar interdependencies between epithelium and mesenchyme from embryonic rabbit incisors. Isolated cervical loop tissues (Slavkin and Bavetta, 1968b) or cell isolates (Slavkin et al., 1968b) in recombination on the chick chorioallantoic membrane (CAM) generated an entire tooth germ in vitro; a PAS-positive basement membrane or extracellular matrix between heterotypic cells was generated by 48 hours. In situ a basement membrane between epithelium and adjacent undifferentiated mesenchyme separates the two principal tissues during odontogenesis.

As the basement membrane thickens (0.1–4.0 μ), increasing numbers of mesenchymal cells within the dental papilla mesenchymal cell population migrate and condense toward the basement membrane (Slavkin et al., 1969b).

It is curious that only cells in intimate association with the basement membrane advance cell differentiation. This led to the suggestion that the selective migration of epithelial and mesenchymal cells toward one another and subsequent differentiation to columnar protein secretory-type cells were mediated by properties intrinsic to the extracellular matrix, surface properties of the cells, or both. Since the elegant work of Holtfreter (1948) and P. Weiss (1950), it appeared increasingly apparent that the mechanism(s) of regulation and control of cell movements and differentiation could be sought in the surface properties of cells or their respective substratum.

Light microscopic observations of serial sections representative of 24- to 26-day embryonic maxillary and mandibular incisor tooth germs showed the basement membrane, associated with the oral epithelial cells, to be a continuous interface between invaginating tooth progenitor epithelial and adjacent mesenchymal cells. Histological stains employed in these studies showed that dentinogenesis preceded amelogenesis. The PAS-

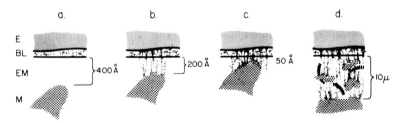

FIG. 9. An illustration summarizing electron microscopic observations of the interface during progressive cellular differentiation in embryonic rabbit odontogenesis. (a) During early epithelial–mesenchymal interactions the extended cell process of the mesenchymal cell (M) extends into the extracellular matrix region (EM), but does not approximate the basal lamina (BL) in association with the epithelia (E). (b) As both cell types differentiate, microfibrils are observed on the undersurface of the basal lamina and on the outer cell surface of the leading edge of the mesenchymal cell process; the heterotypic cells approximate one another. (c) Often very close relationships are observed in situ during cell interaction. (d) Subsequently, the extracellular matrix also differentiates and the apparent distance between heterotypic cells is greatly increased; membrane-bound cellular material is repeatedly observed in the forming extracellular organic matrix (dentine).

positive basement membrane in the cervical loop region, interposed between dental papilla and inner enamel epithelia, was the progenitor material for the subsequent formation of the dentine organic matrix.

In vivo, the cervical matrix represents an increasingly heterogeneous
interface between mesodermally derived odontoblasts and ectodermally
derived ameloblasts; both cell types contribute to the formation of the
extracellular matrix (Gaunt and Miles, 1967). Therefore, the metachromatic interface interposed between epithelial and mesenchymal secretory-
type cells possesses two functional surfaces: an epithelial surface and a
mesenchymal surface (see Fig. 9). The observations reported in these experiments of specific cellular aggregation and differentiation suggested that
properties of the matrix enhanced these phenomena. The surface of the
matrix material which was in contact with those cells demonstrating differentiation was of mesenchymal origin (Slavkin *et al.*, 1969c); the surface

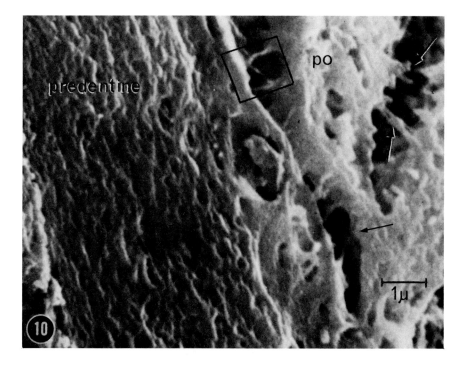

FIG. 10. A stereoscan electron photomicrograph of a 5-μ thick histological section
showing the relationships between (arrow) mesodermally derived preodontoblasts (po)
and the extracellular matrix (predentine) interposed between this type of epithelial–
mesenchymal interacting system. The enclosed area (rectangle) is enlarged in Fig. 11.
12,800 ×.

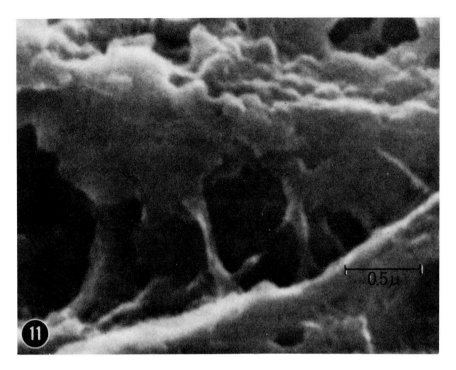

Fig. 11. This stereoscan electron photomicrograph is able to resolve the numerous cytoplasmic processes which extend into the extracellular matrix. 41,100 ×.

facing the odontoblast progenitor cells *in situ* (see Figs. 10 and 11). This factor may be considered crucial although additional information appears necessary. We assumed the matrix constituents were representative of both epithelial and mesenchymal synthetic exports (Slavkin *et al.*, 1968a).

The fine structure of the cervical matrix must be evaluated in terms of the inclusions noted (Slavkin *et al.*, 1969c). Although cells per se were not observed within the microdissected cervical matrix, membrane-bound bodies were noted (see Fig. 12). Such inclusions could be directly responsible for the inductive behavior of the matrix. Other electron microscopic studies of the progenitor extracellular matrix associated with dentinogenesis (Takuma, 1967) have demonstrated cell processes within this material. During embryonic odontogenesis, Pannese (1962) and Reith (1967) found that the basal lamina which separates the epithelial cells from the connective tissue elements (extracellular matrix) is disrupted and penetrated by epithelial microvilli. It was implied that the microvilli may be structural devices engaged in the exchange of developmental information.

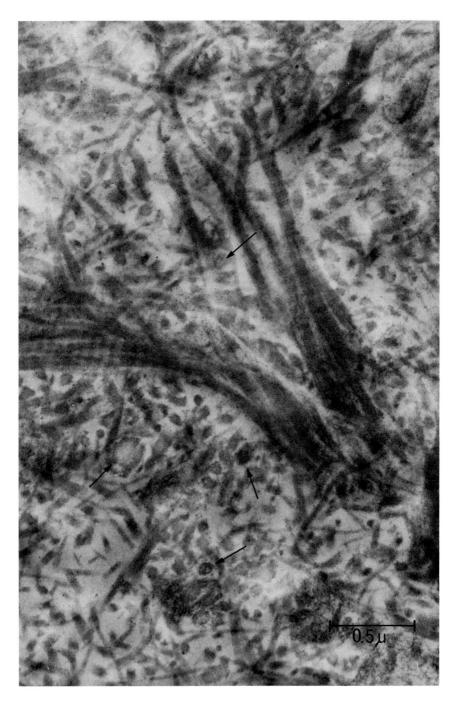

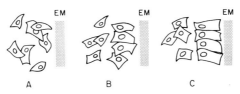

FIG. 13. The extracellular organic matrix (EM) (10 μ thick) associated with embryonic odontogenic epithelial–mesenchymal interactions, is found to be an inductive substratum. This diagram illustrates the temporal events (A–C) in which homotypic cell suspensions (tooth epithelium, tooth mesenchyme, and skin dermal fibroblasts), inoculated within the perimeter of the isolated cervical matrix, selectively aggregate and align at the surface of the substratum. Previously, homotypic cell suspensions did not differentiate *in vitro*. In these studies the cell suspensions, spherical in shape after mild trypsinization, become tall columnar cells with a PAS-positive secretory product when in juxtaposition to the extracellular matrix substratum.

During the 10-day culture period, cervical loop epithelial and mesenchymal cells and dermal fibroblasts migrated in contact with the extracellular matrix material, aligned and subsequently differentiated as columnar protein secretory-type cells (see Fig. 13). Skin epidermal cells did not differentiate when combined with the matrix. It was concluded that the cervical matrix, a semisolid fibrous extracellular material, possesses a morphogenetic property capable of inducing epithelial or mesenchymal cells to differentiate analogous to embryonic odontogenesis *in situ*. The fractionation of the matrix material and subsequent assays of the various fractions for biological activity appear essential prior to such conclusions. The isolation and characterization of an extracellular matrix RNA within this substratum (Slavkin *et al.*, 1969) and the inclusion of nucleotide sugars in the cervical matrix provide fractions to be tested *in vitro*.

C. OBSERVATIONS OF THE COLLAGEN AND NONCOLLAGENOUS PROTEIN COMPLEXES: CORNEA

In recent years numerous investigators have suggested that the sulfated protein–polysaccharide complexes of connective tissue are directly associated with collagen fibrils (Heringa *et al.*, 1956; Balazs, 1965; Meyer, 1966; Schubert, 1966). More recently morphological evidence has been

FIG. 12. During the formation of an extracellular organic matrix, in this case predentine, numerous and varied forms of collagen fibrils and fibers are noted. In addition to the collagenous constitutnets (36% on a dry weight basis), 64% of the total protein in the embryonic rabbit cervical organic matrix is noncollagenous. The matrix also contains various membrane-bound objects which may be derived by the merocine type of tropocollagen secretion (arrows). The section is stained with lead citrate and uranyl acetate. 46,800 ×.

presented demonstrating such associations in cartilage (Smith *et al.*, 1967; Smith and Serafini-Francessini, 1968). With specific reference to the cornea, Balazs (1965) postulated on the basis of anatomical and physiological properties of the corneal stroma that "the interfibrillar glycosaminoglycan matrix is not a random structure filling the space between collagen fibers, but, rather, a well-defined, complex molecular chain system providing rigid bridges between the fibers and thereby being responsible for the maintenance of the regular array of collagen fibers." Recently, Smith and Frame (1969) showed that the ground substance filaments in Araldite sections conform with Balazs' concept of the disposition of the corneal glycosaminoglycans and display the orthogonal association with the collagen fibrils postulated earlier by Meyer (1966). What might these ground substance filaments be?

In the absence of direct chemical data, Smith and Frame (1969) found it reasonable to consider these ground substance filaments as corneal noncollagenous protein-polysaccharide. Such an interpretation seems quite reasonable in considering some biochemical data. The hexosamine content of rabbit corneal stroma is 1.5% of the dry weight (Anseth, 1961). The glycosaminoglycan, identified by Meyer *et al.* (1953) as keratan sulfate, accounts for 50–60% of the total polysaccharides (Anseth and Laurent, 1961). The galactosaminoglycans are chondroitin sulfates in which the hexosamine/sulfur ratio varies from 0.25 to 0.64 (Anseth and Laurent, 1961). The poorly sulfated moiety, described by Davidson and Meyer (1954) as chondroitin, and the more highly sulfated moiety of chondroitin-4-sulfate are present in equal amounts.

It seems reasonable to conclude that all the sulfated polysaccharides of the corneal stroma are, *in situ*, covalently bound to noncollagenous protein. If the extracellular matrix is first treated with proteolytic enzymes the protein chains are split and one or more polysaccharide chains are left, attached to the peptides (Meyer, 1966). Such residual peptides are constant features of the corneal polysaccharides examined by Mathews and Cifonelli (1965) and Seno *et al.* (1965). Earlier evidence presented by Woodin (1954) showed the corneal protein–polysaccharide complex to contain 42% noncollagenous protein; more recently Kern and Brassil (1967) suggested that two distinct complexes exist: one containing the keratan sulfate and the other the galactosaminoglycans. The functional significance of these relationships are, as yet, evasive.

D. Tropocollagen, Fibrils, and Fibers

Collagen fibers are made by ordering tropocollagen molecules and fibrils. When such cross linkages are formed *in vivo* is not known (Piez, 1968).

It should be emphasized that most of our knowledge of collagen fibrillogenesis has been obtained from *in vitro* studies, often in nonphysiological conditions. Theoretically, cross linkages are not required to produce fibrous precipitates. An attractive interaction of some type between molecules is not necessary, nor is it required in theoretical considerations of fiber precipitates because ordering of fibrous molecules results directly from a change in entropy in a closed system. Calculations, however, show that fibrous ordering occurs (can occur) at almost all concentrations of solute when there is high intermolecular attraction. Ordering will occur when there is negative interaction or repulsion, but occurs over a narrower concentration range. Collagen fibrils and fibers, therefore, can be considered as the resultant of a simple statistical mechanism which depends only upon molecular asymmetry.

Tropocollagen molecules, shown to be synthesized (see review of collagen biosynthesis by Gould, 1968; Chvapil and Hurych, 1968) in fibroblasts or fibroblast-like cell populations (osteoblasts, odontoblasts, chondroblast), can be isolated by dissolving native collagen fibers in cold neutral salt solutions and can be reassembled in an analogous ordered phase by raising the temperature or by dialyzing out the salt (see recent review of connective tissue research edited by Hall, 1968). A variety of agents have been shown to prevent fiber formation in very low concentrations (arginine, aspartic and glutamic acids, and guanidine, just to mention a few). Interfibrillar attraction is, therefore, sensitively related to substances in the solution phase, particularly those which alter the charge or electrical interaction of fibers. Perhaps fiber–fiber bonds (intermolecular bonding) form in collagen fiber formation as a result of displacement of water bonds at somewhat elevated temperatures. Indeed, the mechanism of fiber formation from soluble precursor is related to the intramolecular structure of tropocollagen. Subtle variations in temperature conceivably will change the solute–solvent interaction and, therefore, influence the distribution of material between these two forms (based upon the speculations of Fessler, 1960). Studies of collagen in various media clearly show that the rate regulation of collagen fiber formation is dependent, at least in part, on the solution environment. The relative rate of fiber precipitation is diminished by increasing the ionic strength of the environment.

Electron microscopic studies of fibril formation have agreed with biophysical studies. Both have shown that large fibril formation (determined by measurements of the diameter) are favored by precipitation at low temperatures and pH, but high ionic strength at neutral pH also causes large fibers to form. Fiber formation *in vitro* from solutions of tropocollagen have suggested many ways in which molecules interact and become firmly attached (Piez, 1968). Those forces shown to have influence *in vitro*

should also participate during *in vivo* collagen fibrillogenesis. Direct correlation of fibrillogenesis in developing tissues has rarely been made. Contemporary considerations appear to confirm that the sequence of events
attending fibrillogenesis *in vivo* does not contradict predictions derived from
the kinetic mechanism of *in vitro* fiber formation (see Elden for review,
1968).

Collagen fibers in tissues grow to a much greater width than those
developed *in vitro*. Membranes associated with connective tissue contain
fibrils whose diameters range from 300–800 Å. Very small microfibrils
have been observed in spaces between fibrils, while larger ones (0.2–0.9 μ)
have also been seen (Fig. 12). The longitudinal periodicity of fibrils range
from 500 to 800 Å. Attempts to categorize collagen fibers into groups based
upon diameter, morphology, and time elapsed since initial formation have
suggested that primary fibrils, 100–200 Å in width, do not possess the
characteristic regular cross bands of collagen (640 Å spacing). Large fibers
are made up by accretion of primary fibrils vis-a-vis mature fibrils (300–
500 Å), which together form enlarged fibers (see Wasserman, 1954). In
addition to this lateral growth, fibers are believed to form by longitudinal
accretion. Such evidence supports the concept of fibrillogenesis in which
tropocollagen molecules are added stepwise to a growing lattice.

It is most important at this point to acknowledge that within the diameter of a collagen fiber, the arrangement of fibril components is not sym-
metrical. Small diameter fibrils are repeatedly observed within larger
fibrils.

In discussing tropocollagen assembly into collagen fibers, it is my intention to introduce the concepts obtained from *in vitro* analyses in order to
complement the *in situ* observations of collagen in developing systems.
The various morphological observations of embryonic epithelial–mesenchymal interactions have stressed that unknown molecular features,
differences, or complementarities and distribution patterns on the outer
cell surface and in the extracellular matrix are responsible for differential
cell adhesiveness, cell recognition, preferential cell affinities, cell migration,
and preferential paths of migration. This is a simplistic approach to a very
complex problem which, admittedly, must draw upon information from a
broad range of scientific fields. In this context, a model of interactions
between intercellular mucopolysaccharides and collagen is of extreme
interest (Mathews, 1965). This interest emerges from the assumption
that structural and physiological consequences of interactions between
various tissues and outer cell surfaces and extracellular matrices may be
of primary significance to the ordering of cells (histogenesis) and, thereby,
the organization of tissues into developmental patterns which generate an
organism (Grobstein, 1967; Thorp and Dorfman, 1967). Other develop-

mental aspects of the significance of "ectobiology" have been discussed by Kalckar (1965). I also refer the reader to Lippman's hypothesis concerning the effect of nucleotide pool feedback on cell differentiation (1968) and the theoretical considerations of Heinmets (1968), which concern the mechanisms of cell recognition based upon outer cell surface materials and the possible feedback mechanisms of cell differentiation mediated by products within the extracellular matrix.

The type of interaction phenomena that characterize mixtures of soluble collagen and acid mucopolysaccharides has also been widely reported for mixtures of many proteins and anionic polyelectrolytes (see discussion by Mathews, 1968). Our current knowledge of collagen structure (Rich and Crick, 1961) and of the main chemical and structural features of native chondroitin sulfate–protein (CS–protein) macromolecules in connective tissue (see review by Mathews, 1968) provides a basis for speculation as to the possible biological significance of the various *in vitro* experimental results.

One aspect of molecular organization of connective tissue, specifically those specialized connective tissues which become extracellular organic matrices and subsequently mineralize (bone, dentine, cartilage), is the interaction between newly synthesized tropocollagen and a basic unit of CS–protein macromolecules. The basic unit of CS–protein macromolecule in cartilage consists of a 4000-Å long protein core to which sixty 1000-Å long chondroitin sulfate chains (molecular weight ca. 50,000) are covalently linked. The chondroitin sulfate side chains are aligned along the axis of the collagen fibril (Mathews, 1968). In a dilute solution, the requirement of the chondroitin sulfate moieties will lead to maximum opportunities for interaction under conditions in which the protein core of the CS–protein molecule is also aligned parallel to the collagen fibrils (Mathews, 1968). Accretion of collagen fibrils to make fibers and accretion of CS–protein with collagen fibrils would provide for additional growth of the extracellular matrix. Additional noncollagenous proteins other than the CS–protein molecule can also become involved and give further growth as well as variations in a matrix (see observations by Slavkin *et al.*, 1968a). The character of all the interactions will depend upon the type of tissues synthesizing these macromolecules, the stage of development, the species of the organism and the qualitative and quantitative aspects of the carbohydrate material and the protein molecules. Matrices might be characterized by the number of noncollagenous polypeptides, the relative ratio of mucopolysaccharide/protein, the kinds of glycosaminoglycans present, the number of covalent bonds established, etc. These values will greatly affect the properties of the extracellular matrix. For example, a low degree of interactions between collagen and CS–protein will determine the loss of mucopolysaccharides by diffusion from the tissue and the likelihood of subsequent mineralization. Since hyaluronic acid does not link with protein normally; as a side chain component its capacity for linkage with protein is much less than that of CS–protein. It is not surprising to find that hyaluronic acid is the major mucopolysaccharide in highly hydrated and semifluid connective tissues (vitreous humor, synovial fluid, and Wharton's jelly). These assumptions may prove to be false or insignificant with time: however, they provide a contemporary biologist with a point of departure into experimentation.

E. Problems in Extracellular Matrix Protein Patterning: Self-Assembly

One of the most puzzling and interesting aspects of collagen deposition is the geometric ordering shown by fibrils or bundles of fibrils in a variety of locations in vertebrates [cornea, dentine, bone, cartilage, basement lamella (membrane), and tendon] (see Figs. 6, 7, and 12). In the geometric ordering shown by fibrils in the lamina propria and basement lamella, the fibrils often are disposed in layers with their long axes parallel in each layer but running at right angles to one another in adjacent layers. This orthogonal grid arrangement is well illustrated in the basement lamella of amphibian larvae (P. Weiss and Ferris, 1956). How might such a structure be achieved if collagen formation is completely an extracellular phenomenon?

Information transfer between tissues, cells, and molecules has occupied a great deal of contemporary biological thinking. Within the "dogma" that links DNA, RNA, and protein synthesis, and within the universality of the genetic code and colinearity between nucleotide and amino acid sequences, how a polypeptide chain is synthesized and released from the ribosome has been extensively considered. A polypeptide chain may contain an impressive amount of information; once the primary structure is established (amino acid sequence) the chain can take on higher configurations without further direction from the genome. Genetic control of primary structure determines secondary, tertiary, and even quaternary structure.

Several reviews have recently discussed the formation of collagen and other fibrous proteins and the possible role of "self-assembly" in the formation of these complex structures (C. Cohen, 1966a,b). There is now very little doubt that some structures in animal cells are formed by self-assembly of subunits.

Briefly stated, once information is given for specifying structural proteins, what more is needed to build recognizable cell structures? To make a cell organelle or a complex of protein mucopolysaccharides into an extra-cellular organic matrix, is information required beyond that which specifies the component molecules? Can such molecules spontaneously assemble into larger structures under "the proper environmental conditions"? The idea that larger structures can most efficiently be built up by a repetition of small ones is teleologically attractive. First, this concept reduces the amount of information required. Second, in building something that contains a large number of small subunits, whether considering the assembly of amino acids that go into a protein or the individual tropocollagen monomers that make up collagen fibers, there is much less chance of error if a subassembly system is used for the process. Most polymerization processes that form large structures are equilibrium processes tending to conform with the lowest free energy and do not involve covalent bond formation. That self-assembly occurs could be a guiding concept in current research on collagen structure.

Cohen (1966a,b) dealt with the structural role played by α-helices and superhelices made of more than one α-helix (the coiled-coil form). She suggested that this form is subjected to little conformational change and would confer stability on charged polypeptide chains in aqueous environments. This approach, therefore, is suitable for explaining the construction of stiff rods such as are found in collagen. It is well known that collagen can be isolated, dissolved into monomeric units, and reconstituted from solutions as fibrous material resembling, although not the same as, native collagen. The basic monomer, tropocollagen, consists of a three-chain coiled-coil, 2800 Å long and 15 Å wide, and has a molecular weight of ca. 300,000. The tropocollagen molecule may be considered to have a head and tail. When tropocollagen units are aggregated they do not critically align laterally; rather they overlap by a quarter of their length in successive layers. This appears to be responsible for the distinctive banding pattern of native collagen.

Unlike the generalization mentioned previously, tropocollagen molecules are composed of subunits held together by ester-like bonds. Petruska and Hodge (1964) suggested that formation of chains (polypeptides) by subunits of different lengths could provide a vernier mechanism which would determine the length of the assembled tropocollagen. According to this scheme, two of the chains in tropocollagen would each contain five subunits, and the third chain would contain seven slightly smaller subunits. Subsequently, subunits could be added until all chains had reached the same length. Inherent in all studies of the formation of native collagen fibrils from tropocollagen macromolecules is to disclose how macromolecules of approximately 2800 Å in length can combine to build fibrils with a period of approximately 640 Å.

Several critical aspects of this research should be considered. Is the amino acid sequence of mammalian tropocollagen macromolecules similar? If so, one might expect that the primary, secondary, tertiary, and quaternary structures of tropocollagen are similar. What then orders tropocollagen to assemble in such a way as to give 100% light transparency to the cornea, the orthogonal pattern to the basal lamella between epidermis and dermis, and the organic matrix properties to cartilage, bone, and dentine which allow for subsequent mineralization and calcification? Self-assembly does not adequately explain tropocollagen aggregation and subsequent extracellular matrix specificity. Collagen is not formed by simple quaternary associations of monomers. Covalent bonds definitely hold together the subunits of tropocollagen (see review by Piez, 1968). Furthermore, in the mammalian body native collagen possesses covalent cross links, apparently essential for elastic and tensile properties (Piez, 1968).

Studies on the control of cellular and extracellular form may be at a crossroads. Studies of simple systems have yielded great insights into what might be considered the rough determinants of form: The energetic and kinetic considerations which lead to the polymerization of large molecules, the kinds of designs which, being minimal energy states, are formed readily by self-assembly. Simple mechanisms, dependent only on the subunits themselves, may participate in collagen formation.

Students of biology interested in such questions must still account for the abundance of genetic information and still consider self-assembly. As cell complexity increases so does the super-abundance or redundancy of genetic material. The DNA content of *Escherichia coli* suggests that its genome contains enough information to code for 2800 different protein monomers. The DNA content of most eucaryotic cells is from 100 to 1000 times as great as that in bacteria. What is all this redundant information for? Indeed, a differentiated eucaryotic cell is not distinguished by the number of genes derepressed; rather, the size and structural complexity of synthetic capabilities, mitosis, meiosis, specialized organelles, intracellular compartmentalization, and extremely complicated interconnections with other cells of similar or dissimilar developmental origin characterize metazoan cellular differentiation. It remains to demonstrate the participation of genetic information and/or self-assembly in the generation of biological form and properties intrinsic to form.

ACKNOWLEDGMENTS

I wish to dedicate this contribution to Professor Lucien A. Bavetta, whose inspiration, friendship, and many contributions to the original work reported here have been invaluable. The author wishes to express his indebtedness to Drs. Allerton, Deshmukh, Petrushka and Schneir for reading the manuscript and for their many critical discussions.

I also wish to show my appreciation to Mssrs. P. Bringas, P. Flores, R. LeBaron, R. Selmont, and R. Croissant for their competent technical services and Mrs. Rory Dixon for typing the manuscript. The original work cited in this chapter has been supported by Research Grants DE-02848-02 and DE-0094-08 from the National Institute of Dental Research. The author is a recipient of a Research Career Development Award from the National Institute of Health (DE-41739-03).

REFERENCES

Abercrombie, M., and Ambrose, E. J. (1962). The surface properties of cancer cells: a review. *Cancer Res.* **22**, 525–548.

Abercrombie, M., and Heaysman, J. E. M. (1954). Observations on the social behavior of cells in tissue culture. II. Monolayering of fibroblasts. *Exp. Cell Res.* **6**, 293–306.

Allerton, S. E., Beierle, J. W., Power, D. R., and Bavetta, L. A. (1970). Abnormal extracellular components in Wilm's tumor. *Cancer Res.* **30**, 679–683.

Ambrose, E. J. (1967). Possible mechanisms of the transfer of information between small groups of cells. *In* "Cell Differentiation" (A. V. S. DeReuck and J. Knight, eds.), pp. 101–110. Little, Brown, Boston.

Amos, H. (1961). Protamine enhancement of RNA uptake by cultured chick cells. *Biochem. Biophys. Res. Commun.* **5**, 1–4.

Amos, H., and Kearns, K. E. (1962). Synthesis of bacterial protein by cultured chick cells. *Nature (London)* **195**, 806–808.

Amos, H., and Moore, M. O. (1963). Influence of bacterial ribonucleic acid on animal cells in culture. I. Stimulation of protein synthesis. *Exp. Cell Res.* **32**, 1–13.

Anseth, A. (1961). Studies on corneal polysaccharides III. Topographic and comparative biochemistry. *Exp. Eye Res.* **1**, 106–115.

Anseth, A., and Laurent, T. C. (1961). Studies on corneal polysaccharides. I. Separation. *Exp. Eye Res.* **1**, 25–38.

Baitsell, G. A. (1925). On the origin of the connective-tissue ground substance in the chick embryo. *Quart. J. Microsc. Sci.* **69**, 571–589.

Balazs, E. A. (1965). Amino sugar containing macromolecules in the tissues of the eye and ear. *In* "The Amino Sugars" (E. A. Balazs and R. W. Jeanloz, eds.), Vol. 2A. Academic Press, New York.

Barnard, P. J., Weiss, L., and Ratcliffe, T. (1969). Changes in the surface properties of embryonic chick neural retina cells after dissociation. *Exp. Cell Res.* **54**, 293–301.

Beierle, J. W. (1968). Cell proliferation: enhancement of extracts from cell surfaces of polyoma virus transformed cells. *Science* **161**, 798–799.

Benedetti, E. L., and Emmelot, P. (1967). Studies on plasma membranes. IV. The ultrastructural localization and content of sialic acid in plasma membranes isolated from rat liver and hepatoma. *J. Cell Sci.* **2**, 499–512.

Bernfield, M. R. (1970). Collagen synthesis during epitheliomesenchymal interactions. *Develop. Biol.* **22**, 213–231.

Blakley, R. L., and Vitols, E. (1968). The control of nucleotide biosynthesis. *In* "Annual Review of Biochemistry" (P. D. Boyer, ed.), pp. 201–224. Annual Reviews, Palo Alto, California.

Bucher, N., and Swaffield, M. (1966). Nucleotide pools and 6-^{14}C-orotic acid incorporation in early regenerating rat liver. *Biochem. Biophys. Acta* **129**, 445–459.

Carter, S. B. (1965). Principles of cell motility: the direction of cell movement and cancer invasion. *Nature (London)* **208**, 1183–1187.

Chvapil, M., and Hurych, J. (1968). Control of collagen biosynthesis. *In* "International Review of Connective Tissue Research" (D. A. Hall, ed.), pp. 68–196. Academic Press, New York.

Cohen, C. (1966a) Design and structure of fibrous proteins. *In* "Principles of Bimolecular Organization" (G. E. W. Wolstenholme and M. O'Connor, eds.), pp. 101–129. Churchill, London.

Cohen, C. (1966b). Architecture of the alpha-class of fibrous proteins. *In* "Molecular Architecture in Cell Physiology" (T. Hayashi and A. G. Szent-Gyorgyi, eds.), pp. 169–190. Prentice-Hall, Englewood Cliffs, New Jersey.

Cohen, S. (1965). Growth factors and morphogenetic induction. *In* "Developmental and Metabolic Control Mechanisms and Neoplasia" (The Anderson Tumor Institute, Univ. Texas Med. School, eds.), pp. 251–272. Williams and Wilkins, Baltimore, Maryland.

Cook, G. M. W., Heard, D. H., and Seaman, G. V. F. (1962). Electrokinetic characterization of Ehrlich's ascites carcinoma cells. *Exp. Cell. Res.* **28**, 27–29.

Curtis, A. S. G. (1961). Timing mechanisms in the specific adhesion of cells. *Exp. Cell Res. Suppl.* **8**, 107–122.

Curtis, A. S. G. (1964). The mechanism of adhesion of cells to glass: a study by interference reflection microscopy. *J. Cell Biol.* **20**, 199–215.

Curtis, A. S. G. (1966). Cell adhesion. *Sci. Progr. (London)* **54**, 61–86.

Dalton, A. J., and Haguenau, F. (1968). "The Membranes." Academic Press, New York.

Dan, K. (1960). Cyto-embryology of echinoderms and amphibia. *Int. Rev. Cytol.* **9**, 321–367.

Davidova, S. Ya., and Shapot, U. S. (1970). Liporibonucleoprotein complex as an integral part of animal cell plasma membranes. *Fed. Eur. Biol. Soc. Lett.* **6**, 349–351.

Davidson, E. A., and Meyer, K. (1954). Chondroitin, a new mucopolysaccharide. *J. Biol. Chem.* **211**, 605–611.

Davis, B. D., and Warren L. (1967). "The Specificity of Cell Surfaces." Prentice–Hall, Englewood Cliffs, New Jersey.

Defendi, V., and Gasic, G. (1963). Surface mucopolysaccharides of polyoma virus transformed cells. *J. Cell. Comp. Physiol.* **62**, 23–31.

DeHaan, R. L. (1963). Migration patterns of the precardiac mesoderm in the early chick embryo. *Exp. Cell Res.* **29**, 544–560.

Dische, Z. (1964). Glycans of the lens capsule—a model of basement membrane. *In* "Small Vessel Involvement in Diabets Mellitus" (M. D. Siperstein, A. R. Colwell, and K. Meyer, eds.). Amer. Inst. Biol. Sci., Washington, D. C.

Dodson, J. W. (1967). The differentiation of epidermis. II. Alternative pathways of differentiation of embryonic chick epidermis in organ culture. *J. Embryol. Exp. Morph.* **17**, 83–105.

Dulbecco, R. (1965). Interaction of viruses with the genetic material of the host cells. *In* "Reproduction: Molecular, Subcellular and Cellular" (M. Locke, ed.), pp. 95–106. Academic Press, New York.

Eagle, H., Piez, K. A., and Fleischman, R. F. (1957). The utilization of phenylalanine and tyrosine for protein synthesis by human cells in tissue culture. *J. Biol. Chem.* **228**, 847–861.

Eagle, H., Piez, K. A., Fleischman, R. F., and Lyama, V. T. (1959). Protein turnover in mammalian cell cultures. *J. Biol. Chem.* **234**, 592–597.

Ebert, J. D. (1965). "Interacting Systems in Development." Holt, New York.

Edds, M. V., and Sweeny, P. (1960). Chemical and morphological differentiation of the basement lamella. *In* "Molecular and Cellular Structure" (D. Rudnick, ed.), pp. 111–138, Ronald, New York.

Elden, H. R. (1968). Physical properties of collagen fibers. *In* "International Review o Connective Tissue Research" (D. A. Hall, ed.), pp. 283–348. Academic Press, New York.

Fawcett, D. W. (1962). Physiologically significant specializations of the cell surface. *Circulation* **26**, 1105–1125.

Fessler, J. H. (1960). Structural function of mucopolysaccharides in connective tissue. *Biochem. J.* **76**, 124–132.

Fleischmajer, R., and Billingham, R. E. (1968). "Epithelial–Mesenchymal Interactions." Williams and Wilkins, Baltimore, Maryland.

Galanti, N., and Gasic, G. (1967). Sobre la naturaleza del factór agregante de células de esponja (*Haliclona variabilis*). *Biologica* **40**, 28–38.

Garber, B., and Moscona, A. A. (1964). Aggregation *in vivo* of dissociated cells. I. Reconstruction of skin in the chorioallantoic membrane from suspensions of embryonic chick and mouse skin cells. *J. Exp. Zool.* **155**, 179–202.

Gasic, G., and Gasic, T. (1962). Removal and regeneration of the cell coating in tumor cells. *Nature (London)* **196**, 4850–4852.

Gaunt, W. A., and Miles, A. E. W. (1967). Fundamental aspects of tooth morphogenesis. *In* "Structural and Chemical Organization of Teeth" (A. E. W. Miles, ed.), Vol. I, pp. 151–198. Academic Press, New York.

Gesner, B. M., and Ginsburg, V. (1964). Effect of glycosidase on the fate of transfused lymphocytes. *Proc. Nat. Acad. Sci. U. S.* **52**, 750–755.

Ginsburg, V. (1964). Sugar nucleotides in carbohydrate synthesis. *Advan. Enzymol.* **26**, 35–38.

Goel, S. C., and Jurand, A. (1968). Electron microscopic observations on the basal lamina of chick limb buds after trypsin and EDTA treatment. *J. Cell Sci.* **3**, 373–380.

Gould, B. S. (1968). Collagen biosynthesis at the ribosomal level. *In* "International Review of Connective Tissue Research" (D. A. Hall, ed.), pp. 35–67. Academic Press, New York.

Greenlee, T. K., Ross, R., and Hartman, J. L. (1966). The fine structure of elastic fibers. *J. Cell Biol.* **30**, 59–71.

Grillo, H. C., McLeenan, J. E., and Wolfort, F. G. (1969). Activity and properties of collagenase from healing wounds in mammals. *In* "Repair and Regeneration" (J. E. Dunphy and H. W. Van Winkle, Jr., eds.), pp. 185–200. McGraw-Hill, New York.

Grobstein, C. (1955). Tissue interaction in the morphogenesis of mouse embryonic rudiments *in vitro*. *In* "Aspects of Synthesis and Order in Growth" (D. Rudnick, ed.), pp. 233–256. Princeton Univ. Press, Princeton, New Jersey.

Grobstein, C. (1956). Trans-filter induction in tubules in mouse metanephrogenic mesenchyme. *Exp. Cell Res.* **10**, 424–440.

Grobstein, C. (1961). Cell contact in relation to embryonic induction. *Exp. Cell. Res. Suppl.* **8**, 234–245.

Grobstein, C. (1967). Mechanism of organogenetic tissue interaction. *Nat. Cancer Inst. Monogr.* **26**, 279–299.

Grobstein, C. (1969). Epithelio-mesenchymal relations relevant to wound healing and regeneration. *In* "Repair and Regeneration" (J. E. Dunphy and H. W. Van Winkle, eds.), pp. 57–70. McGraw-Hill, New York.

Grobstein, C., and Cohen, J. H. (1965). Collagenase: effect of the morphogenesis of embryonic salivary epithelium *in vitro*. *Science* **150**, 626–628.

Gross, J., Lapiere, C. M., and Tanzer, M. L. (1963). Organization and disorganization of extracellular substances: the collagen system. *In* "Cytodifferentiation and Macromolecular Synthesis" (M. Locke, ed.), pp. 176–202. Academic Press, New York.

Gross, P. R. (1968). Biochemistry of differentiation. *In* "Annual Review of Biochemistry" (P. D. Boyer, ed.), pp. 631–660. Annual Reviews, Palo Alto, California.

Gustafson, T., and Wolpert, L. (1963). The cellular basis of morphogenesis in sea-urchin development. *Int. Rev. Cytol.* **15**, 139–214.

Hall, D. A., ed., (1968). "International Review of Connective Tissue Research." Academic Press, New York.

Harrison, R. G. (1914). The reaction of embryonic cells to solid structures. *J. Exp. Zool.* **4**, 239–281.

Hay, E. D., and Revel, J. P. (1963). Autoradiographic studies of the origin of the basement lamella in amblystoma. *Develop. Biol.* **7**, 152–168.

Hay, E. D., and Revel, J. P. (1969). "Fine Structure of the Developing Avian Cornea." Karger, Basel.

Heard, D. H., and Seaman, G. V. F. (1960). The influence of pH and ionic strength on the electrokinetic stability of the human erythrocyte membrane. *J. Gen. Physiol.* **43**, 635–654.

Heinmets, F. (1968). Cell–cell recognition and interaction. *Curr. Mod. Biol.* **1**, 299–313.

Heringa, G. C., Kroon, D. B., Ruyter, J. H. C., and Smits, G. (1956). Facts and ideas concerning the mucopolysaccharides of the connective tissues. *In* "Contemporary Rheumatology" (J. Goslings and H. van Swaay, eds.). Elsevier, Amsterdam.

Holtfreter, J. (1948). Concepts on the mechanism of embryonic induction and its relation to parthenogenesis and malignancy. *Symp. Soc. Exp. Biol.* **2**, 17–48.

Holtzer, H. (1963). Comments on induction during cell differentiation. *Coll. Ges. Physiol. Chem.* **13**, 128–143.

Holtzer, H. (1968). Induction of chondrogenesis: a concept in quest of mechanisms. *In* "Epithelial–Mesenchymal Interactions" (R. Fleischmajer and R. E. Billingham, eds.), pp. 152–164. Williams and Wilkins, Baltimore, Maryland.

Humphreys, T. (1963). Chemical dissolution and *in vitro* reconstruction of sponge cell adhesions. *Develop. Biol.* **8**, 27–47.

Humphreys, T. (1967). The cell surface and specific cell aggregation. *In* "The Specificity of Cell Surfaces" (B. D. Davis and L. Warren, eds.), pp. 195–210. Prentice-Hall, Englewood Cliffs, New Jersey.

Ito, S. (1965). The enteric surface coat on cat intestinal microvilli. *J. Cell Biol.* **27**, 475–491.

James, D. W. (1969). Wound remodelling. *In* "Repair and Regeneration" (J. E. Dunphy and H. W. Van Winkle, Jr., eds.), pp. 169–184. McGraw-Hill, New York.

Johnston, M. C. (1965). The neural crest in vertebrate cephalogenesis: a study of the migrations and derivatives. Univ. Rochester, Ph.D. thesis.

Kahl, F. R., and Pearson, R. W. (1967). Ultrastructural studies of experimental vesiculation. II. Collagenase. *J. Invest. Dermatol.* **49**, 616–631.

Kalckar, H. M. (1965). Galactose metabolism and cell "sociology." *Science* **150**, 385–413.

Kallman, F., and Grobstein, C. (1965). Source of collagen at epithelio-mesenchymal interfaces during inductive interaction. *Develop. Biol.* **11**, 169–183.

Kallman, F., and Grobstein, C. (1966). Localization of glucosamine-incorporating materials at epithelial surfaces during salivary gland epithelio-mesenchymal interaction *in vitro*. *Develop. Biol.* **14**, 52–67.

Kallman, F., Evans, J., and Wessel, N. W. (1967). Anchor filament bundles in embryonic feather germs and skin. *J. Cell Biol.* **32**, 236–240.

Kern, H. L., and Brassil, D. (1967). Fractionation of the mucoprotein of the bovine corneal stroma. *Arch. Biochem. Biophys.* **118**, 115–121.

Kemp. R. B., Jones, B. M., Cunningham, I., and James, M. C. M. (1967). Quantitative investigation on the effect of puromycin on the aggregation of trypsin- and versene-dissociated chick fibroblast cells. *J. Cell Sci.* **2**, 323–340.

Koch, W. E. (1967). *In vitro* differentiation of tooth rudiments of embryonic mice. I. Transfilter interaction of embryonic incisor tissues. *J. Exp. Zool.* **165**, 155–169.

Kollar, E. J., and Baird, G. R. (1969). The influence of the dental papilla on the development of tooth shape in embryonic mouse tooth germs. *J. Embryol. Exp. Morph.* **21**, 131–148.

Koningsberg, I. R., and Hauschka, S. D. (1965). Cell and tissue interactions in the reproduction of cell type. *In* "Reproduction: Molecular, Subcellular and Cellular" (M. Locke, ed.), pp. 243–290. Academic Press, New York.

Kornfeld, S., Kornfeld, R., Neufield, E., and O'Brien, P. (1964). The feedback control of sugar nucleotides biosynthesis in liver. *Proc. Nat. Acad. Sci. U. S.* **52**, 371–379.

Kraemer, P. M. (1966). Regeneration of sialic acid on the surface of Chinese hamster cells in culture. I. General characteristics of the replacement process. *J. Cell. Physiol.* **68**, 85–90.

Kuroda, Y. (1968). Preparation of an aggregation-promoting supernatant from embryonic chick liver cells. *Exp. Cell Res.* **49**, 626–637.

Lash, J. W. (1968). Chondrogenesis: genotypic and phenotypic expression. *J. Cell. Physiol. Suppl.* **72**, 35–46.

Lazarow, A., and Speidel E. (1964). The chemical composition of the glomerular basement membrane and its relationship to the production of diabetic complications. *In* "Small Vessel Involvement in Diabetes Mellitus" (M. D. Siperstein, A. R. Colwell, and K. Meyer, eds.). Am. Inst. Biol. Sci., Washington, D. C.

Levak-Svajger, B., and Moscona, A. A. (1964). Differentiation in grafts of aggregates of embryonic chick and mouse cells. *Exp. Cell. Res.* **36**, 692–695.

Levine, E. M., Becker, Y., Boone, C. W., and Eagle, H. (1965). Contact inhibition, macromolecular synthesis and polyribosomes in cultured human diploid fibroblasts. *Proc. Nat. Acad. Sci. U. S.* **53**, 350–356.

Lilien, J. E. (1968). Specific enhancement of cell aggregation *in vitro*. *Develop. Biol.* **17**, 657–678.

Lillien, J. E. (1969). Toward a molecular explanation for specific cell adhesion. *In* "Current Topics in Developmental Biology" (A. A. Moscona and A. Monroy, eds.), pp. 169–195. Academic Press, New York.

Lilien, J. E., and Moscona, A. A. (1967). Cell aggregation: its enhancement by a supernatant from cultures of homologous cells. *Science* **157**, 70–72.

Lippman, M. (1965). A proposed role for mucopolysaccharides in the initiation and control of cell division. *Trans. N. Y. Acad. Sci.* **27**, 342–360.

Lippman, M. (1968). Glycosaminoglycans and cell division. *In* "Epithelial–Mesenchymal Interactions" (R. Fleishmajer and R. E. Billingham, eds.), pp. 208–229. Williams and Wilkins, Baltimore, Maryland.

Locke, M. (1964). "Cellular Membranes iin Development." Academic Press, New York.

Loewenstein, W. R. (1967). On the genesis of cellular communication. *Develop. Biol.* **15**, 503–520.

Low, F. N. (1968). Extracellular connective tissue fibrils in the chick embryo. *Anat. Rec.* **160**, 93–108.

Mandel, P. (1964). Free nucleotides in animal tissues. *Progr. Nucl. Acid Res.* **3**, 299–334.

Mandelstam, J. (1960). The intracellular turnover of protein and nucleic acids and its role in biochemical differentiation. *Bacteriol. Rev.* **24**, 289–308.

Manson, L. A. (1968). "Biological Properties of the Mammalian Surface Membrane." Wistar Inst. Press, Philadelphia, Pennsylvania.

Marcus, P. I., and Schwartz, V. G. (1968). Monitoring molecules of the plasma membrane: renewal of sialic acid-terminating receptors. *In* "Biological Properties of the Mammalian Surface Membrane" (L. A. Manson, ed.), pp. 143–151. Wistar Inst. Press, Philadelphia, Pennsylvania.

Margoliash, E., Schenck, T. R., Hargie, M. P., Borokas, S., Richter, W. R., Barlow, G. H., and Moscona, A. A. (1965). Characterization of specific cell aggregating materials from sponge cells. *Biochem. Biophys. Res. Commun.* **20**, 383–388.

Mathews, M. B. (1965). The interaction of collagen and acid mucopolysaccharides. A model for connective tissue. *Biochem. J.* **96**, 710–716.

Mathews, M. B. (1968). The macromolecular organization of connective tissue. *In* "The Chemical Physiology of Mucopolysaccharides" (G. Quintarelli, ed.), pp. 189–198. Little, Brown, Boston, Massachusetts.

Mathews, M. B., and Cifonelli, J. A. (1965). Comparative biochemistry of keratosulphates. *J. Biol. Chem.* **240**, 4140–4145.

Meyer, K. (1966). Problems of the structure and chemistry of the mucopolysaccharides and mucoproteins of connective tissues. *In* "Biochimie et Physiologie du Tissu Conjonctif" (P. Comte, ed). Societe Ormeco, Lyon

Meyer, K., Linker, A., Davidson, E. A., and Weissmann, B. (1953). The mucopolysaccharides of bovine cornea. *J. Biol. Chem.* **205**, 611–616.

Michelazzi, L., Baldini, A., Novelli, A., and Nanni, G. (1965). Immune response induced by RNA-immuno-carrier extracted from heterologous immune sera. *Nature (London)* **205**, 194.

Moscona, A. A. (1961). Rotation-mediated histogenetic aggregation of dissociated cells. *Exp. Cell Res.* **22**, 455–475.

Moscona, A. A. (1962). Analysis of cell recombinations in experimental synthesis of tissues *in vitro. J. Cell. Comp. Physiol. Suppl.* **60**, 65–80.

Moscona, A. A. (1963). Studies of cell aggregation: demonstration of materials with selective cell binding activity. *Proc. Nat. Acad. Sci. U. S.* **49**, 742–747.

Moscona, A. A. (1968). Cell aggregation: properties of specific cell-ligands and their role in the formation of multicellular systems. *Develop. Biol.* **18**, 250–277.

Moscona, M. H., and Moscona, A. A. (1965). Control of differentiation in aggregates of embryonic skin cells: suppression of feather morphogenesis by cells from other tissues. *Develop. Biol.* **11**, 402–423.

Moscona, M. H., and Moscona, A. A. (1966). Inhibition of cell aggregation *in vitro* by puromycin. *Exp. Cell Res.* **41**, 703–706.

Mukerjee, H., Sri Ram, J., and Pierce, G. B. (1965). Basement membranes. V. Chemical composition of neoplastic basement membrane mucoprotein. *Amer. J. Pathol.* **46**, 49–58.

Niu, M. C. (1963) The mode of action of ribonuclei acid. *Develop. Biol.* **7**, 379–393.

Niu, M. C. Cordova, C. C., and Niu, L. C. (1961). Ribonucleic acid-induced changes in mammalian cells. *Proc. Nat. Acad. Sci. U. S.* **47**, 1689–1700.

Niu, M. C., Niu, L. C., and Guha, A. (1968). The entrance of exogenous RNA into the mouse ascites cell. *Proc. Soc. Exp. Biol. Med.* **128**, 550–555.

Okazaki, K., Fukuski, T., and Dan, K. (1962). Cyto-embryological studies of sea urchins. IV. Correlation between shape of ectodermal cells and the arrangement of the primary mesenchyme cells in sea urchin larvae. *Acta Embryol. Morphol. Exp.* **5**, 17.

Pannese, E. J. (1962). Observations on the ultrastructure of the enamel organ. III. Internal and external enamel epithelia. *J. Ultrastruct. Res.* **6**, 186–204.

Parshley, M. S. (1965). Effect of inhibitors from adult connective tissue on growth of a series of human tumore *in vitro. Cancer Res.* **25**, 387–401.

Peachey, L. D. (1968). "Conferences on Cellular Dynamics." New York Acad. Sci., New York.

Pease, D. C. (1966). Polysaccharides associated with the exterior surface of epithelial cells: kidney, intestine, brain. *J. Ultrastruct. Res.* **15**, 555–588.

Pethica, B. A. (1961). The physical chemistry of cell adhesion. *Exp. Cell Res. Suppl.* **8**, 123–140.

Petruska, J. A., and Hodge, A. J. (1964). A subunit model for the tropocollagen macro-molecule. *Proc. Nat. Acad. Sci. U. S.* **51**, 871–876.

Peirce, G. B. (1966). The development of basement membranes of the mouse embryo. *Develop. Biol.* **13**, 231–249.

Pierce. G. B., Beals, T. F., Ram, J. S., and Midgely, A. R. (1964). Basement membranes. IV. Epithelial origin and immunologic cross reactions. *Amer. J. Pathol.* **45**, 929–961.

Piez, K. A. (1968). Cross-linking of collagen and elastin. *In* "Annual Review of Bio-chemistry" (P. D. Boyer, ed.), pp. 547–570. Annual Reviews, Palo Alto, California.

Rambourg, A., and Leblond, C. P. (1967a). Staining of basement membranes and asso-ciated structures by the periodic acid-Schiff and periodic acid-silver methenamine techniques. *J. Ultrastruct. Res.* **20**, 306–309.

Rambourg, A., and Leblond, C. P. (1967b). Electron microscope observations on the carbohydrate-rich cell coat present at the surface of cells in the rat. *J. Cell Biol.* **32**, 27–53.

Rambourg, A., Neutra, M., and Leblond, C. P. (1966) Presence of a "cell coat" rich in carbohydrate at the surface of cells in the rat. *Anat. Rec.* **154**, 41–72.

Reith, E. J. (1967). The early stages of amelogenesis as observed in molar teeth of young rats. *J. Ultrastruct. Res.* **17**, 503–526.

Revel, J. P. (1964). A stain for the ultrastructural localization of acid mucopolysac-charides. *J. Microsc.* **3**, 535–544.

Revel, J. P., and Hay, E. D. (1963) Autoradiographic studies of the origin of the base-ment lamella. Ambystoma. *Develop. Biol.* **7**, 152–168.

Revel, J. P., and Ito, S. (1967). The surface components of cells. *In* "The Specificity of Cell Surfaces" (B. D. Davis and L. Warren, eds.), pp. 211–234. Prentice-Hall, Englewood Cliffs, New Jersey.

Rich, A., and Crick, F. H. C. (1961). The molecular structure of collagen. *J. Mol. Biol.* **3**, 483–506.

Robertson, J. D. (1964). Unit membranes: a review with recent new studies of ex-perimental alterations and a new subunit structure in synaptic membranes. *In* "Cellular Membranes in Development" (M. Locke, ed.), pp. 1–82. Academic Press, New York.

Rosenberg, M. D. (1962). Long range interactions between cell and substratum. *Proc. Nat. Acad. Sci. U. S.* **48**, 1342–1349.

Rosenberg, M. D. (1968). Interaction between artificial and natural membranes. *In* "Conferences on Cellular Dynamics" (L. D. Peachey, ed.), pp. 234–243. New York Acad. Sci., New York.

Rubin, H. (1966). Fact and theory about the cell surface in carcinogenesis. *In* "Major Problems in Developmental Biology" (M. Locke, ed.), pp. 317–340. Academic Press, New York.

Schubert, M. (1966). Structure of connective tissues, a chemical point of view. *Fed. Proc. Fed. Amer. Soc. Exp. Biol.* **25**, 1047–1052.

Seno, N., Meyer, K., Anderson, B., and Hoffman, P. (1965) Variations in keratosulphates. *J. Biol. Chem.* **240**, 1005–1010.

Shen, L., and Ginsburg, V. (1968). Release of sugars from HeLa cells by trypsin. *In* "Biological Properties of the Mammalian Surface Membrane" (L. A. Manson, ed.), pp. 67–71. Wistar Inst. Press, Philadelphia, Pennsylvania.

Sjostrand, F. S. (1967). "Electron Microscopy of Cells and Tissues: Instrumentation and Techniques," Vol. I. Academic Press, New York.

Slavkin, H. C. (1970). Cell aggregation: molecular specificity in outer cell surface materials. *Transpl. Proc.* **2**, 199–201.

Slavkin, H. C., and Bavetta, L. A. (1968a) Morphogenetic expressions during odontogenesis: a tool in developmental biology. *Clin. Orthop. Rel. Res.* **59**, 97–109.

Slavkin, H. C., and Bavetta, L. A. (1968b) Epithelio-mesenchymal interactions during embryonic odontogenesis. *J. Dent. Res.* **47**, 779–785.

Slavkin, H. C., LeBaron, R. D., Bringas, P., Bavetta, L. A. (1968a). Protein biosynthesis in embryonic odontogenic extracellular matrices. *Amer. Zool.* **8**, 788.

Slavkin, H. C., Beierle, J. W., and Bavetta, L. A. (1968b). Odontogenesis: cell–cell interactions *in vitro. Nature (London)* **217**, 269–270.

Slavkin, H. C., Bringas, P., and Bavetta, L. A. (1969a). Ribonucleic acid within the extracellular matrix during embryonic tooth formation. *J. Cell. Physiol.* **73**, 179–190.

Slavkin, H. C., Bringas, P., LeBaron, R. D., Cameron, J., and Bavetta, L. A. (1969b). The fine structure of the extracellular matrix during epithelio-mesenchymal interactions in the rabbit embryonic incisor. *Anat. Rec.* **165**, 237–255.

Slavkin, H. C., Bringas, P., Cameron, J. LeBaron, R., and Bavetta, L. A. (1969c). Epithelial and mesenchymal cell interactions with extracellular matrix material *in vitro. J. Embryol. Exp. Morphol.* **22**, 395–405.

Slavkin, H. C., Flores, P., Bringas, P., and Bavetta, L. A. (1970). Epithelial-mesenchymal interactions during odontogenesis. I. Isolation of several intercellular matrix low molecular weight methylated RNAs. *Develop. Biol.* **23**, 276–296.

Smith, J. W., and Frame, J. (1969). Observations on the collagen and protein-polysaccharide complex of rabbit corneal stroma. *J. Cell Sci.* **4**, 421–436.

Smith, J. W., and Serafini-Francassini, A. (1968). The distribution of the proteinpolysaccharide complex in the nucleus pulposus matrix in young rabbits. *J. Cell Sci.* **3**, 33–40.

Smith, J. W., Peters, T. J., and Serafini-Francassini, A. (1967). Observations on the distribution of the proteinpolysaccharide complex and collagen in bovine articular cartilage. *J. Cell Sci.* **2**, 129–136.

Steinberg, M. S. (1964). The problem of adhesive selectivity in cellular interactions. *In* "Cellular Membranes in Development" (M. Locke, ed.), pp. 321–366. Academic Press, New York.

Steinberg, M. S. (1970). Does differential adhesion govern self-assembly processes in histogenesis? Equilibrium configurations and the emergence of a hierarchy among populations of embryonic cells. *J. Exp. Zool.* **173**, 395–434.

Takeuchi, J. (1966). Growth promoting effect of acid mucopolysaccharides on Ehrlich ascites tumors. *Cancer Res.* **26**, 797–802.

Takuma, S. (1967). Ultrastructure of dentinogenesis. *In* "Structure and Chemical Organization of Teeth" (A. E. W. Miles, ed.), Vol. I, pp. 325–370. Academic Press, New York.

Tiedemann, H. (1967). Inducers and inhibitors of embryonic induction: their chemical nature and mechanism of action. *In* "Morphological and Biochemical Aspects of Cytodifferentiation" (E. Hagen, W. Wechsler, and P. Zilliken, eds.), pp. 8–21. Karger, Basel.

Tiedemann, H. (1968). Factors determining embryonic differentiation. *J. Cell. Physiol. Suppl.* **72,** 129–144.

Thorp, D. E., and S. Dray (1968). The cell-migration-inhibition correlate of delayed hypersensitivity. *J. Immunol.* **101,** 469–480.

Throp, F. K., and Dorfman, A. (1967). Differentiation of connective tissues. *In* "Current Topics in Developmental Biology" (A. A. Moscona and A. Monroy, eds.), pp. 151–190. Academic Press, New York.

Toivonen, S (1967). Mechanism of primary embryonic induction. *In* "Morphological and Biochemical Aspects of Cytodifferentiation" (E. Hagen, W. Wechsler, and P. Zilliken, eds.), pp. 1–7. Karger, Basel.

Urist, M. R. (1969). Mesenchymal cell reactions to inductive substrates for new bone formation. *In* "Repair and Regeneration" (J. E. Dunphy and H. W. Van Winkle, Jr., eds.), pp. 229–262. McGraw-Hill, New York.

Ward, P. D., and Ambrose, E. J. (1969). Electrophoretic and chemical characterization of the charged groups at the surface of murine CL 3 ascites leukemia cells. *J. Cell Sci.* **4,** 289–298.

Warren, L., and Glick, M. C. (1968). The metabolic turnover of the surface membrane of the L cell. *In* "Biological Properties of the Mammalian Surface Membrane" (L. A. Manson, ed.), pp. 3–16. Wistar Inst. Press, Philadelphia, Pennsylvania.

Wasserman, F. (1954). Fibrillogenesis in the regenerating rat tendon with special reference to growth and composition of the collagenous fibril. *Amer. J. Anat.* **94,** 399–437.

Weiss, L. (1967a). "The Cell Periphery, Metastasis, and other Contact Phenomena." Wiley, New York.

Weiss, L. (1967b). Studies on cell deformability. III. Some effects of EDTA on sarcoma 37 cells. *J. Cell Biol.* **33,** 341–347.

Weiss, L. (1968). Some comments on RNA as a component of the cell periphery. *In* "Biological Properties of the Mammalian Surface Membrane" (L. A. Manson, ed.), pp. 73–77. Wistar Inst. Press, Philadelphia, Pennsylvania.

Weiss, L., and Mayhew, E. (1966). The presence of ribonucleic acid within the peripheral zones of two types of mammalian cell. *J. Cell Physiol.* **68,** 345–360.

Weiss, L., and Meyhew, E. (1967). Ribonucleic acid within the cellular peripheral zone and the binding of calcium to ionogenic sites. *J. Cell. Physiol.* **69,** 281–292.

Weiss, P. (1934). *In vitro* experiments on the factors determining the course of the outgrowing nerve fiber. *J. Exp. Zool.* **68,** 393–448.

Weiss, P. (1945). Experiments on cell and axon orientation *in vitro:* the role of colloidal exudates in tissue organization. *J. Exp. Zool.* **100,** 353–386.

Weiss, P. (1950). Perspectives in the field of morphogenesis. *Quart. Rev. Biol.* **25,** 177–198.

Weiss, P. (1961). Guiding principles in cell locomotion and cell aggregation. *Expt. Cell Res. Suppl.* **8,** 260–281.

Weiss, P. (1962). From cell to molecule. *In* "Molecular Control of Cellular Activity" (M. M. Allen ed.), pp. 1–72. McGraw-Hill, New York.

Weiss, P., and Ferris, W. (1956). The basement lamella of amphibian skin. Its reconstruction after wounding. *J. Biophys. Biochem. Cytol.* **2,** 275–281.

Weiss, P., and Garber, B. (1952). Shape and movement of mesenchyme cells as functions of the physical structure of the medium. Contributions to quantitative morphology. *Proc. Nat. Acad. Sci. U. S.* **38,** 264–280.

Weiss, P., and Taylor, A. C. (1960). Reconstitution of complete organs from single cell suspensions of chick embryos in advanced stages of differentiation *Proc. Nat. Acad. Sci. U. S.* **46,** 1177–1185.

Wessels, N. K., and Cohen, J. H. (1968). Effects of collagenase on developing epithelia *in vitro:* lung, ureteric bud, and pancreas. *Develop. Biol.* **18,** 294–309.

Wessels, N. K., and Evans, J. (1968). The ulltrastructure of oriented cells and extracellular materials between developing features. *Develop. Biol.* **18,** 42–61.

Weston, J. A. (1963). A radiogutographic analysis of the migration and localization of trunk neural crest cells in the chick. *Develop. Biol.* **6,** 279–310.

Woodin, A. M. (1954). The properties of a complex of the mucopolysaccharides and proteins of the cornea. *Biochem. J.* **58,** 50–57.

Yamada, E. (1955). The fine structure of the renal glomerulous of the mouse. *J. Biophys. Biochem. Cytol.* **1,** 551–561.

Yamada, T. (1967). Cellular synthetic activities in induction of tissue transformation. *In* "Cell Differentiation" (A. V. S. DeReuck and J. Knight, eds), pp. 116–127. Little, Brown, Boston.

CHAPTER 8

Synthesis, Localization, and Renewal of Lipids in Mammalian Tissues

Sandra Sabatini-Smith

I. Introduction.. 277
II. Fatty Acids and Triglycerides.................................. 279
    A. Chemistry and Occurrence.................................. 279
    B. Biosynthesis.. 280
    C. Ultrastructural Localization and Turnover................. 282
III. Cholesterol.. 293
    A. Biosynthesis.. 294
    B. Subcellular Distribution and Ultrastructural Localization.. 296
    C. Turnover... 300
IV. Sphingolipids.. 302
V. Phospholipids... 305
    A. Introduction... 305
    B. Phosphatidylcholine (Lecithin)........................... 306
    C. Phosphatidylinositol..................................... 310
    D. Phosphatidylethanolamine (Cephalin)...................... 316
VI. Brown Adipose Tissue... 317
VII. Summary... 321
    References... 321

I. Introduction

The lipids constitute a heterogenous group of compounds which were originally classified according to their solubilities in organic solvents. In mammalian tissues the lipids of metabolic and structural significance include triglycerides, cholesterol, phospholipids (phosphatidylcholine, phosphatidylethanolamine, phosphatidylserine, phosphatidylinositol), sphingosine, and gangliosides, together with their products of catabolism,

277

TABLE I
LIPID COMPOSITION OF MAMMALIAN MEMBRANES[a]

	Percent total lipid in			
Lipid	Human myelin	Human erythrocyte, plasma membrane	Rat liver mitochondria	Rat liver microsomes
Cholesterol	25	25	5	8
Phospholipids	32	56	95	92
Phosphatidylcholine	11	23	48	64
Phosphatidylethanolamine	14	20	28	17
Phosphatidylserine	7	11	0	0
Phosphatidylinositol	0	2	8	11
Cardiolipin	0	0	11	0
Sphingolipids	31	18	0	0
Other	12	1	0	0

[a] Data from Masoro (1968).

glycerol, and the unesterified long-chain fatty acids. Table I summarizes the lipid composition of certain mammalian membranes.

The first advances in lipid chemistry were made in 1823 when Chevruel (Morton, 1965) stated that lipids were composed of fatty acids and that following hydrolysis, glycerol was released. During the period from 1860 to 1890, Fischer (Morton, 1965) elucidated the structure of certain lipids. Knoop (1904) subsequently described ω-phenyl-β-oxidation of unesterified fatty acids. Before the advent of isotopes, Knoop conceived the idea of marking a fatty acid with a phenyl ring, which is not oxidized in the body but is excreted after conjugation with glycine. After synthesizing a series of ω-phenyl fatty acids having from 2 to 5 carbons in the side chain, the metabolites isolated from the urine proved to be one to two substances depending on the length of the side chain in the acid administered. When the side chain contained an odd number of carbons, the nonoxidizable residue was excreted as hippuric acid. From acids with an even number of carbons, phenaceturic acid was formed and excreted. From these results Knoop reasoned that the fatty acids were degraded by loss of 2 carbon atoms at a time and that when two more could not be removed without rupture of the phenyl ring, the residue was conjugated with glycine and excreted as hippuric acid. This process is known as β-oxidation since the β-carbon becomes the terminal, carboxyl carbon after each oxidative step. His original theory made no attempt to follow the two carbon molecules to their final oxidation to carbon dioxide and water. It is now known that the 2-carbon fragment formed in stepwise degradation of fatty acid is acetyl coenzyme A, which normally condenses with oxalacetate and enters the citric acid cycle. The enzymes of this cycle, as well as those of fatty acid oxidation, are localized in the mitochondria.

For many years, tissue lipids were considered as metabolically inactive depots, functioning only during severe caloric deprivation. However, Schoenheimer (1942), summarizing a decade of scientific investigations in his laboratory, clearly demonstrated that in mice fed deuterium-labeled fatty acids, more than 50% of the fatty acids present in the liver had been synthesized within 1 day, compared to approximately 1 week for the depot fat. Since the total mass of depot fat remained constant, a considerable quantity of lipid must have been mobilized during this period. These investigations first illustrated the dynamic state of body fats and form the basis of our present understanding of lipid metabolism.

It is the specific aim of this chapter to summarize the synthesis, localization, and molecular renewal of lipids which are of major significance in mammalian tissues.

II. Fatty Acids and Triglycerides

A. CHEMISTRY AND OCCURRENCE

The fatty acids of mammalian tissues are primarily straight-chain, aliphatic monocarboxylic acids containing an even number of carbon atoms. However, in recent years, small quantities of hydroxy and keto acids, as well as acids with branched chains and odd numbers of carbon atoms, have been found im mammals (Masoro, 1968). These acids are considered minor components of the organism and will be properly discussed when their occurrence is of relevance to specific complex lipids. The fatty acids of mammals are usually considered to belong to one of two classes: the saturated acids and the unsaturated acids.

Palmitic acid, a 16-carbon acid, is a major constituent of adipose tissue and other tissue triglycerides representing approximately 25% of the fatty acids present. It is also the major fatty acid of phosphatidylcholine (lecithin). *Stearic acid*, an 18-carbon saturated acid, is found in appreciable quantities in the triglyceride of adipose tissue, and is the predominant constituent in sphingolipids, gangliosides, and most phospholipids. *Palmitoleic acid*, a 16-carbon monounsaturated acid, is widely distributed in liver or adipose tissue triglycerides; and liver phospholipids contain from 3 to 8

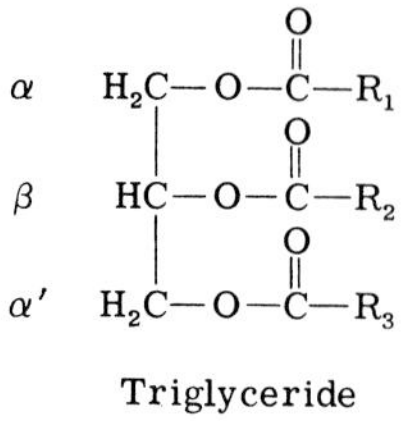

$$\alpha \quad H_2C-O-\overset{\overset{\textstyle O}{\|}}{C}-R_1$$
$$\beta \quad HC-O-\overset{\overset{\textstyle O}{\|}}{C}-R_2$$
$$\alpha' \quad H_2C-O-\overset{\overset{\textstyle O}{\|}}{C}-R_3$$

Triglyceride

FIG. 1. General structure and notation of triglycerides.

moles % palmitoleic acid. *Oleic acid*, an 18-carbon monounsaturated acid, is the predominant fatty acid in nature comprising 50% of the total fatty acid of adipose tissue triglyceride. Most lipid esters contain greater than 10 moles % of this acid. *Linoleic acid*, an 18-carbon diunsaturated acid, is of quantitative importance in a variety of mammalian lipids, comprising 10 moles % of the fatty acids in adipose tissue triglycerides, 15 moles % of the plasma free fatty acids, and 60 moles % of the fatty acids in ester linkage with plasma cholesterol. It is also present in phospholipids, and in the case of cardiolipin, linoleic acid constitutes more than 80 moles % of the fatty acid in ester linkage. *Linolenic acid*, 18-carbon triunsaturated acid, is present in the lipids of mammals but ordinarily not as a major component. *Arachidonic acid*, a 20-carbon tetraunsaturated acid, is found in the phospholipids and adipose tissue triglycerides. As an indication of its abundance, approximately 8 moles %, of hepatic lipids is arachidonic acid.

The triglycerides, which are fatty acid esters of glycerol are the most abundant subclass of neutral lipids found in nature. A general formula is shown in Fig. 1. Most of the triglycerides in mammalian tissues are non-randomly mixed glycerides. In general, the α position consists of palmitic acid, the shorter and more unsaturated fatty acids tend to occupy the β position, and oleic acid is in excess in the α' position (Masoro, 1968).

B. BIOSYNTHESIS

The importance of certain fatty acids was demonstrated by the work of Burr and Burr (1929) which showed that the rigid exclusion of fat from a diet of rats induced cessation of growth, scaly skin, kidney damage, and impaired reproduction. All these abnormalities could be prevented or cured by oral supplements of small amounts of linoleic or arachidonic acid. Linolenic acid has been shown to stimulate the growth of fat-deficient animals, but it is unable to cure the dermal symptoms of the deficiency

(Holman, 1951; Witten and Holman, 1952). In addition, Bernhard and Schoenheimer (1940) and Bernhard *et al.* (1942) demonstrated that the linoleic acid occurring in animal organs was not synthesized but taken up with food by the animals. Thus, the findings of Burr and Burr were gradually accepted, and the term "essential" was eventually used for all polyunsaturated fatty acids, although this term should include only those substances which are active both for growth and for maintainence of dermal integrity. Arachidonic acid is synthesized in the liver from linoleic acid by simple chain extension (Nunn and Smedley-MacLean, 1938). This thesis was advanced following their findings that the livers of fat-deficient rats contained no arachidonic or higher unsaturated fatty acids; but supplementation of the diet with linoleic acid resulted in a production of arachidonate, verifying the theory of the biosynthesis of the polyenoic acids in mammalian organisms. Mead *et al.* (1953) studied the incorporation of carboxyl-labeled acetate into the polyenoic acids and confirmed the findings of Bernhard and Schoenheimer (1940) that acetic acid is not incorporated into linoleic acid of the lipids of weanling rats. Arachidonic acid, on the other hand, was derived from acetate and presumably an exogenous C_{18} precursor. Further work on the metabolism of essential fatty acids gave no evidence for the conversion of oleate to linoleate, and a distribution of the label of arachidonic acid isolated from rats after feeding experiments showed again that this acid was synthesized in the rat by condensation of linoleate with acetate (Mead *et al.*, 1956; Steinberg *et al.*, 1956).

Brain tissue incorporates ^{14}C-acetate into polyenoic acids with a higher uptake of labeled acetate occurring in tissue slices than is obtained in feeding experiments (Klenk, 1957). It is interesting that under the same conditions no uptake of ^{14}C can be found in other lipid elements such as cholesterol, sphingosine, and cerebrosides.

Enzymes for the *de novo* synthesis of fatty acids are present both within the mitochondria and in the extramitochondrial regions of the cell. The enzyme systems of the two intracellular sites are quite similar; yet differences must exist since the end product of the extramitochondrial system is mainly palmitic acid, while that of the mitochondrial system is primarily stearic acid. Moreover, the extramitochondrial enzyme system is by far the most active one and is probably the system chiefly responsible for the *de novo* generation of fatty acids. The metabolism of fatty acids has been reviewed by Lynen (1955), Kennedy (1957), and Stumpf (1969).

Over the years there has been considerable controversy regarding the tissue sites of fatty acid biosynthesis within the mammalian organism. Before 1950, it was strongly felt that only the liver was capable of this biosynthetic reaction. However, evidence soon accumulated establishing unequivocally that many tissues beside the liver were capable of fatty acid biosynthesis, and particular emphasis was placed on the role of adipose tissue. Indeed, by the early 1960's it was rather generally accepted that adipose tissue was the primary site of fatty acid biosynthesis and that the liver played only a minor role. In recent years, however, further evidence has indicated that adipose tissue may be far less important, and that the liver and gastrointestinal tract are the sites of substantial fatty acid biosynthesis. It has also become clear that there are important sites of fatty acid biosynthesis not yet fully considered. For example, it seems that the lung may be an important site and it is also quite possible that there is substantial activity in the bone marrow (Wakil, 1961; Patkin and Masoro, 1964).

C. ULTRASTRUCTURAL LOCALIZATION AND TURNOVER

The initial work by Schoenheimer and colleagues (1942) introduced revolutionary concepts which have been abundantly confirmed by subsequent investigators, namely, that the body fats are in a state of rapid flux, being continually broken down and then reconstituted from the metabolic pool. The time required for complete renewal of any lipid fraction varies from one species to another and from one organ to another. The lipids of the body are constantly subject to a variety of highly complex chemical processes which includes synthesis, interconversion, and degradation. In Schoenheimer's original experiments the rate of fatty acid synthesis in the liver was so rapid it was not possible to determine a half-time exactly; however, the trend of the curve indicated that more than one half of the fatty acids present in the liver of the normal animals had been synthesized within 1 day. By contrast, the half-time for depot fat was approximately 7 days (Bernhard and Schoenheimer, 1940).

Thompson and Ballou (1954) studied the turnover of lipid and protein fractions in female rats administered 100 mCi of tritium oxide for 5 weeks. The saturated fatty acids exhibited apparent biological half-lives of 200, 130, and 60 days in the carcass, skin, and abdominal fat, respectively. By contrast, the unsaturated fatty acids exhibited biological half-lives of 300, 250, and 70 days in the carcass, skin, and abdominal fat, respectively. These calculations are only approximations since they are based on only two points on a retention curve, and it should be emphasized that the biological half-lives determined in any study will not be representative of the total material isolated in each fraction. For example, all the unsaturated fatty acids from the skin would not be expected to exhibit a biological half-life of 250 days. Whether these relatively inert components represent chemical species distinct from the more rapidly catabolized components or whether the same compounds may exhibit different turnover rates, depending on their functional involvement within the organism, remains to be determined. It is of interest to note that the biological half-life for a given fraction may vary significantly within the same animal, depending upon the tissue of origin. Thus, while for any given tissue the unsaturated fatty acids exhibited a longer half-life than the saturated fatty acids, the half-life of either of these fractions may vary by a factor of three of four among different tissues. It is evident that a given compound or group of compounds within the body may not be considered independently of location or function.

Using the technique of light microscopic autoradiography Wirsén (1965) studied the distribution of 1-^{14}C-palmitic acid in skeletal muscle in pectoralis muscle of the pigeon. The albumin-bound fatty acid was injected intravenously and samples were removed at 3, 6, and 15 minutes. In the 3-minute experiments the distribution of isotope was somewhat diffuse, although regions with the white fibers showed a distinctly weaker activity. The difference between red and white fibers became further accentuated in the 6- and 15-minute experiments, with the white fibers showing only slightly more activity than background. It has been demonstrated that white fibers have a high glycogen content and seem to depend more on glycolysis than do the red fibers with their higher capacity for lipolysis and oxidation. Thus, it appears that in each fiber type the uptake of fatty acids from the plasma will proceed at different rates in cells with different metabolic qualities. Boberg (1969) studied the turnover of plasma palmitate in the unanesthetized rat. The mean half-life of this acid was estimated to be 17 seconds with no significant difference found between fed and fasted animals.

Stein and Stein (1963) studied the comparative uptake and distribution of isotopically labeled free fatty acids in the perfused rat heart. When the fatty acids complexed to serum albumin were introduced in pairs, equal extractions were found, indicating that under these conditions the heart did not discriminate between the different fatty acids studied. In contrast to the indiscriminate uptake of different fatty acids from the perfusion medium, their intracellular distribution between neutral lipid and phospholipid varied quite markedly. Of the neutral lipids, over 96% of the fatty acids incorporated were found in the triglyceride fraction. In this fraction the incorporation of palmitic acid exceeded that of its competitors: stearic, oleic, and linoleic acids. Of the phospholipids, the phosphatidylcholine fraction contained over 70% of the fatty acids incorporated; stearic and linoleic acid incorporation exceded the others.

More precise information concerning the localization and transport of fatty acids has been afforded from a series of papers by the Steins utilizing

TABLE II
DISTRIBUTION OF GRAINS OVER CYTOPLASMIC STRUCTURES IN MUSCLE CELLS OF
RAT HEARTS PERFUSED CONTINUOUSLY WITH 9,10-OLEIC ACID-^{3}H[a,b]

	Perfusion time (min)					
	¼	1	2	5	10	20
Structure	Distribution of grain counts (%)					
Mitochondria	30.8	39.3	38.1	36.3	34.2	35.4
Sarcoplasmic reticulum[c]	65.6	43.3	39.0	39.0	30.4	27.4
Lipid droplets	1.2	13.5	18.4	23.7	33.4	35.2
Myofibrils	2.4	3.9	4.5	1.0	2.0	2.0
Total counts	325	230	262	198	209	278

[a] All hearts except those labeled for ¼ minute, were washed by perfusion for 30 seconds.

[b] Data from Stein and Stein (1968).

[c] Includes the transverse tubular system.

electron microscopic autoradiography (Stein and Stein, 1967a,b; 1968; 1969). In all these experiments temporal analyses were made following *in vivo* injection of the labeled lipid precursor in intervals varying from 1 minute up to approximately 30 minutes. Salient features from this elegant series of articles are summarized below.

Working rat hearts were perfused with Krebs-Henseleit bicarbonate buffer, pH 7.4, containing 9,10-^{3}H-oleic acid for varying intervals of time from 15 seconds to 20 minutes. Samples of cardiac tissue were fixed in sodium cacodylate-buffered glutaraldehyde. Table II shows the distribution of grains over cytoplasmic structures seen following development and fixation of radioautographs. Figures 2–5 illustrate the radioautographic reaction at 15 seconds, 1, 5, and 20 minutes. Concentration of silver grains over lipid droplets and mitochondria is particularly prominent with longer intervals of perfusion. Under these conditions approximately 80% of the label was recovered as tri- and diglycerides. By contrast, if the same experiment was carried out at 4°C, 79% of the label could be recovered as free fatty acids. Under these circumstances there was a prominent absence of label concentration over the lipid droplets, adding further evidence that the lipid seen in the form of droplets is in the esterified form. The lack of label over myofibrils would indicate a rather selective nonrandom channeling of fatty acids into the cell (Stein and Stein, 1968). This is in contrast to previous studies performed at the light microscopic level where it was not

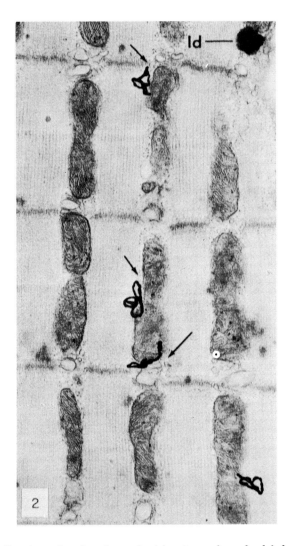

FIG. 2. Radioautographs of sections of rat heart muscle, pulse labeled by perfusion with ³H-oleic acid 15 seconds and fixed by perfusion with osmium tetroxide. The radioautographic reaction is seen over the sarcoplasmic reticulum (arrows); the lipid droplets (ld) are not labeled. 20,000 ×. (Stein and Stein, 1968, Fig. 3.)

possible to visualize adequately a distribution of silver grains (Wirsén, 1965).

This experiment would suggest that the site of fatty acid esterification is localized in the sarcoplasmic reticulum and mitochondria. Enzymes

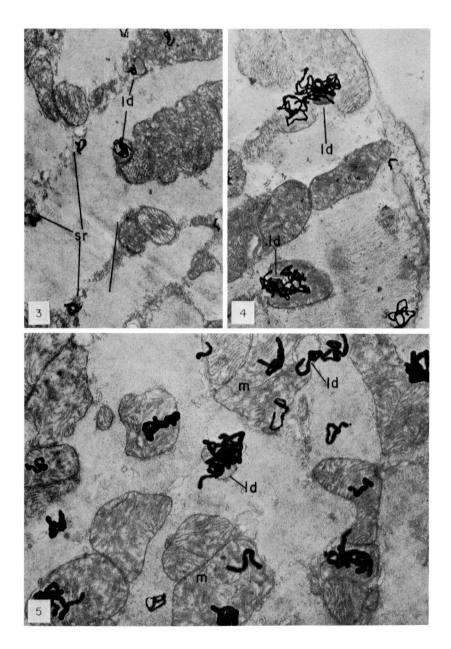

FIGS. 3, 4, and 5. Radioautographs of sections of heart labeled with ³H-oleic acid for 1 minute (Fig. 3), 5 minutes (Fig. 4), and 20 minutes (Fig. 5). Concentration of silver grains is seen over lipid droplets (ld) and mitochondria (m) at the longer intervals of perfusion. sr is the sarcoplasmic reticulum. Fig. 3, 12,000 ×; Fig. 4, 16,000 ×; Fig. 5, 21,600 ×. (Stein and Stein, 1968, Figs. 13, 14, and 15.)

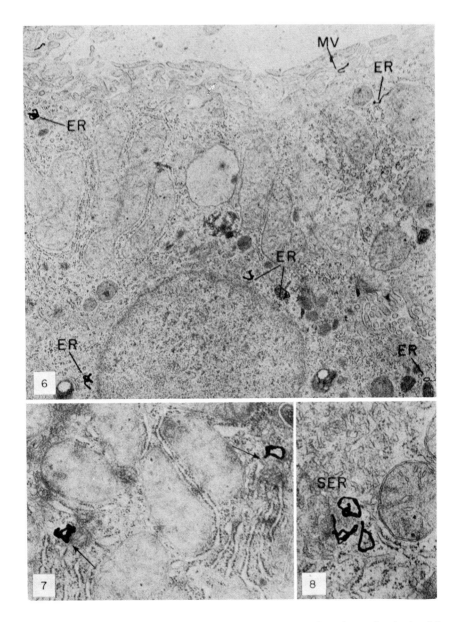

Figs. 6, 7, and 8. Radioautographs of liver biopsies from fasted rats 2 minutes following the injection of ³H-palmitate. The silver grains are seen over the endoplasmic reticulum (ER) and microvilli (MV) (Fig. 6); in the transition regions between the rough and smooth endoplasmic reticulum (arrows) (Fig. 7); and over the smooth endoplasmic reticulum (SER) (Fig. 8). Fig. 6, 12,800 ×; Fig. 7, 20,800 ×; Fig. 8, 24,000 ×. (Stein and Stein, 1967a, Figs. 3, 4, and 5.)

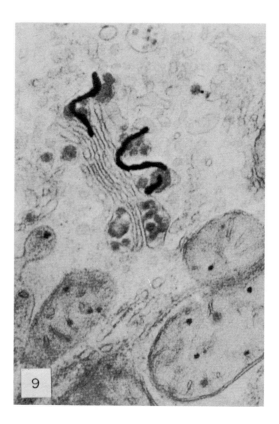

Fig. 9. Liver of fasted rats 10 minutes following injection of ³H-palmitate illustrating radioautographic grains over the Golgi apparatus. 40,000 ×. (Stein and Stein, 1967a, Fig. 19.)

active in the synthesis of triglyceride have been localized within the endoplasmic reticulum (Stein and Sharpiro, 1958) and this structure is analogous to the sarcoplasmic reticulum in cardiac muscle. Recent evidence indicates that fatty acids are transported across vesicles of isolated cardiac sarcoplasmic reticulum and that the lability of such preparations is due to a loss of free fatty acids into the medium (Sarzala and Drabikowski, 1969). The origin of mitochondrial triglyceride is not known; it may occur by translocation of performed triglycerides or *in situ* synthesis from free fatty acids. Recent evidence would suggest that at least in the case of phospholipids, ¹⁴C-oleic acid can be incorporated into phosphatidylethanolamine by the isolated inner mitochondrial membrane while this fatty acid is incorporated into phosphatidylcholine equally but to a much lesser extent by both the inner and outer isolated mitochondrial membrane (Nachbaur

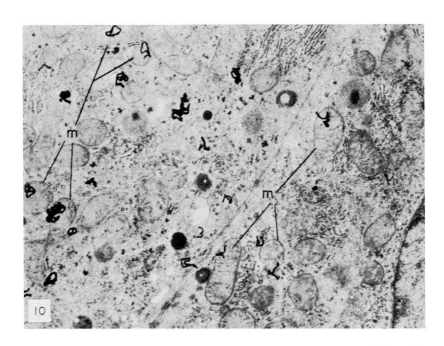

Fig. 10. Liver of fasted rats 20 minutes following injection of ³H-palmitate. Note the many mitochondria (m) labeled. 12,800 ×. (Stein and Stein, 1967a, Fig. 18.)

et al., 1969). By contrast, Wilgram and Kennedy (1963) found very low levels of enzyme activity involved in lipid synthesis and concluded that mitochondrial phospholipids are formed in the endoplasmic reticulum and subsequently transported to the mitochondria.

In parallel experiments, Stein and Stein (1967a) followed the intracellular movement of ³H-glycerol and ³H-palmitate in rat liver with electron microscopic autoradiography and found a rapid incorporation of glycerol at the earliest time interval, 2 minutes. In liver samples biopsied from control rats at 2 minutes, the recovered ³H-palmitate was distributed 25.0, 57.1, and 17.9% among fatty acids, triglycerides, and phospholipids, respectively. On electron microscopic autoradiography it was apparent that concentrations of the label were seen over the microvilli, the elements of smooth endoplasmic reticulum, and in transition areas between the smooth and the rough endoplasmic reticulum at the earliest time interval (Figs. 6–8). Electron micrographs at 10 and 20 minutes revealed an increase in the intensity of label over the mitochondria and Golgi apparatus (Figs. 9 and 10).

If these animals were pretreated with ethanol to increase the rate of

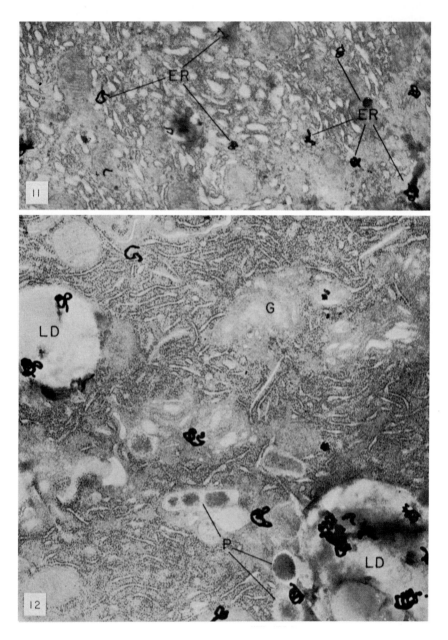

Figs. 11, 12, 13, and 14. Radioautographs of rat lactating mammary gland 1 minute after injection of ³H-oleic acid. The silver grains are seen over the rough endoplasmic reticulum (ER) and mitochondria (Fig. 11). Concentrations of silver grains are seen over intracellular (Figs. 12 and 13) and intraluminal (Figs. 13 and 14) lipid droplets (LD). N is the nucleus. The intraluminal lipid droplets exhibit electron opaque boundaries (arrows) and elements of the rough endoplasmic reticulum adhere to the lipid droplet. The granules (P) in the Golgi vesicles (G) are not labeled. Fig. 11, 12,800 ×; Fig. 12, 20,000 ×; Fig. 13, 9,600 ×; Fig. 14, 17,200 ×. (Stein and Stein, 1967b, Figs. 2, 3, 4, and 5.)

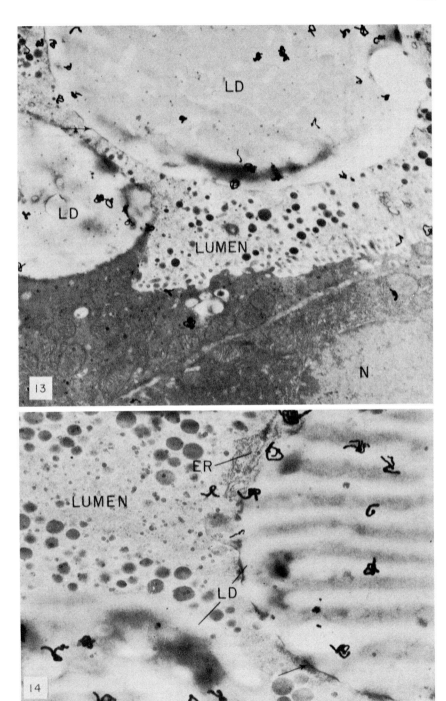

esterification, lipid droplets of varying sizes were seen in the same general vicinity. Liver biopsies taken 20 minutes following injection of ³H-palmitate distributed 2.5, 75.0, and 22.5 among fatty acids, triglycerides, and phospholipids, respectively. Autoradiographic reaction persisted over the endoplasmic reticulum, lipid droplets, and mitochondria. At this time, the label was apparent over the Golgi apparatus; the Golgi vesicles were filled with electron-opaque particles varying in size from 400 to 209 μ in diameter.

Table III summarizes the relative distribution of liver subcellular radioactivity as performed by grain counts at 2 and 20 minutes following injection of ³H-palmitate into control rats. It can be seen there is a rise in grain concentration over the mitochondria and the Golgi apparatus 20 minutes after injection of the isotope. The increase in activity seen over the Golgi apparatus at later time intervals and in the absence of significant amounts of free fatty acids would tend to support the theory that the lipids are esterified in the endoplasmic reticulum, delivered to the Golgi apparatus, and secreted by the Golgi apparatus in vesicles or granules which are discharged at the cell surface. This hypothesis has been proposed to occur in numerous cells (Farquhar, 1961; Caro and Palade, 1964; Nadler et al., 1964).

Since the lactating mammary gland is considered to be one of the most active sites of lipid synthesis and milk secretion is composed mainly of triglycerides, this tissue would represent an ideal model for the study of the formation and release of triglycerides (Stein and Stein, 1967b). Indeed, in mammary biopsies taken 1 minute following the intravenous injection of 9,10-³H-palmitic acid or 9,10-³H-oleic acid, 90% of the recovered radioactivity was in the form of triglyceride and silver grains were seen over the rough endoplasmic reticulum (Fig. 11), intracellular and intraluminal lipid droplets (Figs. 12–14), and some mitochondria. The granules and Golgi vesicles are not labeled. At this same time interval approximately 4% of the label was biochemically recovered in the phospholipid fraction. At the 10-minute interval the autoradiographic raction was concentrated over the lipid droplets, some of these being adjacent to the Golgi region, and occasional grains found over the Golgi vesicles. One hour after injection the radioactivity was concentrated in lipid droplets both in the apical portion of the cell and in the lumen. These droplets showed an attenuated rim of cytoplasm on their luminal surface.

The mode of release of lipid into the lumen has been debated and two hypotheses exist, both of which are probably true. One theory suggests there is no loss of cytoplasm (Bargmann and Knoop, 1959), while the other proposes there is a loss of intracellular content since clearly identifiable elements of the endoplasmic reticulum could be seen adhering to some

TABLE III

DISTRIBUTION OF GRAINS OVER LIVER SUBCELLULAR STRUCTURES AFTER INJECTION
OF 9,10-PALMITIC ACID-³H INTO RATS FASTED FOR 16 HOURS[a]

| Time after injection (min) | Distribution of grains | | | | | Total grains counted |
	Endoplasmic reticulum[b] (%)	Mitochondria (%)	Golgi region (%)	Tissue space (%)	Nucleus (%)	
2	87	6	1	4	2	243
20	65	16	11	6	2	297

[a] Data from Stein and Stein (1967a).
[b] Includes cytoplasmic matrix.

of the released lipid droplets (Grynfeltt, 1937). In contrast to the liver, the mammary gland secretes lipid primarily in the form of triglycerides and as such, this lipid does not appear to pass through the Golgi apparatus. This organelle is thought to complex liver lipids and would suggest that quite different modes of uptake as well as secretion may be found in various tissues.

III. Cholesterol

In addition to the easily hydrolyzable compounds discussed above, the fat solvents extract a certain amount of lipid which does not become soluble during hydrolysis. This nonsaponifiable matter includes a group of structurally related compounds termed the steroids. The steroids are all derivatives of the aromatic hydrocarbon, cyclopentanophenathrene.

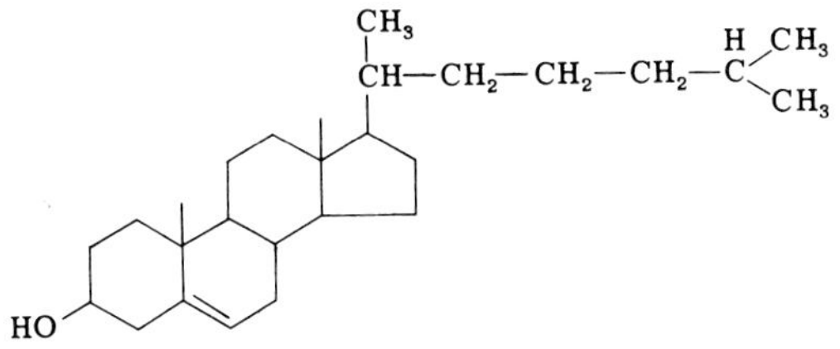

Cholesterol

FIG. 15. Chemical formula for cholesterol.

Cholesterol, the major animal steroid, was originally isolated from gall-stones by the French chemist, Fourcroy, in 1775 (Downes, 1962). It is now known that this compound is only one of a series of sterols and occupies a central position for the further biosynthesis of estrogen, androgens, and adrenal corticosteroids. Cholesterol occurs in blood and all animal cells in both the free form and esterified with long-chain fatty acids (Fig. 15).

A. Biosynthesis

The concept of lipid biosynthesis from 2-carbon compounds was first suggested by Raper (1907); however, experimental evidence was not obtained until 20 years later by MacLean and Hoffert (1926). The significance of this investigation was not fully appreciated until the 1940's (Schoenheimer, 1942), and by 1948, the suggested role of acetate in cholesterol metabolism was well established. The subsequent and continuing contributions of Popják, Bolch, and colleagues have elucidated the complete

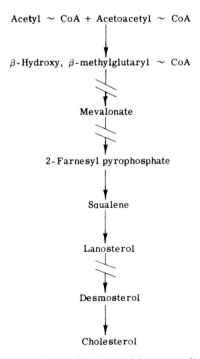

Fig. 16. Synthesis of cholesterol in mammalian tissues.

pathways for cholesterol biosynthesis from acetate (Bloch, 1948; Clayton and Bloch, 1956; Popják and Cornforth, 1960; Bloch, 1965). The current schema of the formation of cholesterol is partially presented in Fig. 16.

Interest has centered upon hepatic cholesterol synthesis primarily because of early experimental findings of Bloch and Rittenberg (1945) and Anker (1948) which demonstrated that the isotopic concentration of liver cholesterol was significantly greater than carcass cholesterol in rats that had been fed deuterium-labeled acetate for 8 days. Bolch *et al.* (1946) were unable to demonstrate *in vitro* conversion of acetate to cholesterol in any tissues other than the liver. The subsequent experiments of Srere (1950) indicated that rats eviscerated and deprived of hepatic circulation for 5 hours were able to convert approximatly 50% of the uniformly labeled ^{14}C-acetate into cholesterol. Furthermore, a significant incorporation occurred in those rats which were also ovariectomized and adrenalectomized. *In vitro*, the most active tissues were found to be the skin and liver of the adult and the skin and brain of the day-old rat. According to their findings, slices of adult brain were totally unable to synthesize cholesterol.

More recently, the investigations by Dietschy and Siperstein (1967) indicate that virtually every tissue is capable of synthesizing cholesterol *in vitro* (see Table IV). In these experiments rats were maintained on a low cholesterol diet supplemented daily with oleic acid for 6 weeks. Tissue slices were incubated in Krebs bicarbonate buffer containing 1 μCi acetate-2-^{14}C and 5 μmoles sodium acetate for 2 hours. Following extraction of the unsaponifiable lipids, the 3β-hydroxy sterols were precipitated with digitonin, a steroid saponin. Digitonide formation has been used extensively for the isolation of cholesterol and other 3β-hydroxy sterols in the presence of cholesterol esters, resulting in the precipitation of a 1:1 molecular complex. In recent years the alkaloid tomatine has been used to precipitate cholesterol in a manner similar to that obtained with digitonin, and some investigators feel that this reaction is preferable for analytical work (Masoro, 1968). Following digitonin precipitation, five major groups of sterols were then separated by either thin layer or gas–liquid chromatography and the amount of radioactivity present was determined.

It is apparent from the data in Table IV that those tissues in group A synthesized sterols most actively. Surprisingly, the ileum, which has the second highest incorporation rate of any tissues tested, synthesized sterols at 65% the rate found in the liver. The tissues in group B have relatively low synthetic rates, or approximately 6% that of hepatic synthesis. Finally, muscle and brain tissue, while they definitely synthesize some sterol, do so at the exceedingly slow rate of less than 1 mμmole acetate-2-^{14}C/ gm/2 hr (less than 0.6% of the hepatic rate).

It is assumed that the conversion of acetate-2-^{14}C- into sterols represents

TABLE IV
Control Rates of Sterol Synthesis in Rat[a]

Group	Tissue	Total DP-sterols[b]	Percent converted to cholesterol	Percent converted to lanosterol
A	Liver	179.0 ± 97.5	92.0	1.5
	Ileum	114.3 ± 55.1	83.5	3.5
	Transverse colon	56.2 ± 31.6	79.5	2.5
	Stomach	35.7 ± 10.5	87.5	3.0
B	Esophagus	17.4 ± 7.3		
	Jejunum	15.2 ± 10.0	83.0	3.5
	Testis	8.7 ± 2.7	15.0	55.0
	Lung	6.7 ± 0.2	60.5	2.5
	Adrenal	5.0 ± 1.1		
	Skin	4.9 ± 1.8	38.5	13.0
	Kidney	3.8 ± 3.1	79.0	3.5
	Duodenum	3.6 ± 1.6		
	Spleen	3.5 ± 0.7	63.0	6.5
C	Smooth muscle	0.9 ± 0.3		
	Heart muscle	0.7 ± 0.2		
	Skeletal muscle	0.5 ± 0.2		
	Brain	0.5 ± 0.4		

[a] Data from Dietschy and Siperstein (1967).

[b] Values are mμmoles (mean for 4 rats ± 1 SD) of acetate-2-^{14}C converted to digitonin-precipitable sterols per gram of tissue during a 2-hour incubation.

the inherent rate of synthesis for each tissue. However, the possibility exists that the rate of entry of acetate into the cell or the activation of acetyl-CoA may be the limiting factors in certain tissues.

B. Subcellular Distribution and Ultrastructural Localization

A portion of cholesterol biosynthesis was originally thought to occur in the microsomal fraction of mammalian cells (Tchen and Bloch, 1955). However, since recent work has demonstrated that rat liver plasma membrane breaks up during homogenization, it was not possible to define a specific organelle as the site of synthesis. Plasma membranes contain appreciable amounts of cholesterol (Coleman and Finean, 1965) and could participate in the synthetic process. The method of Michell and Hawthorne (1965) minimizing the vesicular formation of plasma membranes combined with the procedure of Dallner (1963) separating the granular and agranular endoplasmic reticulum has largely circumvented this problem. Chesterton (1966; 1968) has demonstrated that within 2 minutes following intravenous administration of mevalonate-2-^{14}C, 12% of the radioactivity is found as cholesterol. After 30 minutes 80% can be isolated as free cholesterol and 7% esterified cholesterol. The subcellular distribution of ^{14}C-cholesterol and various precursors was studied by the use of fairly specific enzyme markers. A significant amount of ^{14}C-cholesterol was found in the nuclear fraction and the endoplasmic reticulum. Since nuclei are known to contain relatively small amounts of cholesterol (Schotz et al., 1953), the major portion of ^{14}C-cholesterol in that fraction is supposedly associated with the plasma membrane. This could indicate that cholesterol is transferred from the endoplasmic reticulum to the plasma membrane after synthesis. Since ^{14}C-squalene and ^{14}C-lanosterol do not accumulate it is highly unlikely that significant synthesis of cholesterol occurs per se within the plasma membrane. Jones and Fawcett (1966) have described evidence which suggests the presence of cholesterol biosynthetic activity in the agranular membranes of rat liver cells. The above data suggest that the conversion of squalene to cholesterol occurs in the endoplasmic reticulum as a whole and is not confined to either the granular or the agranular membranes. The possibility of some cross contamination exists since these preparations were not examined for purity with the electron microscope. ^{14}C-cholesterol esters are also associated with the endoplasmic reticulum, indicating that this is the primary site of cholesterol esterification.

The intracellular location of cholesterol is a topic of considerable interest, but one which has not received thorough investigation. One of the major questions which must be resolved is the extent to which both free and esterified sterols are maintained within the cell, either associated with cellular membranes or in lipid vacuoles. From studies on tissue culture cells it appears that cholesterol is confined almost entirely to membrane structures (Mackenzie et al., 1964; 1967). It was concluded that under normal conditions most culture cells probably will not exhibit accumulation of sterols in lipid particles, but under certain circumstances cells can be forced to accumulate excess steroid which is probably not membrane associated. Bailey (1967) showed that L-cells grown in a medium containing added free cholesterol would form cholesterol microcrystals intracellularly. Ninety-three percent of the total lipid in the plasma membrane of L-cells

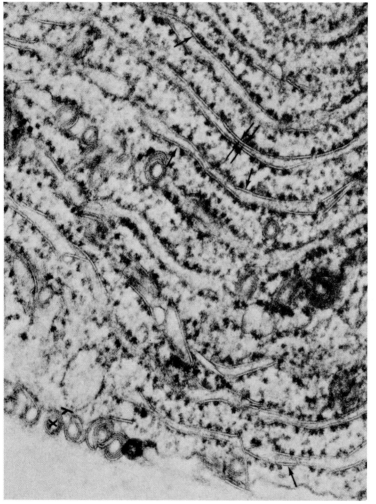

Fig. 17. Portion of a pancreatic acinar cell in which membranes have been altered (arrows). Intracellular and extracellular whorled digitonin–cholesterol complexes are present with several located between basement membrane and plasma membrane in the upper left corner. Densitometric tracings were taken between points X and Y to estimate distances. 85,000 ×. (Williamson, 1969, Fig. 13.)

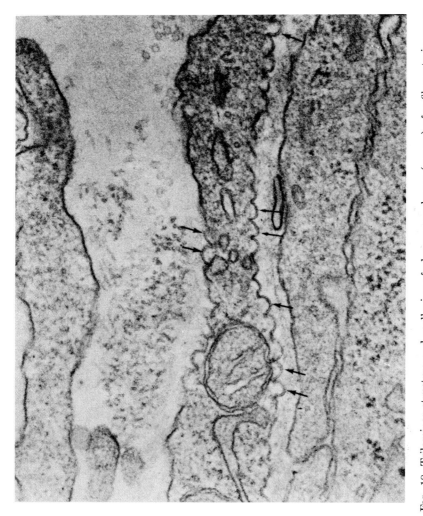

Fig. 18. Trilaminar structure and scalloping of plasma membrane (arrows) of a fibrocyte in mouse intestinal mucosa following digitonin treatment. 72,500 ×. (Williamson, 1969, Fig. 1.)

can be removed as free cholesterol. By the combined use of autoradiography and electron microscopy Robertson (1967) demonstrated the incorporation of exogenous labeled free cholesterol into lipid vacuoles in cultured human arterial cells. These experiments also indicated a progressive movement of labeled free cholesterol from cell membrane ghosts into the microsomal cell sap. Even less is known about the intracellular distribution of esterified cholesterol. It has been estimated that 65–86% of the total cholesterol in cultured human arterial cells is esterified.

Williamson (1969) has devised a method for the ultrastructural localization of free cholesterol in extracellular and intracellular compartments. In brief, tissues are fixed in 3% glutaraldehyde in 0.1 M cacodylate buffer, pH 7.4, for 2 hours at 25°C. Following two rinses in cacodylate buffer (20 minutes), the tissues are immersed in saturated solutions of digitonin for 2–4 hours. After postfixation in 1% osmium tetroxide the tissues are dehydrated in acetone, embedded in Araldite, and stained with uranyl acetate and lead citrate. Figure 17 illustrates the cholesterol–digitonin complex in a pancreatic acinar cell. The most easily recognized and most frequently observed digitonin–cholesterol complexes were multilamellar cylindrical structures 400–1300 Å in diameter and up to 1.3 μ in length. These structures were observed in the cytoplasm of every cell type examined with the exception of erythrocytes. They were not associated with Golgi vesicles or smooth endoplasmic reticulum. Trilaminar unit membrane structure was focally enchanced in many cellular organelles including plasma membranes (Fig. 18), lysosomes, cytoplasmic vacuoles, and secretory granules. Altered membranes were demonstrable in every cell type examined but varied considerably in thickness and were often deeply scalloped into segments 400–800 Å wide.

C. Turnover

The classic tracer studies of Schoenheimer provide a framework for new concepts concerning a dynamic state of body constituents in the study of the metabolism of cholesterol. The original experiment of Rittenberg and Schoenheimer (1937) indicated that the synthesis of cholesterol in the mouse carcass proceeds with a half-time of approximately 21 days following the administration of deuterium oxide. Subsequently, Thompson and Ballou (1954) studied the metabolic turnover of lipid and protein fractions in rats receiving 100 mCi of tritium oxide over a period of 5 weeks. The rats were then divided into two groups and sacrificed 4 months and 8 months following the initial injection. Correcting for loss of tritium due to breakdown and dilution as a consequence of growth, these investigators found an apparent biological half-life for the sterols of 100 and 300 days in the skin and carcass, respectively. In these experiments collagen fractions exhibited half-lives of 300 to 1000 days, and the highest concentration of tritium was found in the brain lipids.

The permanence of cerebral lipids has been the subject of considerable controversy over the years. Much of this data has been ambiguous primarily due to the relative uncertainty concerning the influence of the blood-brain barrier. Initial experiments indicated that cholesterol was unable to enter the brain (Waelsch et al., 1941; Bloch et al., 1943; Folch-Pi, 1955). More recent experiments do not fully corroborate these conclusions. Following injection of 1-day-old chicks with cholesterol-^{14}C-4, appreciable radioactivity is present in the brain after 40 days (Davison et al., 1958). Similar results were obtained by Kritchevsky and Defendi (1961; 1962) when tritium-labeled cholesterol, sitosterol, and lanosterol were injected directly into yolk sacs of newly hatched chicks. The amount of radioactive cholesterol in brain and liver was determined on days 50, 85, and 120. In the brain, the amount of cholesterol and sitosterol seemed to reach a constant level by the eighty-fifth day, while lanosterol radioactivity was still falling. Autoradiography revealed a localization of the labeled sterols in the white matter of the cerebellum and the optical vesicle and in Kupfer cells of the liver. A significant incorporation of the label was seen in erythrocytes and a lesser amount in the aorta.

In a series of experiments Davison et al. (1959a,b) found that following administration of ^{14}C-cholesterol appreciable amounts of sterol were found in 30 days, followed by a slow fall to a constant level after 100 days. The most persistent radioactivity was found in white matter, whereas turnover of ^{14}C was observed mainly in gray matter of brain. Thus, the successful incorporation of cholesterol into the central nervous system led Davison to suggest that the metabolic processes involving brain cholesterol take place at different rates and in different morphological compartments. Early time measurements of Smith and Eng (1965) estimated that half-life data from brain myelin and spinal cord myelin were shorter than 14 days. An increment measured between 2 weeks and 6 months indicated a longer half-life.

More recently, Gautheron et al. (1969) have studied the radioautographic localization of cholesterol in the central nervous system following intracerebral injection of labeled mevalonate. Rats were sacrificed at various intervals: 5 minutes; 1 hour; 3 days; 2.5 and 9 months. In radioautographs of brain slices performed soon after injection, two kinds of cholesterol-synthesis localization were distinguished. First, the slight blackening suggested that all anatomical brain structures are able to synthesize cholesterol. Second, it appeared that all heavily myelinated anatomical structures close to the site of injection were highly darkened, indicating poor diffusion of the mevalonate. In long-term experiments a high density of labeling was also recovered in heavily myelinated areas such as the white matter of the cerebellum, corpus callosum, chiasma opticum, and commissura anterior. These structures appeared more homogeneously blackened than in short-term experiments. These experiments yielded results similar to those obtained in cholesterol transfer experiments demonstrating that three cholesterol compartments occur in adult rat brain (Chevallier, 1967): 79% of cholesterol is turned over; 24–25% is exchangeable with plasma cholesterol; and 2.5% is turned over by *in situ* synthesis.

Studies on the turnover of plasma cholesterol in man have been carried out by Goodman (1967) in which he finds that the turnover of total plasma cholesterol conforms to a two-pool model. This means that the various tissue pools of cholesterol would fall into two groups in terms of the rates at which they equilibrate with plasma cholesterol. One pool is apparently in fairly rapid equilibrium with plasma cholesterol, exhibiting a half-time of approximately 5 days, and probably includes erythrocytes, and liver cholesterol, together with some of the cholesterol in the viscera (spleen, kidney, intestine). The second pool is in fairly slow equilibrium with plasma cholesterol, exhibiting a half-time of 52 days, and includes most of the cholesterol in peripheral tissues, particularly skeletal muscle.

IV. Sphingolipids

Characterization of the sphingolipids has been reviewed by Ledeen (1969); it is apparent that a variety of compounds is now known, and no doubt others will be found. The biosynthesis of sphingolipids has been the subject of rather comprehensive study, and the general steps for the assembly of smaller entities are well understood (for a review in nervous tissue see Eichberg *et al.*, 1969). The sphingolipids are a heterogeneous group of compounds which have in common either the 18-carbon amino alcohol, sphingosine, or a closely related compound. Although sphingosine is the most abundant compound of its type in the sphingolipids in animals, dihydrosphingosine and the C_{20} homolog of sphingosine can replace it in some animal sphingolipids. None of these, however, are present in mammals in appreciable levels as free compounds, but rather are components of sphingomyelin, glycosyl ceramides (cerebroside), cerebroside sulfate, and gangliosides. In all these lipids sphingosine is present as *N*-acylsphingosine compounds which are called ceramides.

Approximately 10% of the lipid phosphorus in brain is in the form of sphingomyelin, while from 10 to 25% is present in erythrocytes, lung, kidney, and spleen. In most other tissues, approximately 5 to 10% of the lipid phosphorus is in this form (Masoro, 1968). The fatty acids in amide linkage in sphingomyelin are mainly long-chain saturated and unsaturated acids of unusual structure. Stearic, lignoceric, and nervonic acids comprise greater than 75% of the fatty acids in brain sphingomyelin.

The gangliosides are distinguished from the other sphingolipids by the presence of sialic acid in the carbohydrate chain. They are found in very high concentrations in the neurons of the central nervous system and have also been isolated from spleen and erythrocytes. Four major gangliosides have been isolated from human brain and specific disease states have been related to the dramatic increase in one or more of these gangliosides in brain either in white or gray matter (Tay-Sachs disease, gargoylism) (Ledeen, 1966).

Ceramide galactoside (cerebroside) was the first glycosyl ceramide to be discovered. Large amounts are found in white matter of the central nervous system and approximately 4% of the wet weight of the brain are cerebrosides. Cerebrosides are found in most, if not all, mammalian tissues though in much lower quantities. An inherited lipidosis in which glucose cerebrosides accumulate in spleen, liver, and lymph nodes is called Gaucher's disease. It has recently been shown that these cerebrosides function immunological as haptens, but the possible significance of this to the pathophysiology of mammals is not yet known (Carter et al., 1965; Brady, 1966).

In addition to the cerebrosides, the brain contains sulfate esters of ceramide galactoside in the ratio of 4:1. Although most abundant in the brain, cerebroside sulfates are found in low concentrations in other tissues such as liver, lungs, skeletal muscle, and heart.

The turnover rate of sphingolipids in human tissues varies with the chemical nature of the lipid, the tissue, and the subcellular structure in which it is located. Although mammals are capable of biosynthesizing and metabolizing sphingolipids, the complete enzymatic pathways are not completely known. Smith (1967) has calculated half-lives of 30 and 300 days for sphingomyelin in brain mitochondria and myelin, respectively (Table V).

Kishimoto et al. (1965a,b) have studied the turnover of cholesterol and the fatty acids of gangliosides, cerebrosides, and sulfatides in the developing rat brain. Seven-, thirteen-, and twenty-two-day-old rats were administered a single injection of acetate-1-^{14}C intraperitoneally and then sacrificed at intervals from 4 hours to 275 days. The brains were then analyzed for the incorporation of radioisotope into the fatty acids of

TABLE V

HALF-LIVES OF VARIOUS LIPIDS INTO BRAIN MITOCHONDRIA AND MYELIN[a]

Lipid	Mitochondria $T_{1/2}$, (days)	Myelin $T_{1/2}$, (days)
Phosphatidylinositol	2	35
Phosphatidylcholine	14	60
Phosphatidylserine	21	120
Phosphatidylethanolamine	30	210
Cholesterol	60	210–240
Sphingomyelin	30	300
Cerebroside		>365

[a] Data from Smith (1967).

gangliosides, cerebrosides, and sulfatides. In these experiments, a new analytical method for determining gangliosides was adopted. In each age group the palmitate ganglioside reaches a maximum value at approximately 4 hours, as compared to 2–10 days for the stearate ganglioside. Stearate was found to be the major acid of gangliosides comprising between 83 and 91% of the total acids present. In these experiments the highest specific activity was seen in the group of 13-day-old rats; at an age in which ganglioside deposition has slowed down considerably, 22 days, there was still significant incorporation of the isotope. Their data indicate that the palmitate of gangliosides is made *de novo* from acetate while the stearate of these lipids is made by elongation of palmitate which has entered a free fatty acid pool following degradation from the complex lipid.

The gangliosides are localized primarily in the gray matter of the central nervous system and the highest levels of bound acetylcholine have been found in association with this fraction. Because of the similar distribution and the physical properties of the gangliosides, this class of lipids has been implicated in the presynaptic release and binding of neurohormones (Burton and Howard, 1967). These experiments indicated that the binding of acetylcholine was due primarily to the phosphatidylcholine present, that neither cholesterol nor gangliosides alone could bind acetylcholine. However, both gangliosides and cholesterol had a marked effect on the ability of phosphatidylcholine to bind acetylcholine. Higher concentrations of gangliosides exhibited a marked inhibitory effect on this binding. Under these circumstances, choline was bound to an extent equal that of acetylcholine.

The incorporation of labeled acetate into cerebrosides and sulfatides was found to increase with time indicating a more complex course of accumulation (Kishimoto et al., 1965a,b) and a higher specific activity found in the 22-day-old rats. These turnover studies are primarily concerned with the fatty acid portion of the lipid and the possibility exists that other residues turn over with the gangliosides turning over at a more rapid rate (Radin et al., 1957). Studies with tritium-labeled acetate indicate that the sphingosine residue undergoes turnover and suggests the existence of a cerebroside fraction possessing a high turnover rate (Hajra and Radin, 1963). The data of Smith (1967) would indicate a long half-life (> 365 days) for cerebrosides from rat brain myelin (Table V).

V. Phospholipids

A. INTRODUCTION

The ubiquitous occurrence and unique physical properties of the phospholipids have provoked a number of important ideas concerning the function of these compounds in living cells. Possessing marked solubility in

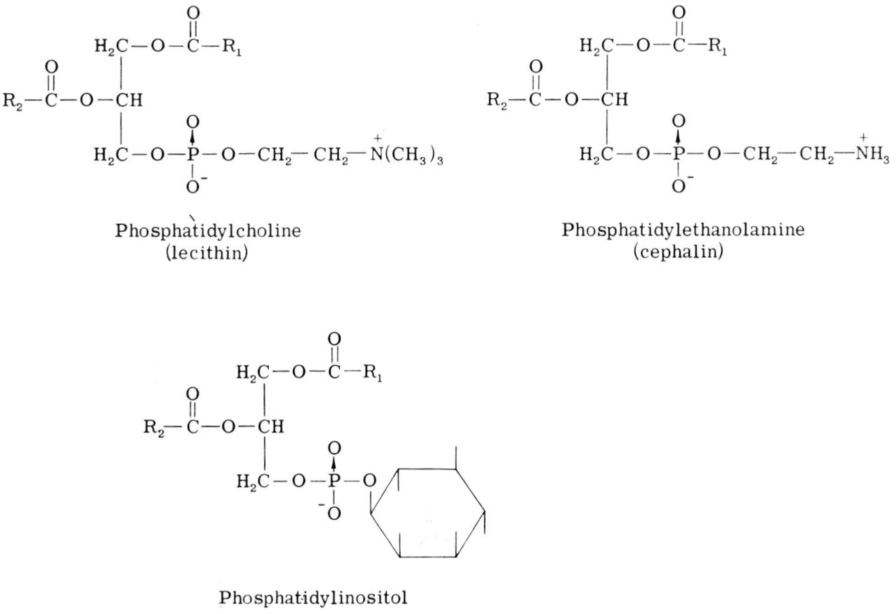

Phosphatidylcholine
(lecithin)

Phosphatidylethanolamine
(cephalin)

Phosphatidylinositol

FIG. 19. Chemical structures of phosphatidylcholine, phosphatidylethanolamine, and phosphatidylinositol.

both nonpolar solvents and water, the phospholipids play special roles in the mitochondrial cytochrome complex of respiratory enzymes, the stability of chylomicra and other membranes, ion transport, and secretory processes. An excellent review of the chemistry, metabolism, and function of the phospholipids has been collated by Ansell and Hawthorne (1964). Figure 19 illustrates the structures of the three most abundant phospholipids: phosphatidylcholine (lecithin), phosphatidylinositol, and phosphatidyl-ethanolamine (cephalin).

A first step in the elucidation of the biosynthetic pathways of phospholipids was the observation of Kornberg and Pricer (1953) that liver microsomes catalyzed the acylation of glycerol-3-phosphate to diacyl glycerol-3-phosphate, a lipid heretofore unknown as a biosynthetic intermediate substance.

B. Phosphatidylcholine (Lecithin)

1. *Biosynthesis*

The original work of Kennedy and Weiss (1955; 1956) and Weiss and Kennedy (1956) clearly defines the *in vitro* pathway for phospholipid biosynthesis, a problem which had been the subject of much speculation for decades. Investigating the mechanism of the incorporation of phosphorylcholine into the lecithin of isolated rat liver mitochondria, these investigators found that significant incorporation occurred only when the enzyme preparation was incubated with large quantities of adenosine triphosphate (5 μM). When the amorphous adenosine triphosphate was recrystallized, no activation occurred. It was later found that the amorphous adenosine triphosphate was contaminated with less than 1% cytidine triphosphate. Upon the addition of 0.5 μM cytidine triphosphate the amount of lecithin synthesized increased threefold. The discovery of the requirement of cytidine triphosphate for the conversion of phosphorylcholine to lecithin was the first demonstration of the specific role of a cytidine nucleotide in a major metabolic reaction.

2. *Subcellular Occurrence and Turnover*

As shown in Table I, phosphatidylcholine is the major phospholipid constituent of most membranes: 23, 48, and 64% in plasma membrane, rat liver mitochondria, and rat liver microsomes, respectively. To date, the biosynthesis of phospholipid molecules has been intensively investigated and fairly well understood; however, the biogenesis of specific cell structures from macromolecules remains relatively unknown. Dallner *et al.* (1966a,b) have studied the biochemical and ultrastructural development of the endoplasmic reticulum of rat hepatocytes during a period of rapid cell differentiation, from 3 days before to 8 days after birth. Ultrastructural studies 3 days before birth reveal that hepatocytes comprise approximately 1/3 of the total cell population with the endoplasmic reticulum consisting primarily of randomly dispersed rough-surfaced tubular elements, whose cavities appear slightly distended with an amorphous material. The attached ribosomes appear in the usual patterns, tightly packed at small intervals. The surrounding cytoplasmic matrix contains a large population of free ribosomes. Smooth endoplasmic reticulum occurs only in small randomly scattered vesicles. Biochemical studies indicate that at this time the phospholipid content of the liver is 12 mg/gm rising rapidly after birth to 20 mg/gm. At birth, the cell population becomes more homogeneous; the endoplasmic reticulum is greatly enlarged, and its elements are predominantly rough-surfaced with little change in the appearance and frequency of the smooth-surfaced endoplasmic reticulum. Three days after birth, the cell population of liver is comparable to that seen in adults, and the hepatocytes have almost reached the appearance of fully differentiated cells. The cytoplasm now contains numerous large lipid droplets.

The incorporation of ^{32}P into the individual phospholipids was studied in order to determine whether different rates of phospholipid production were operative during these periods. With the exception of phosphatidylethanolamine, which appears to be turning over quite rapidly, the percentage of radioactivity found in the individual phosphatides closely parallels the percentage of phosphatides in the lipid fraction. In all these age groups phosphatidylcholine represents approximately 44% of the total phospholipid. During this time, however, there are marked changes in the percentage composition of the fatty acids in the phospholipids: palmitic acid decreases 50%; oleic acid decreases 66% at day 5, and by day 90 is the same as newborn; arachidonic acid increases 30% at day 5, and by day 90 is the same as newborn.

Since the capacity of fetal liver to synthesize lipids is very high (Popják, 1954), Dallner *et al.* (1966a,b) concluded that the synthesis of membrane lipids is linked in some way to at least certain membrane proteins. Without proteins in the system, phospholipid synthesis stops after a short initial period. These products appear to be used exclusively for the biogenesis of various membranes since they are not further metabolized. These data suggest that the rate-limiting factor is not phospholipid synthesis, but the amount of membrane protein available.

Miller and Cornatzer (1966) found a marked increase in phosphatidylcholine P/mg microsomal protein during pre- and postnatal development;

the concentration of total and individual phospholipid P/mg mitochondrial protein does not change during development. Studies with ^{32}P into the phospholipid fractions of both liver mitochondria and microsomes indicate a relatively constant rate of synthesis during development. These authors concluded that the self-replicating machinery for the phospholipid mitochondrial membrane is well developed 12 days before birth.

Considerable uncertainty exists as to the origin of mitochondrial phospholipids. For example, Wilgram and Kennedy (1963) concluded that phosphatidylcholine is synthesized by the microsomes and subsequently transferred to the mitochondria. On the other hand, it has recently been shown that the phospholipid precursors, choline and acetate, can be incorporated *in vivo* into membrane phospholipids by rat liver mitochondria (Bygrave, 1969). In these experiments adult male rats were injected with ^{14}C-choline or ^{14}C-acetate. At subsequent intervals the livers were removed and purified microsomal, mitochondrial, outer mitochondrial, and inner mitochondrial membrane fractions were prepared. Following injection of ^{14}C-choline, the specific activities of the microsomal fraction, the outer mitochondrial membrane fraction, and whole mitochondria were approximately equivalent, reaching a maximum value at 6 hours and falling to minimum at 33 hours. The total specific activity of the inner membrane was lower, peaking at 12 hours and falling to minimum 18 hours after injection. If ^{14}C-acetate was injected the appearance of the curves were different. The data indicate that the apparent turnover of phosphatidyl-

TABLE VI

PHOSPHOLIPID TURNOVER IN MITOCHONDRIA[a]

	Turnover (hours)		
Lipid	Inner membrane	Outer membrane	Total mitochondria[b]
Phosphatidylcholine			
^{14}C-Acetate	5	11	14
^{14}C-Choline	3	16	15
Phosphatidylethanolamine			
^{14}C-Acetate	6	20–40	15

[a] Data from Bygrave (1969).
[b] Probably overestimated since peak incorporation occurs between the 6- and 12-hour interval.

choline constituents varies widely. As shown in Table VI, if choline is used as a marker, the turnover of phosphatidylcholine is 3, 16, and 8 hours for the inner membrane, the outer membrane, and the microsomal fraction, respectively. However, if acetate is used as a marker, the turnover times are 5, 11, and 30 hours for the inner membrane, outer membrane, and microsomal fraction, respectively.

Original studies concluded that mitochondria turned over *in toto* with a half-life of approximately 10 days (Fletcher and Sanadi, 1961). However, it is clear from the data of Pascaud (1964), Gurr *et al.* (1965), and Taylor *et al.* (1967) that some mitochondrial lipids can turn over with a half-life of several hours. Taylor *et al.* (1967) suggested that there are present in mitochondria different phospholipid components which exhibit turnovers of both long and short duration. From the data of Bygrave (1969) it appears that the inner mitochondrial membrane turns over faster than that of the outer mitochondrial membrane. The outer mitochondrial membrane and whole mitochondria appear indistinguishable.

Nachbaur *et al.* (1969) studied the incorporation of ^{14}C-oleic acid into rat liver mitochondrial phospholipids. The degree of purification was monitored by enzyme markers and electron microscopy. Under these conditions the inner membrane + matrix contained 31% phosphatidylcholine while the outer membrane contained approximately 50%. The outer membrane incorporated twice as much ^{14}C-oleic acid into phosphatidylcholine compared to the inner membrane + matrix. However, the incorporation into phosphatidylethanolamine was several fold greater.

It is of interest to note that the phospholipid components of mitochondrial membranes turn over faster than the protein component (Brunner and Neupert, 1968). This has previously been noted for microsomal membranes (Omura *et al.*, 1967) and may well represent a property of all biological membranes. The previous work cited (Dallner *et al.*, 1966a,b) would be compatible with a multistep assembly of membrane components allowing for phospholipid turnover independent of protein turnover.

Lewis and Majerus (1969) have recently demonstrated that human platelets represent a metabolically active source of *de novo* synthesis of phosphatidylcholine and certain other phospholipids to a lesser extent. While the amount of total phospholipids synthesized from glycerol is small compared to the total lipid content of the platelets, one cannot negate this as an important function of platelets. When platelets were incubated with thrombin there was a fivefold decrease in the incorporation into phosphatidylcholine over a 30-minute incubation period. The mechanism of this thrombin effect is not known; however, there exists the possibility it may act directly on one or more of the enzymes involved in phospholipid synthesis.

3. Ultrastructural Localization

Stein and Stein (1969) studied the incorporation of ^{3}H-choline into rat liver phosphatidylcholine by electron microscopic autoradiography. In these experiments rats were fed either a synthetic diet deficient in choline or the same diet supplemented with 0.6 gm/kg choline chloride (4–5 days).

Ultrastructurally, the livers of choline-deficient rats contained increased amounts of glycogen and lipid compared to control animals. The increased deposition of glycogen was probably due to the high sucrose content of the diet. The deposition of lipid occurred in the form of multiple droplets varying in size from a fraction of a micron to a few microns, which were not bounded by membrane. The endoplasmic reticulum, mitochondria, and lysosomes did not appear different. The Golgi cisternae were often dilated, and contained 50–80 mμ lipoprotein granules which were less abundant than in normal liver.

Five minutes following the intravenous injection of ^{3}H-choline into choline-deficient rats the autoradiographic reaction was uniformly distributed throughout the cytoplasm of the liver cell. Grains were found over the microvilli of the sinusoidal border and bile canaliculi. Grain counts indicated that 33.8, 28.6, and 13.0% of the radioactivity was present over the rough endoplasmic reticulum, smooth endoplasmic reticulum, and mitochondria, respectively. The occasional grains noted over the nuclei generally were associated with the nuclear membrane. Usually the central portion of the lipid droplets was not labeled; however, grains were associated with the droplet boundary. Sixty minutes after injection the distribution of activity was essentially the same.

Liver slices incubated in vitro with an excess of nonlabeled choline indicated that 80% of the microsomal phosphatidylcholine was present in the linoleyl fraction. It was not morphologically possible to distinguish this pool as the specific source of biliary phosphatidylcholine but other biochemical data would suggest that it is (Balint et al., 1965). It is possible that a specific carrier system exists for selectively binding and transporting this form of phosphatidylcholine to the bile. A protein carrier has been proposed for the exchange of phosphatidylcholine within the liver organelles (Wirtz and Zilversmit, 1968).

C. PHOSPHATIDYLINOSITOL

1. Biosynthesis

From the observations of Kennedy and Weiss (1955), other investigators looked in vain for an inositol kinase and the presence of CDP-inositol to induce the formation of phosphatidylinositol. Through no evidence was found for either, Agranoff *et al.* (1957) demonstrated that cytidine nucleotides significantly stimulated inositol incorporation into lipid phase, as a function of time. This observation led these investigators to postulate the formation of CDP-diglyceride and its subsequent cleavage by inositol to phosphatidylinositol and cytidine monophosphate. The sequence of reactions has been studied extensively in kidney (Agranoff *et al.*, 1958), liver (Paulus and Kennedy, 1960), and brain (Thompson *et al.*, 1963; Benjamins and Agranoff, 1969) and can be summarized as follows:

$$\text{CTP} + \text{diacyl glycerol-3-phosphate} \rightarrow \text{CDP-diglyceride} + \text{PPi}$$

$$\text{CDP-diglyceride} + \text{myoinositol} \rightarrow \text{phosphatidylinositol} + \text{CMP}$$

It is only in recent years that phosphotidylinositol has been recognized as a constituent of brain. Earlier work on the incorporation of radioactive precursors into brain inositides (Dawson, 1954; McMurray *et al.*, 1957) is difficult to interpret, since no distinction was made between phosphatidylinositol and the di- and triphosphoinositides. Thompson *et al.* (1963), taking advantage of the fact that a mixture of chloroform and methanol extracted only phosphatidylinositol, studied the biosynthesis of this lipid in aqueous dispersions of brain microsomes and confirmed the findings of Paulus and Kennedy (1960) in liver and kidney microsomes.

Thompson and his colleagues (Thompson *et al.*, 1960; Strickland *et al.*, 1960) also obtained evidence for a second biosynthetic pathway, not involving phosphatidic acid as an intermediate. In these experiments brain homogenates were incubated with ^{14}C- or ^{32}P-glycerophosphate in the presence of ATP, Mg^{++}, and CoA. Labeling of phosphatidylinositol was greatly increased by CDP-choline and to a lesser extent by cytidine triphosphate. In the presence of either nucleotide, the specific activity of phosphatidic acid dropped below that of phosphatidylinositol.

Much less is known concerning the biosynthesis of the polyphosphoinositides. Most workers assume that phosphotidylinositol is the precursor, with successive phosphorylations forming the di- and triphosphoinositides (Wagner *et al.*, 1962). Using rabbit brain slices, Brockerhoff and Ballou (1962) found that following isolation of the phosphoinositides and subsequent cleavage by phosphatase the ^{32}P specific activity of the 1-phosphate was greatest in phosphatidylinositol > di- > triphosphatidylinositol. This would be expected if biosynthesis is by successive phosphorylation of phosphatidylinositol. Subsequently Garbus *et al.* (1963) and Galliard and Hawthorne (1963) have shown that liver or kidney mitochondria rapidly incorporated ^{32}P into diphosphoinositide and trace amounts of triphosphoinositide. Labeling was markedly reduced by inhibitors of oxidative phosphorylation, but it is not known whether ATP or a precursor of ATP is the phosphate donor.

2. *Distribution*

Phosphatidylinositol comprises approximately 5 to 10% of the lipid P in most mammalian tissues; the polyinositides seem to be characteristic of nervous tissue. An exception to this is the work of Lo Chang and Sweeley (1963), who calculated the content of inositol lipids from dog adrenal tissue as follows: 9% phosphatidylinositol, 1% diphosphoinositide, 3% triphosphoinositide (% inositide P/total lipid P). Traces of higher inositides are present in heart, lung, and kidney (Wagner *et al.*, 1963).

3. *Functional Activity*

M.R. Hokin and Hokin (1953) demonstrated that the addition of acetylcholine to *in vitro* pancreas slices would cause a marked stimulation of ^{32}P-orthophosphate into total phospholipid. Later studies showed that the greatest turnover occurred in phosphatidylinositol; this was a selective increase in phospholipid turnover and not merely a reflection of increased tissue metabolism or stimulation of secretion (L.E. Hokin and Hokin, 1956; 1958). Subsequent autoradiographs have revealed that this increment in ^{32}P incorporation into phosphatidylinositol was associated primarily with the rough endoplasmic reticulum and the Golgi membranes (Hokin and Heubner, 1967). Hokin (1969) offers the following explanation for phosphatidylinositol turnover associated with protein secretion in pancreas. When protein synthesis is stimulated, the zymogen granule membrane coalesces with the plasma membrane and discharges its contents by reverse pinocytosis. The zymogen granule membrane then breaks down releasing the molecular constituents of phosphatidylinositol (inositol, glycerol, fatty acids, and phosphate), undegraded phosphatidylcholine, and other phosphatides. Phosphatidylinositol is then resynthesized in the rough endoplasmic reticulum and Golgi apparatus to replace that portion of the zymogen granule membrane which was secreted. Phosphatidylcholine is reassembled in the endoplasmic reticulum and Golgi apparatus without undergoing degration and resynthesis.

As shown in Table VII, phosphatidylinositol effects have been observed in many other glands on stimulation with natural secretagogues and in synaptic tissue on stimulation with acetylcholine (ACh). The secretion of proteins, polypeptides, or catecholamines by these glands probably involves intracellular protein transport mechanisms similar to those in the pancreas and the phosphatidylinositol effects in these glands play a similar role to that in the pancreas.

TABLE VII

Phosphatidylinositol Effects in Various Tissues

Tissue	Secretory product	Stimulating agent	Ratio of radioactivity of phosphatidylinositol of stimulated to unstimulated tissue	Reference
Pigeon pancreas	Digestive enzymes	ACh, pancreozymin	15.0	Hokin and Hokin (1960)
Parotid gland	Amylase	ACh, adrenaline	5.2	Eggman and Hokin (1960)
Thyroid	Thyroid hormone	Thyrotropin	3.6	Freinkel (1957)
Salt gland	NaCl	ACh	3.2	Hokin and Hokin (1960)
Cat superior cervical ganglion	?	ACh	3.2	L. E. Hokin (1965)
Cerebral cortex	?	ACh	2.4	Hokin and Hokin (1955)
Adrenal medulla	Adrenaline	ACh	2.2	M. R. Hokin et al. (1958a)
Adenohypophysis	ACTH	CRF	1.4	M. R. Hokin et al. (1958b)

In superior cervical ganglion where ACh has been established as the synaptic transmitter, the stimulation in phosphatidylinositol turnover is within the cytoplasm of the cell body (Hokin, 1965). The nerve cell body is in many ways like glandular cells in that it possesses abundant rough-surfaced endoplasmic reticulum localized in the classic Nissl bodies, shows prominent smooth-surfaced Golgi membranes, and exhibits high rates of protein synthesis and biogenic amine formation. There is good evidence that the biogenic amines are packaged in synaptic vesicles in the cell bodies and are transported down the axon. The increased synthesis of phosphatidylinositol in sympathetic ganglia on stimulation by ACh may be involved with an accelerated rate of formation of vesicle membranes and may represent a natural adaptor response to excessive stimulation of the nerve cell.

4. *Turnover*

Yagi and Kotaki (1969) have recently studied the turnover of myoinositol on hepatic phospholipid metabolism. These *in vitro* studies indicate that microsomal incorporation of isotopic myoinositol into phosphatidylinositol reached a peak 1 hour after injection and quickly decreased to the normal level, indicating that most of the phosphatidylinositol synthesized in the earlier stage did not stay in the microsome but moved from these organelles. The slow incorporation of the isotope found after the spike phase was probably due to the labeling of structural or membranous phosphatidylinositol in the microsomes. Since these results indicate the production of transferable phosphatidylinositol in the microsomes, it is possible to presume that the other transferable phosphatides are produced analogously in these organelles.

Although the production of phosphatides in the isolated liver mitochondria has not been clearly established, a rapid labeling of the liver mitochondrial phosphatidylinositol can be observed when young rats are injected with isotopic myoinositol (Yagi and Kotaki, 1969). In contrast to the labeling of microsomal phosphatidylinositol, however, a spike is not observable. There is an initial 3-hour stage of rapid labeling after injection followed by a slow labeling which continues for at least 70 hours.

Despite the rapid incorporation of the isotopic cyclitol into mitochondrial phosphatidylinositol at the intital 3-hour stage, no significant change is detectable in that period in the phosphatidylinositol/phosphatidylcholine ratio. This would imply that the mitochondrion is not an organelle producing extra phosphatidylinositol. Nevertheless, it may be important to consider whether the mitochondrion could produce phosphatides in a way different from that found in microsomes, since there is some evidence

(Pullman and Schatz, 1967) that the mitochondrion is self-replicating in a way similar to cell division. If this were the case, the mitochondrion itself would contain the systems required for the production of major components of their structure. As previously discussed, the findings of Agranoff *et al.* (1958) have demonstrated that an enzyme system in guinea pig kidney mitochondrial preparation catalyzing the incorporation of myo-inositol into inositol phosphatide suggesting the possible production of phosphatidylinositol in these organelles.

Following injection of acetate-1-^{14}C, phosphatidylinositol exhibited a half-life of 2 days in rat brain mitochondrial-rich fraction (also containing axoplasmic fragments, synaptic membranes, and particles) while the half-life for brain myelin was 35 days (Smith, 1967). In these experiments, a number of brain lipids were analyzed both in the mitochondrial-rich fraction and purified myelin, and the half-lives are shown in Table V. These experiments were corrected for the dilution by new myelin, a process which proceeds throughout most of the life of the rat.

Much of the current interest in brain phosphoinositide metabolism stems from the original observation of Dawson (1954) that, in a guinea pig brain dispersion incubated with ^{32}P, inositides (probably phosphatidylinositol) and phosphatidic acid were much more highly labeled than the other phospholipids. L.E. Hokin and Hokin (1958) obtained similar results with brain slices, though specific activities were not recorded. LeBaron *et al.* (1962) studied the labeling of brain phosphoinositide in rats given ^{32}P and found that maximum specific activity occurred at about 4 hours. It seems clear that the inositide fraction of the brain owes its high turnover of ^{32}P *in vivo* and *in vitro* to its content of di- and triphosphoinositide. This has provoked speculation about the role of the higher inositides in cation transport, especially since enzymes capable of removing the monoester phosphate occur in the brain and are activated by sodium and potassium ions.

Hayashi *et al.* (1962) observed the effect of electric convulsions on the equilibration of ^{32}P *in vivo* into rabbit brain lipids. In unstimulated brain, a lipid resembling triphosphoinositol is highly labeled and one resembling phosphatidylinositol less so; however, the identities of the lipids were not established definitely. After the convulsions the triphosphoinositol was not detected, while the radioactivity of the phosphatidylinositol was increased; thus it was thought that a conversion of triphosphoinositide to phosphatidylinositol took place, and the authors suggest that this might occur in physiological stimulation also. Subsequently Larrabee *et al.* (1963a) perfused rat superior cervical ganglia with a medium containing inorganic ^{32}P. Stimulation of the preganglionic nerve supermaximally 5 to 10 times per second for 3 hours increased the labeling of phosphatidylinositol by more than 50%. The labeling of phosphatidic acid, phosphatidylcholine, and phosphatidylethanolamine was unaffected. In these experiments the lipids were identified by chromatography on silica-impregnated paper. Subsequent work indicated that the labeled phosphatidylinositol was located largely in the nerve cell bodies (Larrabee et al., 1963b). Baranov (1960) observed an increase in phosphatidylpeptide turnover as measured by ^{32}P in the superior cervical sympathetic ganglion stimulated with super-maximal square wave shocks.

Durell and Garland (1969) have demonstrated that the addition of $10^{-4}M$ acetylcholine stimulates the phosphodiesteratic cleavage of phospho-inositide in rat brain synaptosomes and hypothesized that this chemical reaction results in increased local permeability with secondary consequences in various tissues: for example, in the neuron, depolarization would occur which could trigger the action potential. Most previous speculations on the mechanisms of chemical transmission are focused on the possibility that a confirmational change in a membrane component or a dissociation of two membrane components triggers the action potential (Nachmansohn, 1963; Watkins, 1965). The experiments of Durell and Garland have been per-formed at concentrations of ACh several orders of magnitude higher than are generally believed to be required to trigger neurons; thus ultimate confirmation of their hypothesis will require considerably more attention to the correspondence with physiological phenomena.

D. Phosphatidylethanolamine (Cephalin)

Phosphatidylethanolamine is another class of phospholipids occurring in quantities second only to phosphatidylcholine. The amine group of this class is less basic than the quaternary ammonium of phosphatidylcholine, and accordingly when both contain similar fatty acids phosphatidylethanol-amine is approximately 100 times less soluble in alcohol. At present, the Kennedy scheme for synthesis for phosphatidylethanolamine would appear to be the only one which can be produced in vitro to give a de novo synthesis of the lipid (Kennedy and Weiss, 1955; 1956). The scheme necessitates the rapid turnover of the cytidine intermediates but since their concentrations in tissues are quite low, this is difficult to measure. Glyceride-glycerol serves as the immediate precursor in phosphatidylethanolamine biosynthesis. The ethanolamine portion of the molecule is available either from dietary sources or is biosynthesized from the amino acids serine and glycine. In general, this group of phospholipids contains larger amounts of unsaturated fatty acids than does the phosphatidylcholine of the same tissue.

As shown in Table I, phosphatidylethanolamine comprises 14, 20, 28, and 17% of the total lipids found in human myelin, plasma membrane, rat liver mitochondria, and rat liver microsomes, respectively.

The in vivo incorporation of L-^{14}C-serine into phospholipids of developing rat brain was studied before and during the stage of active myelination, 3 and 6 days of age, (Abdel-Latif and Abood, 1966). Of the total phospholipids tested, the incorporation of radioactivity into phosphatidylethanolamine was second only to that seen with phosphatidylserine. Similar results were found with liver mitochondria (Hübscher *et al.*, 1959). By contrast, heart homogenates exhibited the greatest incorporation of serine into phosphatidylethanolamine (Marinetti *et al.*, 1962).

Arvidson (1968) found that the incorporation of ^{32}P into phosphatidylethanolamine of rat liver subcellular fractions showed a much higher specific activity when compared with phosphatidylcholine. Differences in the specific activity parallel the degree of unsaturation of the fatty acid present, alluding to a metabolic heterogeneity and a much more rapid turnover of phosphatidylethanolamines. A more rapid turnover of phosphatidylethanolamine was observed by Dallner *et al.* (1966a,b) in the rough endoplasmic reticulum of developing rat liver. Smith (1967) has calculated half-lives for phosphatidylethanolamine of 30 and 210 days in purified brain mitochondria and myelin, respectively.

Nachbaur *et al.* (1969) found that the incorporation of ^{14}C-oleic acid into phosphatidylethanolamine was 2 times greater by the inner membrane + matrix of rat liver mitochondria as compared to the incorporation by the outer membrane. Studying the incorporation of ^{14}C-acetate into phosphatidylethanolamine by various subcellular fractions, Bygrave (1969) found optimal activity by the mitochondria and inner membrane at 6 hours, no change in the outer membrane during this time, and a fall in the microsomal fraction over a period of 18 hours. The specific activity of the whole mitochondria was intermediate between the purified outer and inner membrane fractions throughout the duration of the experiment. As shown in Table VI, the turnover of acetate into phosphatidylethanolamine was 6, 20–40, and 15 hours by the inner membrane, outer membrane, and whole mitochondria, respectively. Thus phospholipid constituents of the inner mitochondrial membrane turn over more rapidly than the other fractions studied. From the work of Stoffel and Schiefer (1968) the enzymes for complex phospholipid formation in mitochondria are located at the outer membrane, and the temporal relationship found by Bygrave (1969) would suggest that the phospholipid constituents are transferred from the outer mitochondrial membrane to the inner membrane.

VI. Brown Adipose Tissue

In 1551, Gesner (Smith and Roberts, 1964) first described the multilocular nature of brown adipose tissue in the intercapsular region of the

marmot. This tissue has subsequently been demonstrated in a number of
species, both hibernators (Chaffee *et al.*, 1964; Chaffee *et al.*, 1966b),
nonhibernators (Brück and Wünnenberg, 1965; Chaffee *et al.*, 1966a),
and human neonates (Dawkins and Scopes, 1965; Silverman *et al.*, 1964).
In most mammals brown adipose tissue accounts for only a very small
portion of the body weight, but in newborn rabbits it averages approximately 5% of the body weight. According to Smith and Roberts (1964)
the distribution of brown adipose tissue consists of

1. a pair of brown fat pads located middorsal deep in the middorsal
   superior cervical region;
2. the intercapsular region with extensions engulfing the vessels of the
   axillary region;
3. that portion of the thorax overlying the aorta, azygous vein, and the
   sympathetic chain; and
4. extensions along the aorta diverging mediodorsally at the level of
   the kidneys coverning the converging iliacs and renal veins.

Joel (1965), Napolitano (1965), and Smith and Horwitz (1969) have
reviewed the biochemistry, fine structure, and physiological function of
brown adipose tissue.

Fat cells from brown adipose tissue can be histologically distinguished
from white adipose tissue by their smaller size (25–40 μ), larger cytoplasmic
volume, and increased vascularity. Characteristically, the lipid is contained
in small inclusions in the cytoplasm (multilocular), as opposed to the large
lipid vacuole (unilocular) seen in while adipose tissue. Furthermore, the
nucleus is more centrally located in the cytoplasm and is generally spherical.
The cytoplasm contains a profusion of mitochondria of varying size and
shape, which exhibit a complex internal structure generally characterized by
closely packed christae. Closely associated with the mitochondria are numerous lipid droplets, and there appears to be an absence of the mitochondrial limiting membrane when these two subcellular particles are in
close opposition. In accordance with these ultrastructural findings, subsequent chemical studies have indicated an unusually high content of the components of the electron transport system (cytochrome content, 2.3 mg/gm
lipid-free dry weight). For these reasons it has been suggested by many
investigators that the primary function of brown adipose tissue is to increase heat production in nonshivering thermogenesis. There appears to
be little subcellular organization as the Golgi apparatus and endoplasmic
reticulum are relatively sparse, though considerable amounts of glycogen
may often be detected.

Steiner and Cahill (1964) estimate the total lipid content to be 30 $\pm$ 3
and 141 $\pm$ 11 mg/mg N in brown and white adipose tissues, respectively.

The nature of the lipid comprising brown adipose tissue was estimated to be 1.3 mg phospholipid/mg N and the remainder being in the form of neutral lipids. In the mouse approximately 75% of the triglycerides contain oleic and linoleic acid (Napolitano *et al.*, 1965). The high phospholipid concentration, compared to white adipose tissue, presumably reflects the greater number of mitochondria. Approximately 68% is in the form of phosphatidylcholine and phosphatidylethanolamine (Spencer and Dempster, 1962).

The turnover of the specific lipids in brown adipose tissue has not been examined in any detail. The autoradiographic study by Cameron and Smith (1964) indicates that after 6–12 hours of acute cold exposure (6°C) the size of the lipid vacuole in brown adipose tissue is minimal and approximately 1/3 that of the control. However, by 24 hours the vacuole returned to control size and remained the same for a period up to 60 days. Parallel with this, a decrease in cell area was found which subsequently returned within 24 hours. By contrast, the cells from white adipose tissue markedly decreased in size for a period of 8 to 16 days. During cold exposure new brown fat cells arise by cytogenesis from vascular associated cells and mitotic division of brown fat cells was not seen. These results have subsequently been confirmed by Hunt and Hunt (1967).

Steiner and Cahill (1964) found that following 9 days of cold exposure, the total lipid content of brown adipose tissue decreased to approximately 37% compared to rats maintained at 20°C. This was associated with a significant change in the nature of the lipid. The neutral lipids decreased from 28.7 to 9.0 mg/mg N while the phospholipid increased from 1.3 to 2.4 mg/mg N. These same investigators studied the conversion of uniformly labeled ^{14}C-glucose into the various lipid fractions 1 hour after administration of the isotope. The specific activities of the neutral lipids, fatty acids, and glyceride-glycerol was increased four-, ten-, and tenfold respectively, as a result of cold exposure, whereas the total lipid content is decreased only threefold. There was no significant change in the specific activity of the phospholipids while total phospholipid content doubled. These authors reported no significant change in the total lipid content of white adipose tissue. The work of Baumber and Denyes (1964) clearly indicates an increased *in vitro* incorporation of ^{14}C from acetate-1-^{14}C into the brown fat lipid of cold-adapted hamsters (3–8) weeks. However, this cannot be offered as definitive proof of increase fatty acid synthesis since no assay of the tissue acetate pool before and after cold exposure was made. In a subsequent study Steiner *et al.* (1968) demonstrated that before and after chronic cold exposure (12 weeks) the neutral lipids, primarily triglycerides, decreased from 98 to 88% of the total tissue lipid and the phospholipids increased from 2.3 to 11.6% following cold exposure. It is

TABLE VIII
Turnover Rates of Lipids in Mammalian Tissues

Class	Lipid	Tissue	$T_{1/2}$ (days)	Reference
I	Triglycerides	Lactating mammary gland	30 minutes	Stein and Stein (1967b)
	Palmitic acid	Plasma	17 seconds	Boberg (1969)
	Glycerol	Plasma	30	Shafrir and Gorin (1963)
	Phosphatidylinositol	Mitochondria	2	Smith (1967)
	Cholesterol	Erythrocytes	5	Goodman (1967)
II	Cholesterol	Cord myelin	14	Smith and Eng (1965)
	Cerebroside	Brain (myelin)	45	Kishimoto et al. (1965a)
	Phosphatidylcholine	Mitochondria	11–23	Smith (1967)
	Cholesterol	Skeletal muscle	52	Goodman (1967)
III	Phosphatidylcholine	Brain myelin	60	Smith (1967)
	Cerebroside fatty acid moiety	Brain	125–156	Burton (1965)
	Saturated fatty acids	Abdominal fat	60	Thompson and Ballou (1954)
		Skin	30	
	Unsaturated fatty acids	Skin	250	Thompson and Ballou (1954)
		Carcass	300	Thompson and Ballou (1954)
		Carcass	20	Schoenheimer (1942)
	Cholesterol	Skin	100	Thompson and Ballou (1954)
		Carcass	300	Thompson and Ballou (1954)
		Brain myelin	210–240	Smith (1967)

difficult at this time to evaluate the activity of the triglyceride cycle though all these studies suggest that in cold-acclimated animals there is an increased rate of lipid synthesis in brown adipose tissue.

Himms-Hagen (1965) reported that following acute cold exposure there is a loss of lipids and edema of the brown adipose tissue; however, during prolonged cold exposure, an increase in wet weight, lipid content, nonlipid material, and water is seen. She also found the rate of fatty acid synthesis from ^{14}C-glucose is markedly increased in brown adipose tissue following prolonged cold exposure. By contrast, Patkin and Masoro (1964) found an unaltered fatty acid synthesis in the brown adipose tissue of cold-acclimated rats. Dawkins and Hull (1964) have also obtained evidence indicating that following cold exposure brown adipose tissue of newborn rabbits has an increased rate of triglyceride lipolysis and most of the free fatty acids formed are reesterified into triglyceride within the brown adipose tissue cell. This data would implicate the lipolysis–fatty acid esterification cycle as an important biochemical mechanism in the thermogenic response of brown adipose tissue following cold exposure.

VII. Summary

It is evident from the original investigations of Schoenheimer (1942) that the lipids in mammalian tissues are constantly subject to a variety of complex chemical processes which includes synthesis, interconversion, and degradation. The specific studies summarized indicate that any given lipid or lipid class may not be considered independently of location or function; correspondingly, the half-life for the renewal of the same lipid may vary as much as three- or fourfold, depending upon the tissue studied and the method used. Table VIII illustrates this point and clearly indicates that all the lipid classes are capable of molecular renewal although the rates may vary widely. The improved techniques of electron microscopic autoradiography combined with sensitive analytical procedures will afford insight into the subcellular events involved in lipid synthesis, secretion, and transport.

REFERENCES

Abdel-Latif, A. A., and Abood, L. G. (1966). *In vivo* incorporation of L-(^{14}C) serine into phospholipids and proteins of the subcellular fractions of developing rat brain. *J. Neurochem.* **13**, 1189–1196.

Agranoff, B. W., Bradley, R. M., and Brady, R. O. (1957). The role of cytidine nucleotides in the formation of inositol-containing lipide. *Biochim. Biophys. Acta* **25**, 445–446.

Agranoff, B. W., Bradley, R. M., and Brady, R. O. (1958). The enzymic synthesis of inositol phosphatide. *J. Biol. Chem.* **233**, 1077–1083.

Anker, H. S. (1948). Synthesis of carbonyl-labeled pyruvic acid. *J. Biol. Chem.* **176**, 1333–1335.

Ansell, C. B., and Hawthorne, J. N. (1964). "Phospholipids—Chemistry, Metabolism and Function." Elsevier, Amsterdam.

Arvidson, G. A. E. (1968). Structural and metabolic heterogeneity of rat liver glycerophosphatides. *Eur. J. Biochem.* **4**, 478–486.

Bailey, J. M. (1967). Cellular lipid nutrition and lipid transport. *In* "Lipid Metabolism in Tissue Culture Cells" (G. H. Rothblat and D. Kritchevsky, eds.), pp. 85–109. Wistar Inst. Press, Philadelphia, Pennsylvania.

Balint, J. A., Kyriakides, E. C., Spitzer, H. L., and Morrison, E. S. (1965). Lecithin fatty acid composition in bile and plasma of man, dogs, rats, and oxen. *J. Lipid Res.* **6**, 96–99.

Baranov, M. N. (1960). Changes in phosphorus metabolism of the superior and nodose ganglia with reference to some functional states of these structures. *Biokhimiya* **25**, 781–786.

Bargmann, W., and Knoop, A. (1959). Uber die Morphologie der Milchskration. Licht und elektronmikroscropische Studien an der Milchdruse der Ratte. *Z. Zellforsch. Mickroskop. Anat. Abt. Histochem.* **49**, 344–388.

Baumber, J., and Deynes, A. (1964). Acetate-1-C^{14} utilization by brown fat from hamsters in cold exposure and hibernation. *Can. J. Biochem.* **42**, 1397–1401.

Benjamins, J. A., and Agranoff, B. W. (1969). Distribution and properties of CDP-diglyceride: Inositol transferase from brain. *J. Neurochem.* **16**, 513–527.

Bernhard, K., and Schoenheimer, R. J. (1940). The inertia of highly unsaturated fatty acids in the animal investigated with deuterium. *J. Biol. Chem.* **133**, 707–720.

Bernhard, K., Steinhauser, H., and Bullet, F. (1942). Investigations on fat metabolism with the aid of D as indicator. I. The question of the fat acids necessary for life (essential fat acids). *Helv. Chim. Acta* **25**, 1313–1318.

Bloch, K. (1948). The biological synthesis of lipides. *Cold Spring Harbor Symp. Quant. Biol.* **13**, 29–34.

Bloch, K. (1965). Biological synthesis of cholesterol. *Science* **150**, 19–28.

Bloch, K., and Rittenberg, D. (1945). An estimation of acetic acid formation in the rat. *J. Biol. Chem.* **159**, 45–58.

Bloch, K., Berg, B. N., and Ritternberg, D. (1943). The biological conversion of cholesterol to cholic acid. *J. Biol. Chem.* **149**, 511–517.

Bloch, K. E., Borek, E., and Rittenberg, D. (1946). Synthesis of cholesterol in surviving liver. *J. Biol. Chem.* **162**, 441–449.

Boberg, J. (1969). Turnover of H^3-labelled palmitate in the unanesthetized rat. *Acta Physiol. Scand.* **76**, 495–502.

Brady, R. O. (1966). Immunochemical properties of the glycolipids. *J. Amer. Oil Chem. Soc.* **43**, 67–69.

Brockerhoff, H., and Ballou, C. E. (1962). On the metabolism of the brain phosphoinositide complex. *J. Biol. Chem.* **237**, 1764–1766.

Brück, K., and Wünnenberg, B. (1965). Unterschungen über die Bedeutung des multilokularen Fettgewbes fur die Thermogenese des neugebarenen Meerschweinchens. *Arch. Ges. Physiol.* **283**, 1–16.

Brunner, G., and Neupert, W. (1968). Turnover of outer and inner membrane proteins of rat liver mitochondria. *Fed. Eur. Biochem. Soc.* **1**, 153–155.

Burr, G. O., and Burr, M. M. (1929). A new deficiency disease produced by the rigid exclusion of fat from the diet. *J. Biol. Chem.* **82**, 345–367.

Burton, R. M. (1965). The role of lipids in the binding and release of neurohormones by subcellular particles. *Ninth Int. Conf. Biochem. Probl. Lipids, Noordwyzik, The Netherlands.*

Burton, R. M., and Howard, R. E. (1967). Gangliosides and acetylcholine of the nervous system. VIII. Role of lipids in the binding and release of neurohormones by synaptic vesicles. *Ann. N. Y. Acad. Sci.* **144**, 411–432.

Bygrave, F. L. (1969). Biosynthesis and turnover of the phospholipid components of the inner and outer membranes of rat liver mitochondria. *J. Biol. Chem.* **244**, 4768–4772.

Cameron, I. L., and Smith, R. E. (1964). Cytological responses of brown fat tissue in cold-exposed rats. *J. Cell Biol.* **23**, 89–100.

Caro, L. G., and Palade, G. E. (1964). Protein synthesis, storage, and discharge in the pancreatic exocrine cell. An autoradiographic study. *J. Cell. Biol.* **20**, 473–495.

Carter, H. E., Johnson, P., and Weber, E. J. (1965). Glycolipids. *Annu. Rev. Biochem.* **34**, 109–142.

Chaffee, R. R. J., Allen, J. R., Cassuto, Y., and Smith, R. E. (1964). Biochemistry of brown fat and liver of cold-acclimated hamsters. *Amer. J. Physiol.* **207**, 1211–1214.

Chaffee, R. R. J., Allen, J. R., Brewer, M., Horvath, S. M., Mason, C., and Smith, R. E. (1966a). Cellular physiology of cold- and heat-exposed squirrel monkeys (*Saimiri sciurea*). *J. Appl. Physiol.* **21**, 151–157.

Chaffee, R. R. J., Pengelley, E. T., Allen, J. R., and Smith, R. E. (1966b). Biochemistry of brown fat and liver of hibernating golden-mantled brown squirrels (*Citellus lateralis*). *Can. J. Physiol. Pharmacol.* **44**, 217–223.

Chesterton, C. J. (1966). The subcellular site of cholesterol synthesis in rat liver. *Biochem. Biophys. Res. Commun.* **25**, 205–209.

Chesterton, C. J. (1968). Distribution of cholesterol precursors and other lipids among rat liver intracellular structures. *J. Biol. Chem.* **243**, 1147–1151.

Chevallier, F. (1967). Dynamics of cholesterol in rats, studied by the isotopic equilibrium method. *In* "Advances in Lipid Research" (R. Paoletti and D. Kritchevsky, eds.), pp. 209–239. Academic Press, New York.

Clayton, R. B., and Bloch, K. (1956). The biological conversion of lanosterol to cholesterol. *J. Biol. Chem.* **218**, 319–325.

Coleman, R., and Finean, J. B. (1965). Some properties of plasma membranes isolated from guinea-pig tissues. *Biochem. J.* **97**, 39P–40P.

Dallner, G. (1963). Studies on the structural and enzymic organization of the membranous elements of liver microsomes. *Acta Pathol. Microbiol. Scan. Suppl.* **166**, 1–94.

Dallner, G., Siekevitz, P., and Palade, G. E. (1966a). Biogenesis of endoplasmic reticulum membranes. I. Structural and chemical differentiation in developing rat hepatocyte. *J. Cell Biol.* **30**, 73–96.

Dallner, G., Siekevitz, P., and Palade, G. E. (1966b). Biogenesis of endoplasmic reticulum membranes. II. Synthesis of constitutive microsomal enzymes in developing rat hepatocyte. *J. Cell Biol.* **30**, 97–117.

Davison, A., Dobbing, J., Morgan, R., and Payling Wright, G. (1958). The deposition and disposal of cholesterol-4-C^{14} in the brain of growing chickens. *J. Neurochem.* **3**, 89–94.

Davison, A., Dobbing, J., Morgan, R., and Payling Wright, G. (1959a). Metabolism of myelin: The persistence of (4-^{14}C) cholesterol in the mammalian central nervous system. *Lancet* **1**, 658–660.

Davison, A., Morgan, R., Wajda, M., and Payling Wright, G. (1959b). Metabolism of myelin lipids: Incorporation of 3-C^{14}-serine in brain lipides of the developing rabbit and their persistence in the central nervous system. *J. Neurochem.* **4**, 360–365.

Dawkins, M. J. R., and Hull, D. (1964). Brown adipose tissue and the response of new-born rabbits to cold. *J. Physiol.* **172**, 216–238.

Dawkins, M. J. R., and Scopes, J. W. (1965). Non-shivering thermogenesis and brown adipose tissue in human new-born infant. *Nature (London)* **206**, 201–202.

Dawson, R. M. C. (1954). The measurement of ^{32}P labelling of individual kephalins and lecithin in a small sample of tissue. *Biochim. Biophys. Acta* **14**, 374–379.

Dietschy, J. M., and Siperstein, M. D. (1967). Effect of cholesterol feeding and fasting on sterol synthesis in seventeen tissues of the rat. *J. Lipid Res.* **8**, 97–104.

Downes, H. R. (1962), "The Chemistry of Living Cells." Harper and Row, New York.

Durell, J., and Garland, J. T. (1969). Acetylcholine-stimulated phosphodiesteratic cleavage of phosphoinositides: Hypothetical role in membrane depolarization. *Ann. N.Y. Acad. Sci.* **165**, 743–754.

Eggman, L. D., and Hokin, L. E. (1960). The relationship between secretory activity and the incorporation of P^{32} into phosphoinositide and phosphatidic acid in salivary glands and pigeon esophageal mucosa *in vitro*. *J. Biol. Chem.* **235**, 2569–2571.

Eichberg, J. Hauser, G., and Karnovsky, M. L. (1969). Lipids of nervous tissue. *In* "The Structure and Function of Nervous Tissue" (G. H. Bourne, ed.), pp. 185–287. Academic Press, New York.

Farquhar, M. G. (1961). Origin and fate of secretory granules in cells of the anterior pituitary gland. *Trans. N. Y. Acad. Sci.* **23**, 346–351.

Fletcher, M. J., and Sanadi, D. R. (1961). Turnover of rat-liver mitochondria. *Biochim. Biophys. Acta.* **51**, 356–360.

Folch-Pi, J. (1955). Composition of the brain in relation to maturation. *In* "Biochemistry of the Developing Nervous System" (H. Waelsch, ed.), pp. 121–136. Academic Press, New York.

Freinkel, N. (1957). Pathways of thyroidal phosphorus metabolism: the effect of pituitary thyrotropin upon the phospholipids of the sheep thyroid gland. *Endocrinology* **61**, 448–460.

Galliard, T., and Hawthorne, J. N. (1963). Rapid labelling of diphosphoinositide in liver mitochondria. *Biochim. Biophys. Acta* **70**, 479–481.

Garbus, J., De Luca, H. F., Loomans, M. E., and Strong, F. M. (1963). The rapid incorporation of phosphate into mitochondrial lipids. *J. Biol. Chem.* **238**, 59–63.

Gautheron, C., Petit, L., and Chevallier, F. (1969). Synthesis of cholesterol in the central nervous system and in radiographic localization. *Exp. Neurol.* **25**, 18–23.

Goodman, D. S. (1967). Studies of turnover of plasma cholesterol. *In* "Proceedings of the 1967 Deuel Conference on Lipids on The Fate of Dietary Lipids" (G. Cowgill and L. W. Kinsell, eds.), pp. 88–92. U. S. Dept. Health, Education, and Welfare, Washington, D. C.

Grynfeltt, J. (1937). Etude de processus cytologique de la sécrétion mammaire. *Arch. Anat. Microscop. Morphol. Exp.* **33**, 177–208.

Gurr, M. I., Prottey, C., and Hawthorne, J. N. (1965). The phospholipids of liver-cell fractions. II. Incorporation of (^{32}P) orthophosphate *in vivo* in normal and regenerating rat liver. *Biochim. Biophys. Acta* **106**, 357–370.

Hajra, A. K., and Radin, N. S. (1963) Isotopic studies of the biosynthesis of the cerebroside fatty acids in rats. *J. Lipid Res.* **4**, 270–278.

Hayashi, K., Kanoh, T., Shimizu, S., Kai, M., and Yamazoe. S., (1962). Studies on the brain phospholipids. I. Incorporation of P^{32} into phospholipids in guinea pig brain slices. *J. Biochem.* **51,** 63–71.

Himms-Hagen, J. (1965). Lipid metabolism in warm-acclimated and cold-acclimated rats exposed to cold. *Can. J. Physiol. Pharmacol.* **43,** 379–403.

Hokin, L. E. (1965). Autoradiographic localization of the acetylcholine-stimulated synthesis of phosphatidylinositol in the superior cervical ganglion. *Proc. Nat. Acad. Sci. U.S.* **53,** 1369–1376.

Hokin, L. E. (1969). Functional activity in glands and synaptic tissue and the turnover of phosphatidylinositol. *Ann. N. Y. Acad. Sci.* **165,** 695–709.

Hokin, L. E., and Heubner, D. (1967). Radioautographic localization of the increased synthesis of phosphatidylinositol in response to pancreozymin or acetylcholine in guinea pig pancreas slices. *J. Cell Biol.* **33,** 521–530.

Hokin, L. E., and Hokin, M. R. (1955). Effects of acetylcholine on the turnover of phosphoryl units in individual phospholipids of pancreas slices and brain cortex slices. *Biochim. Biophys. Acta* **18,** 102–110.

Hokin, L. E., and Hokin, M. R. (1956). The actions of pancreozymin in pancreas slices and the role of phospholipids in enzyme secretion. *J. Physiol.* **132,** 442–453.

Hokin, L. E., and Hokin, M. R. (1958). Phosphoinositides and protein secretion in pancreas slices. *J. Biol. Chem.* **233,** 805–810.

Hokin, L. E., and Hokin, M. R. (1960). Studies on the carrier function of phosphatidic acid in sodium transport. I. The turnover of phosphatidic acid and phosphoinositide in the avian salt gland in stimulation of secretion. *J. Gen. Physiol.* **44,** 61–85.

Hokin, M. R., and Hokin, L. E. (1953). Enzyme secretion and the incorporation of P^{32} into phospholipides of pancreas slices. *J. Biol. Chem.* **203,** 967–977.

Hokin, M. R., Benfey, B. G., and Hokin, L. E. (1958a). Phospholipides and adrenaline secretion in guinea pig adrenal medulla. *J. Biol. Chem.* **223,** 814–817.

Hokin, M. R., Hokin, L. E., Saffran, M., Schally, A. V., and Zimmermann, B. U. (1958b). Phospholipides and the secretion of adrenocorticotropin and of cortico-steroids. *J. Biol. Chem.* **233,** 811–813.

Holman, R. T. (1951). Metabolism of isomers of linoleic and linolenic acids. *Proc. Soc. Exp. Biol. Med.* **76,** 100–102.

Hübscher, G., Dils, R. R., and Pover, W. F. R. (1959). Studies on the biosynthesis of phosphatidyl serine. *Biochim. Biophys. Acta* **36,** 518–528.

Hunt, T. E., and Hunt, E. A. (1967). A radioautographic study of proliferation in brown fat of the rat after exposure to cold. *Anat. Rec.* **157,** 537–545.

Joel, C. D. (1965). The physiological role of brown adipose tissue. *In* "Handbook of Physiology—Section 5: Adipose Tissue" (A. E. Renold and G. F. Cahill, Jr., eds.), pp. 59–85. Amer. Physiol. Soc., Washington, D. C.

Jones, A. L., and Fawcett, D. W. (1966). Hypertrophy of the agranular endoplasmic recticulum in hamster liver induced by phenobarbital (with a review on the functions of this organelle in liver). *J. Histochem. Cytochem.* **14,** 215–232.

Kennedy, E. P. (1957). Metabolism of lipides. *Annu. Rev. Biochem.* **26,** 119–148.

Kennedy, E. P., and Weiss, S. B. (1955). Cytidine diphosphate choline: A new inter-mediate in lecithin biosynthesis. *J. Amer. Chem. Soc.* **77,** 250–251.

Kennedy, E. P., and Weiss, S. B. (1956). The function of cytidine coenzymes in the biosynthesis of phospholipides. *J. Biol. Chem.* **222,** 193–214.

Kishimoto, Y., Davies, W. E., and Radin, N. S. (1965a). Turnover of fatty acids of rat brain gangliosides, glycerophosphatides, cerebrosides, and sulfatides as a function of age. *J. Lipid Res.* **6,** 525–531.

Kishimoto, Y., Davies, W. E., and Radin, N. S. (1965b). Developing rat brain: changes in cholesterol, galactolipids, and the individual fatty acids of gangliosides and glycerophosphatides. *J. Lipid Res.* **6**, 532–536.

Klenk, E. (1957). Incorporation of ^{14}C-labelled acetate into some lipids of nervous tissue. *In* "Metabolism of the Nervous System" (D. Richter, ed.), pp. 396–398. Pergamon, Oxford.

Knoop, F. (1904). Der Abbau aromatischer Fettsauren in Tierkorper. *Beitr. Chem. Physiol. Pathol.* **6**, 150–162.

Kornberg, A., and Pricer, W. E. (1953). Enzymatic synthesis of the coenzyme A derivatives of long chain fatty acids. *J. Biol. Chem.* **204**, 329–343.

Kritchevsky, D., and Defendi, V. (1961). Persistence of sterols other than cholesterol in chicken tissues. *Nature (London)* **192**, 71.

Kritchevsky, D., and Defendi, V. (1962). Deposition of tritium labelled sterols (cholesterol, sitosterol, lanosterol) in brain and other organs of the growing chicken. *J. Neurochem.* **9**, 421–425.

Larrabee, M. G., Klingman, J. D., and Leicht, W. S. (1963a). Effects of temperature, calcium and activity on phospholipid metabolism in a sympathetic ganglion. *J. Neurochem.* **10**, 549–570.

Larrabee, M. G., Nagata, Y., and Leicht, W. S. (1963b). Effects on activity on P^{32} labeling on phosphatidylinositol in a sympathetic ganglion. *Fed. Proc. Fed. Amer. Soc. Exp. Biol.* **22**, 632.

LeBaron, F. N., Hauser, G., and Ruiz, E. E. (1962). The occurrence and metabolism of protein-bound phosphoinositides in several lipid–protein complexes from brain. *Biochim. Biophys. Acta* **60**, 338–349.

Ledeen, R. (1966). The chemistry of gangliosides: A review. *J. Amer. Oil Chem. Soc.* **43**, 57–66.

Lewis, N., and Majerus, P. W. (1969). Lipid metabolism in human platelets. II. *De novo* phospholipid synthesis and the effect of thrombin on the pattern of synthesis. *J. Clin. Invest.* **48**, 2114–2123.

Lo Chang, T. C., and Sweeley, C. C. (1963). Characterization of lipids from canine adrenal glands. *Biochemistry* **2**, 592–604.

Lynen, F. (1955). Lipide metabolism. *Annu. Rev. Biochem.* **24**, 653–688.

Mackenzie, C. G., Mackenzie, J. B., and Reiss, O. K. (1964). Regulation of cell lipid metabolism and accumulation. III. The lipid content of mammalian cells and the response to the lipogenic activity of rabbit serum. *Exp. Cell Res.* **36**, 533–547.

Mackenzie, C. G., Mackenzie, J. B., and Reiss, O. K. (1967). Increase in cell lipid and cytoplasmic particles in mammalian cells cultured at reduced pH. *J. Lipid Res.* **8**, 642–645.

MacLean, I. S., and Hoffert, D. (1926). Carbohydrate and fat metabolism of yeast. III. The nature of the intermediate stages. *Biochem. J.* **20**, 343–357.

McMurray, W. C., Strickland, K. P., Berry, J. F., and Rossiter, R. J. (1957). Incorporation of ^{32}P labeled intermediates into phospholipides of cell-free preparations of rat brain. *Biochem. J.* **66**, 634–644.

Marinetti, G. V., Griffith, M., and Smith, T. (1962). Incorporation of [1-^{14}C] glycerol, [1-^{14}C] acetate, and DL[3-^{14}C] serine into the lipids of rat-heart and liver homogenates. *Biochim. Biophys. Acta* **57**, 543–554.

Masoro, E. J. (1968). "Physiological Chemistry of Lipids in Mammals." Saunders, Philadelphia, Pennsylvania.

Mead, J. F., Steinberg, G., and Howton, D. R. (1953). Metabolism of essential fatty acids. Incorporation of acetate into arachidonic acid. *J. Biol. Chem.* **205**, 683–689.

Mead, J. F., Slaton, W. H., Jr., and Decker, A. B. (1956). Metabolism of the essential fatty acids. II. The metabolism of stearate, oleate, and linoleate by fat deficient and normal mice. *J. Biol. Chem.* **218**, 401–407.

Michell, R. H., and Hawthorne, J. N. (1965). The site of diphosphoinositide synthesis in rat liver. *Biochem. Biophys. Res. Commun.* **21**, 333–338.

Miller, J. E., and Cornatzer, W. E. (1966). Phospholipid metabolism in mitochondria and microsomes of rabbit liver during development. *Biochim. Biophys. Acta* **125**, 534–541.

Morton, L. T. (1965). "A Medical Bibliography." Morrison and Gibb, London.

Nachbaur, J., Colbeau, A., and Vignais, P. M. (1969). Incorporation of fatty acids into the outer and inner membranes of isolated rat liver mitochondria. *Fed. Eur. Biochem. Soc.* **3**, 121–128.

Nachmansohn, D. (1963). The chemical basis of Claude Bernard's observations on Curare. *Biochem. Z.* **338**, 454–473.

Nadler, N. J., Young, B. A., Leblond, C. P., and Mitmaker, B. (1964). Elaboration of thyroglobulin in the thyroid follicle. *Endocrinology* **74**, 333–354.

Napolitano, L. (1965). The fine structure of adipose tissues. *In* "Handbook of Physiology–Section 5: Adipose Tissue" (A. E. Renold and G. F. Cahill, Jr., eds.), pp. 109–123. Amer. Physiol. Soc., Washington, D. C.

Napolitano, L. J., McNary, J. E., and Kloep, L. P. (1965). The release of free fatty acids from brown and white adipose tissues after incubation with ACTH or epinephrine. *Metabolism* **14**, 1076–1083.

Nunn, L. C. A., and Smedley-MacLean, I. (1938). The nature of the fatty acids stored by the liver in the fat-deficiency disease of rats. *Biochem. J.* **32**, 2179–2184.

Omura, T., Siekevitz, P., and Palade, G. E. (1967). Turnover of constituents of the endoplasmic reticulum membranes of rat hepatocytes. *J. Biol. Chem.* **242**, 2389–2396.

Pascaud, M. (1964). Les Phospholipides de la cellule hépatique. Interprétation fontionnelle de leur renouvellement. II. Renouvellement des acides gras des phosphoglycerides. *Biochim. Biophys. Acta* **84**, 528–537.

Patkin, J. K., and Masoro, E. J. (1964). Fatty acid synthesis in normal and cold-acclimated rats. *Can. J. Physiol. Pharmacol.* **42**, 101–107.

Paulus, H., and Kennedy, E. P. (1960). Enzymatic synthesis of inositol monophosphatide. *J. Biol. Chem.* **235**, 1303–1311.

Popják, G. (1954). The origin of fetal lipids. *Cold Spring Harbor Symp. Quant. Biol.* **19**, 200–208.

Popják, G., and Cornforth, J. (1960) The biosynthesis of cholesterol. *Advan. Enzymol.* **22**, 281–335.

Pullman, M. E., and Schatz, G. (1967). Mitochondrial oxidations and energy coupling. *Annu. Rev. Biochem.* **36**, 539–564.

Radin, N. S., Martin, F. B., and Brown, J. R. (1957). Galactolipide metabolism. *J. Biol. Chem.* **224**, 499–508.

Raper, H. S. (1907). The condensation of acetaldehyde and its relation to the biochemical synthesis of fatty acids. *J. Chem. Soc.* **91**, 1831–1838.

Rittenberg, D., and Schoenheimer, R. J. (1937). Deuterium as an indicator in the study of intermediary metabolism. XI. Further studies on the biological uptake of deuterium into organic substances with special reference to fat and cholesterol formation. *J. Biol. Chem.* **121**, 235–253.

Robertson, A. L., Jr. (1967). Transport of plasma lipoproteins and ultrastructure of human arterial intimacytes in culture. *In* "Lipid Metabolism in Tissue Culture

Cells" (G. H. Rothblat and D. Kritchevsky, eds.) pp. 115–128. Wistar Inst. Press, Philadelphia, Pennsylvania.

Sarzala, M. G., and Drabikowski, W. (1969). Free fatty acids as a factor modifying properties of fragmented sarcoplasmic reticulum during ageing. *Life Sci.* **8**, 477–483.

Schoenheimer, R. (1942). "The Dynamic State of Body Constituents." Harvard Univ. Press, Cambridge, Massachusetts.

Schotz, M. C., Rice, L. I., and Alfin-Slater, R. B. (1953). II. Further studies on cholesterol in liver-cell fractions of normal and cholesterol-fed rats. *J. Biol. Chem.* **204**, 19–26.

Shafrir, E., and Gorin, E. (1963). Release of glycerol in conditions of fat mobilization and deposition. *Metabolism* **12**, 580–587.

Silverman, W. A., Zamelis, A., Sinclair, J. C., and Agate, F. J. (1964). Warm nape of the newborn. *Pediatrics* **33**, 984–987.

Smith, M. E. (1967). The metabolism of myelin lipids. *In* "Advances in Lipid Research" (R. Paoletti and D. Kritchevsky, eds.), pp. 241–278. Academic Press, New York.

Smith, M. E., and Eng., L. (1965). Turnover of the lipid components of myelin. *J. Amer. Oil Chem. Soc.* **42**, 1013–1018.

Smith, R. E., and Horwitz, B. A. (1969). Brown fat and thermogenesis. *Physiol. Rev.* **49**, 330–425.

Smith, R. E., and Roberts, J. C. (1964). Thermogenesis of brown adipose tissue in cold-acclimated rats. *Amer. J. Physiol.* **206**, 143–148.

Spencer, W. A., and Dempster, G. (1962). The lipids of mouse brown fat. *Can. J. Biochem. Physiol.* **40**, 1705–1715.

Srere, P. A. (1950). The extrahepatic synthesis of cholesterol. *J. Biol. Chem.* **182**, 629–634.

Stein, Y., and Shapiro, B. (1958). Glyceride synthesis by microsome fractions of rat liver. *Biochem. Biophys. Acta* **30**, 271–277.

Stein, O., and Stein, Y. (1963). Metabolism of fatty acids in the isolated perfused rat heart. *Biochem. Biophys. Acta* **70**, 517–530.

Stein, O., and Stein, Y. (1967a). Lipid synthesis, intracellular transport, storage, and secretion. I. Electron microscopic radioautographic study of liver after injection of tritiated palmitate of glycerol in fasted and ethanol-treated rats. *J. Cell Biol.* **33**, 319–339.

Stein, O., and Stein, Y. (1967b) Lipid synthesis, intracellular transport, and secretion. II. Electron microscopic radioautographic study of the mouse lactating mammary gland. *J. Cell Biol.* **34**, 251–263.

Stein, O., and Stein, Y. (1968). Lipid synthesis, intracellular transport, and storage. III. Electron microscopic radioautographic study of the rat heart perfused with tritiated oleic acid. *J. Cell Biol.* **36**, 63–77.

Stein, O., and Stein, Y. (1969). Lecithin synthesis, intracellular transport, and secretion in rat liver. IV. A radioautographic and biochemical study of choline-deficient rats injected with choline-^{3}H. *J. Cell Biol.* **40**, 461–483.

Steinberg, G., Slaton, W. H., Jr., Howton, D. R., and Mead, J. F. (1956). Metabolism of essential fatty acids. IV. Incorporation of linoleate into arachidonic acid. *J. Biol. Chem.* **220**, 257–264.

Steiner, G., and Cahill, G. F. (1964). Brown and white adipose tissue metabolism in cold-exposed rats. *Amer. J. Physiol.* **207**, 840–844.

Steiner, G., Schönbaum, E., Johnson, G. E., and Sellers, E. A. (1968). Lipid metabolism: effects of immunosympathectomy and acclimation to cold. *Can. J. Physiol. Pharmacol.* **46**, 453–461.

Stoffel, W., and Schiefer, H. G. (1968). Biosynthesis and composition of phosphatides in outer and inner mitochondrial membranes. *Hoppe-Seyler's Z. Physiol. Chem.* **349**, 1017–1026.

Strickland, K. P., Thompson, W., Subrahmanyam, D., and Rossiter, R. J. (1960). Studies of the biosynthesis of brain inositol phosphatide. *Biochem. J.* **76**, 41P–42P.

Stumpf, P. K. (1969). Metabolism of fatty acids. *Annu. Rev. Biochem.* **38**, 159–212.

Taylor, C. B., Bailey, E., and Bartley, W. (1967). Studies on the biosynthesis of protein and lipid components of rat liver mitochondria. *Biochem. J.* **105**, 605–610.

Tchen, T. T., and Bloch, K. (1955). *In vitro* conversion of squalene to lanosterol and cholesterol. *J. Amer. Chem. Soc.* **77**, 6085–6086.

Thompson, R. C., and Ballou, J. E. (1954). Studies of metabolic turnover with tritium as a tracer. IV. Metabolically inert lipide and protein fractions from the rat. *J. Biol. Chem.* **208**, 883–888.

Thompson, W., Subrahmanyam, D., and Strickland, K. P. (1960). Some precursors of brain inositol phosphatide. *Fed. Proc. Fed. Amer. Soc. Exp. Biol.* **19**, 234.

Thompson, W., Strickland, K. P., and Rossiter, R. J. (1963). Biosynthesis of phosphatidylinositol in rat brain. *Biochem. J.* **87**, 136–142.

Waelsch, H., Sperry, W. M., and Stayanoff, V. A. (1941). The influence of growth and myelination on the deposition and metabolism of lipides in the brain. *J. Biol. Chem.* **140**, 885–897.

Wagner, H., Lissau, Ä., Hölzl, J., and Hörhammer, L. (1962). The incorporation of P^{32} into the inositol phosphatides of rat brain. *J. Lipid Res.* **3**, 177–180.

Wagner, H., Hölzl, J., Lissau, Ä., and Hörhammer, L. (1963). Papierchromatographie von Phosphatiden. III. Mitteilung Quantitative papierchromatographische Bestimmung von phosphatiden und phosphatidsäuren in rattenorganen. *Biochem. Z.* **339**, 34–45.

Wakil, S. J. (1961). Mechanism of fatty acid synthesis. *J. Lipid Res.* **2**, 1–24.

Watkins, J. C. (1965). Pharmacological receptors and general permeability phenomena of cell membranes. *J. Theor. Biol.* **9**, 37–50.

Weiss, S. B., and Kennedy, E. P. (1956). The enzymatic synthesis of triglycerides. *J. Amer. Chem. Soc.* **78**, 3550.

Wilgram, G. F., and Kennedy, E. P. (1963). Intracellular distribution of some enzymes catalyzing reactions in the biosynthesis of complex lipids. *J. Biol. Chem.* **238**, 2615–2619.

Williamson, J. R. (1969). Ultrastructural localization and distribution of free cholesterol (3-β-hydroxysterols) in tissues. *J. Ultrastruct. Res.* **27**, 118–125.

Wirsén, C. (1965). Autoradiography of injected albumin-bound 1-C^{14}-palmitate in pigeon pectoralis muscle. *Acta Physiol. Scand.* **65**, 120–125.

Wirtz, K. W. A., and Zilversmit, D. B. (1968). Exchange of phospholipids between liver mitochondria and microsomes *in vitro*. *J. Biol. Chem.* **243**, 3596–3602.

Witten, P. W., and Holman, R. T. (1952). Polyethenoid fatty acid metabolism. VI. Effect of pyridoxine on essential fatty acid conversions. *Arch. Biochem. Biophys.* **41**, 266–273.

Yagi, K., and Kotaki, A. (1969). Effect of massive doses of *myo*-inositol on hepatic phospholipid metabolism. *Ann. N. Y. Acad. Sci.* **165**, 710–725.

CHAPTER 9

Localization, Identification, and Renewal of Carbohydrates in Tissues and Cells*

T. John Leppi†

I. Introduction... 331
II. Histochemistry of Mucins.. 334
    A. Fixation... 336
    B. Staining Procedures.. 337
    C. Alterations of Staining.. 346
    D. Autoradiography... 349
III. Histochemistry of Polysaccharides................................. 353
    A. Fixation... 354
    B. Staining Procedures.. 355
    C. Alterations of Staining.. 361
    D. Autoradiography... 364
    References... 366

I. Introduction

The morphochemical approach to the study of complex carbohydrates has a basic advantage in being more morphologically accurate, even to the cytological level, than most of the chemical methods currently utilized in the characterization of these tissue macromolecules. Although chemical procedures have provided excellent structural, qualitative, and quantitative data on carbohydrates, especially from connective tissues, these methods are of low morphological precision because of their inability to separate and localize regional chemical differences in heterogeneous tissues such as salivary glands and other mucigenic epithelia. Similarly, regional varia-

* Supported by Grant No. AM–11064 of the United States Public Health Service.
† Recipient of a Lederle Medical Faculty Award, 1968–1971.

tions in the content of complex carbohydrates in the extracellular matrices of compact and loose connective tissues cannot be appreciated fully. On the other hand, a characteristic disadvantage in the use of the histochemical approach is the frequent reliance on results obtained from the use of empirical staining methods alone to ascertain the carbohydrate composition of certain tissues. In reality, currently acceptable light microscopic methodology has limited capabilities of differentiating among certain reactive groups by determination of the relative charge of acid radicals and on the relative distances between certain acid groups and hydroxyls on adjacent carbon atoms which have been oxidized to dialdehydes by periodate. Methodology carried to the ultrastructural level must result in stainable products that are capable of diffracting electrons to achieve the desired level of preferential staining. The significance of these electron markers will only be meaningful when they can be altered by methods of proven chemical specificity.

The histochemical localization of complex carbohydrates in epithelial and conncetive tissues is dependent on the presence of acid radicals such as ester sulfate, carboxyl, and to a lesser extent, phosphate. Staining reactions probably result from electrostatic or "salt" linkages formed between the polyanionic carbohydrate and a cationic dye. Hydroxyl groups on adjacent carbon atoms (*vic*-glycols) provide another means for localizing acid carbohydrates through treatment with periodate and subsequent exposure to chromogenic reagents in the classic periodic acid-Schiff (PAS) sequence. In histochemical practice, this procedure affords visualization of epithelial acid mucosubstances but not acid polysaccharides of connective tissues which should react theoretically toward the PAS technique. There is slow periodate consumption by several of the polysaccharides in the test tube because of the vicinal hydroxyls contained in their uronidic moieties. Recent evidence points to an inhibitory phenomenon involving the repulsion of the negatively charged periodate ion from the negative field of the polyanion (Scott and Harbinson, 1968).

The specific identification of a reactive group in tissue carbohydrates can be established through the use of certain blocking and unblocking procedures. Prevention of a staining reaction can result in either neutralization or removal of freely reactive groups. Unblocking usually restores the stainability of previously neutralized groups while stainability is totally lost for those groups removed by the blocking procedure. These techniques have been of critical value in assessing the histochemical properties of most epithelial mucosubstances and selected carbohydrates from connective tissues. In addition to chemical modification of staining, the reactivity of carbohydrate-rich materials can be compared with controls following exposure to enzymes which effectively remove stainable radicals.

In the past, biochemists and histochemists have maintained separate approaches in attempting to understand some of nature's most complex polymers, the heterosaccharides or those containing two or more different carbohydrate units. This insular attitude has given way to a few meaningful correlations between data derived from each discipline. For example, histochemists reported a wealth of evidence for the presence of sulfate ester groups in certain epithelial mucins in addition to the ubiquitous sialic acid moiety which was well characterized by mucin biochemists (see Leppi *et al.*, 1967 for review). At first, the presence of another acid group besides sialic acid in any mucin was refuted, but a gradual and concerted effort on the part of some biochemists to improve the methodology for detecting sulfate in a pure fraction of a particular mucin resulted in the characterization of several mucosubstances containing both acid groups. If further correlations can be made, a more complete dissection of carbohydrate-containing substances should be possible.

The term complex carbohydrates of animal tissues, as referred to throughout this chapter, denotes the two major classes of macromolecules which are distinct chemically because of the nature of their carobyhdrate content with or without a serially repeating unit and their carbohydrate–protein linkage regions. The categories seem to be: (1) the glycoproteins, also known to histochemists as mucins, mucosubstances, and mucosaccharides, and (2) the polysaccharides, also termed glycosaminoglycans or protein–polysaccharides by biochemists. Polysaccharides of connective tissues are chemically well characterized compared to the glycoproteins or mucins of epithelial origin. In the past, it had been assumed that polysaccharides were of mesodermal origin while glycoproteins were products of epithelial cell biosynthetic activity. This categorization may not be entirely accurate in view of recent findings which have demonstrated that some epithelial secretions contain a sulfated carbohydrate (Spicer and Henson, 1967). This material closely resembles polysaccharide on a histochemical basis, although it also shares some of the properties exhibited by sialic acid-containing mucins of epithelial origin. By the same token, all of the complex carbohydrates of connective tissues may not be composed of polysaccharides, but rather contain oligosaccharides typical of glycoproteins (Buddecke, 1966). Biochemically, glycoproteins seem to be a major component in certain connective tissues such as bone, cartilage, skin, tendon, cornea, and the vitreous body. Current histochemical methodology does not permit the unequivocal differentiation between glycoprotein and polysaccharide in connective tissues, although sialic acid has been identified as a normal component of the polysaccharide fraction in ground substance (Quintarelli, 1961).

An unambiguous and consistent terminology of carbohydrate-rich macromolecules is unavailable at present despite several attempts to bring the histochemist and biochemist to a mutual understanding (Jeanloz, 1960; Saunders and Rosan, 1966; Spicer *et al.*, 1965; Meyer, 1966; Stoward *et al.*, 1966). Much of the problem centers on the failure to recognize that histochemical methods for tissue carbohydrates, even if well-controlled, have definite limitations. For example, these techniques cannot provide structural information about the nature of the carbohydrate–protein linkage region. The classic PAS reaction in histochemical practice cannot detect *vic*-glycol groups that may react with periodate in the test tube after a long exposure, since a 10-minute exposure of a tissue section to periodic acid is the usual test. Histochemists should evoke more caution in the interpretation of results from histochemical tests and should attempt to equate the specificity of a given method with terminology that is understood by the biochemist, e.g., if a tissue component is periodate-reactive, this means exposure to periodate for 10 minutes.

A comprehensive recollection of carbohydrate histochemistry is not attempted here since there are excellent reviews that consider polysaccharides (Curran, 1961, 1964; Spicer *et al.*, 1967) and mucins (Quintarelli, 1963; Spicer and Henson, 1967). The purpose of the present discussion will be to indicate those studies which have aided significantly in the histochemical differentiation of carbohydrate-rich substances of certain connective and epithelial tissues at both light and electron microscopic levels of resolution.

II. Histochemistry of Mucins

The carbohydrate moiety of these substances is generally described, in chemical terms, as forming the prosthetic group of a conjugated protein, a glycoprotein. Structural features common to all glycoproteins of animal origin appear to be: (1) a widely varying carbohydrate content of from two to six different types of sugars with *N*-acetylhexosamine and sialic acid as regular members of the oligosaccharide; (2) a lack of serially repeating unit; and (3) the covalency of the carbohydrate–protein linkage (Gottschalk, 1966). Since the glycoproteins of mucous secretions are the only group being considered here, owing to the wide diversity of the composition of glycoproteins from other sources, it should be stressed that glycoproteins of epithelial origin are also heterogeneous and complex by nature and have not given up their secrets easily.

Biochemical knowledge of mucins derives primarily from the studies of Pigman and Gottschalk (1966) and Pigman and Hashimoto (1964) and others on the submandibular glands of ruminants, particularly cattle and sheep. Analyses of relatively pure fractions of mucous secretions from these large salivary glands have aided in understanding the physical and biochemical characteristics of mucin. Since ungulate mucins are well characterized biochemically, the histochemical aspects of these mucins have centered on the differentiation of acid and periodate-oxidizable (vicinal hydroxyl) groups (Leppi and Spicer, 1967; see also Quintarelli and co-workers as cited in this reference). Attention has also been given to correlating periodate reactivity with the biochemically known sugar content of certain ungulate glands. Through these and other studies dealing with attempts to correlate known biochemical composition of a particular mucin with histochemical properties, a better appreciation has been gained for limitations inherent in the morphochemical and analytical approach.

Experience with certain light microscopic histochemical procedures, considered highly specific for tissue carbohydrates, has led to the confirmation of biochemical data from other workers for the types of mucin present in pig colonic mucosa, dog gastric mucosa and submandibular gland, and hagfish skin. The biochemical reports were from Inoue and Yosizawa (1966), Gerard et al., (1967), Bignardi et al., (1964) and Lehtonen et al., (1966) for these sites, respectively. The correlative histochemical data were derived from a number of reports (Leppi and Kinnison, 1967; Spicer et al., 1967; Leppi et al., 1967; Leppi, 1968). Histochemical staining, combined with ^{35}S-sulfate autoradiography and enzymatic modification of staining, provided the morphological addresses of certain acid mucins such as those containing sialic acid and sulfate. For example, the mucous demilunes of dog submandibular gland contained demonstrable sialic acid while the mucous acini exhibited a mucin with an unknown sulfated component. This latter type of epithelial secretion was unfamiliar to biochemists on the basis of available data.

Among the plethora of reports dealing with the differentiation of complex carbohydrates, the studies of Scott, Quintarelli, and co-workers have added new dimensions to this area of histochemistry. In a series of publications dealing with the elucidation of the chemical and histochemical properties of Alcian Blue, they have explored the mechanisms of dye binding to tissue and model polyanions, the effects of chemical blocking and unblocking on such staining, and have correlated known biochemical properties of certain mucins with histochemical staining characteristics (Scott et al., 1964; Quintarelli et al., 1964a,b; Quintarelli and Dellovo, 1965). The development of the "critical electrolyte concentration" method (CEC) as a by-product of the cetylpyridinium fractionation system (Scott, 1960) has been directed specifically at the problem concerning the nature of the interactions between cationic (e.g., the isothiouronium groups of Alcian Blue) groups and the carboxyl, phosphate, and ester sulfate groups of tissue carbohydrates (Scott and Dorling, 1965). The principle of the CEC approach to the localization of tissue polyanions involves the addition of electrolyte (MgCl$_2$) in increasing molarities to a solution of basic dye like Alcian Blue. Studies of polyanions in model systems revealed that substances of low-molecular-weight stain at relatively low concentrations of added electrolyte while those of higher weight stain at higher electrolyte concentrations.

A. FIXATION

The carbohydrate–protein complexes of epithelial origin are easier to retain through a variety of fixative procedures than the similar substances of connective tissues. On a strictly empirical basis, this apparent ease of fixation might be due to the protein content of the glycoproteins in epithelial secretions. The mechanism commonly evoked to explain the fixing event is that the reagents denature and precipitate proteins. Thus, any carbohydrate attached to a protein core presumably can be salvaged for subsequent histochemical procedures. There has been continual dependence on the use of aldehyde-containing fixatives, particularly neutral, buffered formalin in the cold or at room temperature to prepare carbohydrate-rich materials from various epithelia for histochemistry. Staining of an extrinsic protein associated with certain epithelial secretions can be achieved by utilizing formalin- or Carnoy-fixed materials (Spicer, 1962; Lev and Gerard, 1967). The formation of aminealdehyde condensates during fixation, especially with formalin, may be a reversible or incomplete reaction.

Fixation of epithelial mucins by a mixture of aldehydes, such as glutaraldehyde and formaldehyde, probably deserves a wider trial in electron cytochemical studies of complex carbohydrates. As developed by Karnovsky (1965) and extended by Flickinger (1967), these combination fixatives may have the dual capacity to fix quickly due to a faster rate of penetration of the formalin component and fix complex carbohydrate for cytochemical manipulation. Buffered glutaraldehyde works well as a primary fixative as shown in cytochemical investigations of acid mucosubstances in mouse colon (Wetzel et al., 1966). In this study, the penetration of certain iron-containing stains was evaluated and it was shown that buffered formalin or osmium tetroxide as primary fixatives resulted in satisfactory intracellular staining of mucosubstances in the Golgi region.

Recent studies of the microvillar surface coat (fuzz) of cat small intestine have stressed a cautious interpretation of the appearance of carbohydrate-rich sites following different methods of fixation for electron microscopy (Pratt and Napolitano, 1969; Leppi and Pratt, 1969). A wealth of evidence has suggested that complex acid carbohydrates form an important moiety of the surface coat although the exact nature of the carbohydrate portion has not been revealed, be it glycoprotein and/or polysaccharide. The need for stating the conditions of exposure of carbohydrate-rich materials to osmium tetroxide or to any other fixative is emphasized by the studies of Pratt and Napolitano (1969). Fixation of the small intestine by glutaraldehyde in phosphate buffer followed by OsO$_4$ resulted in a fibrillar surface coat covering the microvilli. A structureless zone occurred where the surface coat was usually seen following glutaraldehyde alone or followed by postfixation in OsO$_4$ in carbon tetrachloride. The application of heavy metals did not increase the density of the fuzz. If binding of osmium to the acid carbohydrates of the surface coat did occur, it was thought to be differential since there was greater density of the coat following postfixation by OsO$_4$ in phosphate than after OsO$_4$ in carbon tetrachloride. Although the interactions between OsO$_4$ and complex carbohydrates are not at all understood, the fact has been emphasized that osmium fixes carbohydrate-rich sites effectively for histochemistry (Wetzel et al., 1966; Pratt and Napolitano, 1969; Leppi and Pratt, 1969).

The fixation of choice for carbohydrates of epithelial tissues probably depends on several, individual factors related to the site being studied. Among these could be (1) amount of protein attached to carbohydrate in the particular secretion; (2) degree of hydration of the complex carbohydrate; and (3) the concentration of reactive groups at the site which remain stainable and capable of being characterized histochemically. In the present state of inadequate knowledge on the mechanisms underlying fixation, this is probably a portion of what could be understood about a most critical step in carbohydrate histochemistry.

B. Staining Procedures

1. Light Microscopy

a. *Vicinal Hydroxyl Methods.* The familiar periodic acid-Schiff sequence for the light microscopic demonstration of aldehydes in complex carbohydrates depends on (1) the presence of free, neighboring hydroxyl groups positioned on adjacent carbon atoms; (2) the cleavage of the carbon–carbon bond by the brief action of periodate with resulting dialdehyde formation; and (3) the subsequent demonstration of aldehydes produced by periodate oxidation through application of the colorless Schiff's reagent, a sulfurous acid leucofuchsin solution (Lillie, 1965). The sites of aldehydes are marked by the formation of reddish coloration in tissue section. Despite its wide and accepted use in the histochemistry of carbohydrates, the chemical mechanisms involving the interaction between the Schiff reagent and aldehydes of carbohydrates are poorly understood (Hardonk and van Duijn, 1964; Stoward, 1966c).

The PAS staining alone of epithelial mucins does not provide much information about their carbohydrate content. The use of enzymes such as amylase to rule out the presence of homopolysaccharides like glycogen in mucins, and chemical modifications of staining such as acetylation and phenylhydrazine blockage (Spicer, 1961), all tend to improve the specificity of the PAS reaction in epithelial mucins.

Besides the familiar Schiff reagent, there are other sequences capable of visualizing sites of dialdehyde formation in epithelial carbohydrates. These include (1) phenylhydrazine post-coupled with a diazonium compound to yield a colored formazan (Stoward and Mester, 1964); (2) a sequence employing methanolic thionyl chloride followed by periodate oxidation and exposure to sulfurous acid (Stoward, 1966b); and (3) the use of salicylhydrazide, an aromatic hydrazine, as a reagent capable of forming condensates with either the free dialdehydes, hemialdals, or hemiacetals (Stoward, 1966c). The latter two methods were devised to test their uniqueness as fluorescence histochemical reagents in the localization of periodate-oxidized mucosubstances. In studies on the use of "pseudo"-Schiff reagents, Stoward (1966b) proposed a new interpretation for the mechanism underlying the Schiff reagent as used in histochemistry. Previous explanations held that dialdehydes react with Schiff's reagent through N-sulfinic acids, but Stoward favors that an intermediate alkyl sulfonic acid is formed by the reaction with the sulfurous acid of Schiff's. This combines with basic pararosaniline, the key ingredient of Schiff's, and this then results in the classic magenta color of the positive PAS reaction. Some slight departure from this scheme to explain the interactions between Schiff's reagent and periodate-engendered aldehydes has been proposed by Hardonk and van Duijn (1964).

Spicer (1965) has devised an array of diamine methods utilizing the *meta* and *para* isomers of N,N-dimethylphenylenediamine, used singly or in combination, which have been particularly useful in differentiating between different acid mucosaccharides. Information can also be obtained regarding relative proximities of acid to periodate-induced dialdehyde groups. One of the methods involves exposure of sections to periodate, followed by metadiamine and then staining by a basic dye such as colloidal iron, Alcian Blue, or azure A. Differentiation of mucins is achieved by such a sequence since the basophilia of some acidic mucins is prevented by periodate oxidation and exposure to metadiamine, while the cationic staining of other mucins is unaltered after the same sequence. It is thought that the metadiamine may condense on periodate-engendered aldehydes which, if this disubstituted amine is close enough to the anionic charge of the mucin, may neutralize the electrostatic attraction of cationic dye molecules. This mechanism would imply the presence of vicinal hydroxyls in close proximity to acidic groups of epithelial mucins. The periodic acid–paradiamine technique (Spicer and Jarrels, 1961) does not visualize sugars rich in the hemiacetal or hemialdal configurations such as in polymeric glucose (glycogen), but does detect residues in which the dialdehydic form predominates after periodate oxidation such as fucose or galactose.

b. Basic Dye Methods. Polyvalent cationic stains applied to epithelial mucosubstances can be utilized singly or in combination to differentiate between complex carbohydrates. Certain of the thiazine dyes such as toluidine blue and azure A are capable of combining with anionic groups of polymeric carbohydrate to produce varying degrees of metachromasia depending on the pH of the staining solution and density of negative charges in the substrate. The subject of the metachromatic properties of certain basic dyes has been fully reviewed elsehwere (Curran, 1961, 1964; Spicer *et al.*, 1967). Of the various reagents used widely by histochemists, the copper phthalocyanine dye, Alcian Blue, is the most acceptable in terms of understanding its staining mechanism. The structure of Alcian Blue, which is the soluble form of copper phthalocyanine, has been elucidated by Scott, Quintarelli, and their collaborators (see Section II for references). Through exhaustive testing of this polycationic (up to four isothiouronium groups per molecule) dye on both model and fixed tissue polyanions from a variety of sources, it has been concluded that the major binding force between dye cations and tissue anions is electrostatic in nature. This bonding differs quantitatively from that envisioned for thiazine dyes since Alcian Blue resists extraction from sections during tissue processing more strongly than do some of the metachromatic dyes. Also, there may be more positive charges in the dye which could contribute to a stronger bond.

The addition of different electrolytes in varying amounts to Alcian Blue dye solutions has resulted in the critical electrolyte concentration methodological approach to the study of tissue polyanions (Scott and Dorling, 1965). The degree of Alcian Blue staining of selected epithelial mucins closely parallels the density and strength of the anionic charges within the carbohydrates. In general, application of Alcian Blue containing high (0.5–1.0 *M*) concentrations of electrolyte resulted in alcianophilia of mucins known to contain strongly acidic groups such as ester sulfate. Conversely, alcianophilia, which is present in mucins following exposure to dye solutions containing low salt (0.05–0.4 *M*), was thought to represent staining of weaker acidic groups such as carboxylate. Although this concept of a histochemical fractionation system has provided good correlations between results of tests on pure model and tissue polyanions which are most characteristic of polysaccharides of mesodermal origin, similar correlative data are not generally available for pure substances characteristic of epithelial oligosaccharides. As this technique gains wider use, it should prove to be a fruitful area for meaningful collaboration between morphochemists and biochemists interested in the problems of identifying complex carbohydrates with a high degree of specificity.

In a series of experiments to determine the composition of aldehyde fuchsin as a suitable dye for the histochemical localization of certain reactive groups, Sumner (1965a,b) has demonstrated that the dye is cationic. This property varied with the age of the dye solution to the extent that fresh solutions contained different components than old ones. Sumner's conclusions agree with Spicer and Meyer's (1960) data which indicated that aldehyde fuchsin is a fairly specfic stain for localizing strongly acidic groups such as ester sulfates in epithelial mucins. When fresh solutions of aldehyde fuchsin were used in combination staining with Alcian Blue, the former dye displayed stronger affinity for sulfate groups as verified by ^{35}S-sulfate autoradiography while the latter visualizes the carboxyls of sialic acid as judged by the lability of alcianophilia following sialidase digestion. The histochemical staining results of the combination aldehyde fuchsin–Alcian Blue staining procedure have been correlated with results from ^{35}S-labeling and enzyme digestion techniques applied to various mucins for the simultaneous localization of different acidic groups (Spicer and Duvenci, 1964; Leppi and Spicer, 1966, 1967; Leppi et al., 1967).

Another method for use in the identification of sulfated epithelial mucins is the high iron diamine procedure which is a variant of the diamine methods developed by Spicer (1965). The question of whether or not the reaction was specific for compounds with ester sulfate groups was recently investigated using model substrates with known physical and chemical properties (Gad and Sylvén, 1969). When certain proportions of the meta and para isomers of N,N-dimethylphenylenediamine are mixed together with ferric ions in the form of $FeCl_3$ and the mixture adjusted to pH 1.3–1.5, this dye system, as formulated by Spicer, was found to be highly specific for tissue sulfates. Depending on the charge density of the substrate, the high iron diamine method produced various colored reaction products. If highly charged, dark purple to violet colors were present and if the substrate was less charged with sulfates, the resulting colors were brownish-red or purple.

In histochemical practice, the high iron diamine procedure affords differentiation between sulfate- and sialic acid-containing mucins when Alcian Blue is used as the second basic dye in a combination sequence.

Sulfomucins are stained by the high iron diamine reagent while sialomucins are alcianophilic. As a general rule, ^{35}S-sulfate autoradiography has correlated with the high iron diamine reactivity of mucinous sites just as affinity toward aldehyde fuchsin has indicated the presence of sulfated mucins. Many epithelia exhibit mixtures of these two mucins which are either in different cells or coexist in the same cell. A lower concentration of the two isomers of the diamine and the $FeCl_3$ can also be employed as the low iron diamine reagent which stains sialomucins less selectively, but still stains sulfomucins specifically.

Stoward (1966a) has advanced the use of certain fluorescence–histochemical techniques in the specific differentiation of chemical groups of carbohydrate macromolecules. Toward this goal, a series of methods have been devised which rely on comparisons between results from acceptable histochemical methods and those obtained from the fluorescence of certain reactive groups. If there is agreement of results, the mechanism underlying the fluorescence reaction is then pursued. The application of a basic fluorescent dye such as coriphosphine for the exclusive localization of sulfomucins has shown potential specificity, although, like other staining methods, the presumed dye–substrate complex (i.e., sulfate–coriphosphine) has not been dissected. This will continue to be a strict requirement for the analysis of any histochemical staining reagent and its interactions with complex macromolecules.

c. Combination Methods. This group of techniques is similar to the combined basic dye sequences in that both involve a two-step staining process. However, these combination procedures usually employ a basic dye, usually Alcian Blue (AB) or colloidal iron, followed by the periodic acid-Schiff sequence to distinguish between acidic and neutral mucins in the same tissue section. With AB at pH 2.5 or 1.0, the differentiation between sulfomucins and sialomucins is possible since the dissociation of the carboxyls in sialic acid is suppressed at the lower pH. Thus, most alcianophilia at pH 1.0 is probably due to ester sulfates. In the AB, pH 2.5-PAS sequence, both carboxylate and ester sulfate groups are stained blue to blue-purple while uncharged (neutral) mucins are red. Sialomucins change to a red color in the AB, pH 1.0-PAS sequence while sulfomucins remain blue.

The subject of combined basic dye–vicinal hydroxyl staining methods has been thoroughly reviewed elsewhere (Spicer and Henson, 1967; Spicer *et al.*, 1967).

2. Electron Microscopy

The visualization of complex carbohydrates by this optical system depends on the formation of electron-dense products as a result of the interactions between staining reagents and tissue macromolecules rich in carbohydrate. Simple carbohydrates such as a glycogen were localized by a variety of methods. The staining of glycogen could not be considered specific since attempts to alter stainability resulted in erratic patterns and the staining mechanisms were poorly understood. More recent efforts at improving specificity at the electron level of resolution have been directed toward the characterization of acid carboydrates and those which are periodic acid-Schiff reactive as visualized by light optics.

a. Periodic Acid–Pentafluorophenylhydrazine. Potentially, this method could be equivalent to the PAS method of light microscopy. Although the sequence of reactions postulated by Bradbury and Stoward (1967) for the technique remain theoretical, further work directed at elucidating specificity and mechanism of staining will hopefully reveal its value in the electron microscopic localization of complex carbohydrates. Briefly, tissue sugars are oxidized by periodic acid and resulting dialdehydes are condensed with pentafluorophenylhydrazine (PFPH). Presumably, a hydrazone end product of the condensation is exposed first to ammonium sulfide and then to osmium tetroxide with both steps adding electron density to carbohydrate-rich sites. The final dense product of the full PFPH method may be an "osmium black" of the type suggested by Seligman and associates as cited by Bradbury and Stoward (1967). Positive staining reactions were observed on the microvillar surface coat, cytoplasmic mucus, and in liver cells of the rat. Treatment with diastase prior to PFPH staining resulted in the absence of electron-dense deposits from liver sections, suggesting loss of glycogen. Omission of the periodate oxidation step resulted in a failure of the electron density to develop. Our own experience with the PFPH method on liver cells agreed with these observations, except that intracellular sites which previously contained dense products of the reaction were empty and composed of profiles of smooth membranes following exposure to amylase prior to staining. We also noted, as described for the method, that cold, buffered formalin-fixed tissues are preferable to those fixed with glutaraldehyde. In our hands, nonfrozen sections, prepared by use of the Sorvall TC-2 tissue sectioner, proved superior for the PFPH reaction compared to the use of small tissue blocks as originally described.

b. Periodic Acid–Silver Methenamine. Recent investigations of the carbohydrate-rich "coats" (Rambourg *et al.*, 1966) covering a wide variety of mammalian cells have led to improved specificity of the periodic acid–silver methenamine (PA–silver) technique for periodate-reactive substances (Rambourg and Leblond, 1967; Rambourg, 1967). The adaptation of the

PA–silver method to electron microscopy was reviewed in detail by Rambourg (1967) as well as the pitfalls encountered in the interpretation of staining. Nonspecific deposition of silver on many structures was encountered at first, and much of this was accounted for by the probable presence of free aldehydic groups of glutaraldehyde in tissues. Considerable care is urged in the preparation of reagents for the staining sequence as evidenced by the detailed descriptions found in Rambourg's (1967) improved technique. The current interpretation of PA–silver staining is that reactions of glutaraldehyde-fixed tissues are only considered specific after exposure to periodate. These reactions should be absent in unoxidized control sections, but if reactivity is present in control sections, this is considered nonspecific. After periodate oxidation, silver staining is probably due to the reduction of silver methenamine by the dialdehydes formed as a result of interaction between periodic acid and vicinal hydroxyl groups of carbohydrates.

Despite these improvements in the use of PA–silver as a means to identify periodate-reactive sites with the electron microscope, the desired level of specificity for the reaction has not been attained. Except for comparing sections with and without exposure to periodate, no other modifications of staining have been attempted. Blockade of periodate-engendered staining can be achieved by utilizing phenylhydrazine or acetylation procedures. Presently, the electron histochemical identification of carbohydrate residues in cell coats has been possible in only a few instances, particularly involving sialic acid-containing complexes. The morphochemical technology does not permit differentiation between the larger classes of carbohydrates, the glycoproteins and polysaccharides, except perhaps on the basis that the former are usually PAS positive and the latter are not. Until more chemically based alterations of electron densities thought to represent complex sugars can be applied to thin sections, we shall continue to rely heavily on other data for the composition of carbohydrate-rich cell coats.

c. Colloidal Metallic Methods. The reader is referred to the critical discussion by Zobel and Beer (1965) on the use of heavy metal salts as electron stains. These techniques are directed toward increasing the mass at various chemical sites by the selective attachment of heavy metal atoms or their complexes. The mechanism of staining by coordination complexes formed between the heavy metal-containing ions and chemical groups with nitrogen, sulfur, phosphorus, and especially oxygen atoms is thought to occur as an electrostatic interaction between the positively charged colloidal metallic complexes and the negatively charged ionic groups of the carbohydrate macromolecules (Zobel and Beer, 1965). Specifically, the binding of iron-containing stains is probably more dependent on electrostatic forces than on chelation or complexing mechanisms (Gasic *et al.*, 1968).

The adaptation of the classic Hale's colloidal iron reaction for the light microscopic detection of acid mucosubstances to use in thin sections for the electron microscope has shown considerable promise. The specificity of the reaction has been markedly improved over the years, largely due to the efforts of Mowry (1958; 1963), who has also provided a concise, historical review on the development of the method (Mowry, 1963). Briefly, staining of fixed, frozen, or nonfrozen sections for electron microscopy is accomplished by exposing them to a freshly dialyzed ferric oxide solution at low pH (2.0 or less) prior to embedding in plastic. Exposure of sections to a potassium ferrocyanide–HCl (1:1) solution following iron staining interfered with localization of iron deposits in thin sections because the resulting Prussian blue particles containing ferric ferrocyanide were too large (Curran *et al.*, 1965; Wetzel *et al.*, 1966). This interference may vary depending on the site since Gasic and Berwick (1962) observed fairly uniform iron staining of sialic acid-rich coats in thin sections of cells reacted for the Prussian blue of light microscopy.

The effective penetration of different iron-containing solutions has been compared in mouse colonic mucosa (Wetzel *et al.*, 1966). Aldehyde–fixed, cryostat sections were exposed to either a 0.4% ferric chloride solution, the Rinehart and Abul-Haj modification of the Hale iron solution, or Mowry's (1958) version of the Hale solution. Osmium tetroxide was also used as an initial or poststaining fixative. The final pH of each iron-containing solution was a critical factor since optimum densities appeared between pH 1.4 and 2.4. Optimum staining of intracellular mucin occurred in specimens that had been (1) prefixed in OsO_4 with formalin-fixed material also showing sufficient density of mucin; and (2) exposed to either the Rinehart and Abul-Haj dialyzed iron solution or the 0.4% ferric chloride solution. The stained Golgi zones of the colonic goblet cells are consistent with results from several other electron histochemical and autoradiographic studies, which strongly reinforces the opinion that the Golgi apparatus is intimately involved with the formation of complex carbohydrates.

The use of another positively charged colloidal metal, thorium, has provided excellent intracellular localization of acid mucosubstances in osmium-fixed cat intestinal goblet cells (Revel, 1964). The formation of intracellular densities, particularly in the Golgi zone and presumably indicating sites of interaction between the cationic thorium and polyanionic sugar complexes, has been shown to depend on methacrylate-embedded thin sections being exposed to colloidal thorium at pH 2.0. A marked reduction of staining specificity occurred when the pH was raised to 3.5–4.0. From these results, it was concluded that colloidal thorium can im-part electron density to acid mucosubstances which is denser than that produced by colloidal iron. Attempts to establish the specificity of the colloidal thorium technique are discussed elsewhere (see Section II,C,2).

d. Phosphotungstic Acid. The use of the phosphotungstate radical for the visualization of saccharide moieties in thin sections has been of limited value so far, mainly because the reagent is not cationic as are the colloidal metallic stains and therefore interpretation of stain–carbohydrate interactions are difficult. As devised by Pease (1966a), a method of preparing unfixed tissues for electron microscopy termed "inert dehydration" has probably reduced the amount of complex carbohydrates lost in tissue preparation due to their high solubility in water. The commonly expressed objection to the use of aqueous fixatives for the preservation of protein–sugar macromolecules is, in part, overcome by exposing tissues to a glycol and embedding directly in hydroxypropyl methacrylate. However, most intracellular carbohydrate-containing sites of epithelial cells are not as prone to losing their complex sugar content following aqueous fixation as are the extracellular polysaccharides. Routine electron micrographs obtained from tissues which have been exposed to the regimen described above contain many negative images owing to loss of lipid from membranes which makes interpretation of morphology difficult.

The staining of intracellular mucus of the intestinal tract by phosphotungstic acid (PTA) was confined to cisterns of the rough-surface endoplasmic reticulum, Golgi lamellae, and the main goblet mass of mucus (Pease, 1966b). The nature of the staining mechanism by PTA is thought to involve the formation of multiple hydrogen bonds between the complex phosphotungstate radical and polysaccharide chains at low pH (1.2–1.4). It is argued that, since these chains are long and presumably flexible, there are plentiful sites for hydrogen bonding to occur providing spatial configurations between the polysaccharide chain and the bulky phosphotungstate radical are satisfactory to permit interaction. This interpretation may have some validity in explaining the formation of electron densities in complexing between PTA and long-chain, polymeric, high molecular weight macromolecules like polysaccharides. However, this reasoning may need overhauling when one considers the relatively short sugar chains (2–6 sugars) which comprise the glycoproteins of epithelial mucus. The stearic fit between these oligosaccharide chains and PTA may not occur because this chain length may not be as flexible.

At present, there have been no attempts to establish the specifiicity of PTA staining by enzymatic or chemical modification. Unless this is accomplished, the method will remain highly empirical for complex carbohydrates despite its capacity to produce dense staining as observed with the electron microscope. Some reduction of this empiricism is already apparent since the presumed PTA staining of polysaccharides depends on a low pH environment. This staining is selective up to about pH 3.5 at which point nucleoproteins take up PTA. From pH 5.5 to 8.5, PTA acts as a general protein stain.

C. Alterations of Staining

1. *Enzymes*

The application of certain enzymes to fixed mucins prior to staining is one means of increasing the specificity of a reaction for carbohydrates. Amylase or diastase is often employed to rule out the possibility that the periodic acid-Schiff reactivity of mucins is due to simple polymeric carbohydrate such as glycogen. As a general rule, the PAS staining of mucins is unaltered by amylase or diastase digestion, but in the case of certain ungulate mucins, the PAS reactivity was notably altered by such digestion (Leppi and Spicer, 1967). There was general agreement, however, between the amount of neutral sugars (hexose or deoxyhexose) present in most of the ungulate salivary glands studied and the degree of PAS reactivity and staining by the periodic acid–paradiamine (PAD) method (Spicer and Jarrels, 1961).

Many mucins have been shown histochemically to contain sialic acids in their carbohydrate moiety owing to the stainability of their carboxyl groups. Sialic acids are usually terminally positioned on the oligosaccharides of epithelial carbohydrates and in this position can react easily with basic dyes. Elimination of this carboxyl-dependent basophilia from tissue sections by their exposure to *Vibrio cholerae* sialidase is a valid test for localizing sialic acid (Spicer and Warren, 1960). Brief, mild acid hydrolysis accomplishes the same thing by releasing sialic acid from the oligosaccharide, thus removing the reactive carboxyl component (Neuberger and Marshall, 1966). Sialidase cleaves the α-ketosidic linkage between the terminal neuraminic acid and the adjacent sugar residue (Gibbons, 1963). Prior treatment of various primate and ungulate mucins with sialidase has aided in the differentiation of sulfomucins and sialomucins by the resulting loss of alcianophilia produced by the high iron diamine–Alcian Blue and aldehyde fuchsin–Alcian Blue combination basic dye procedures (Leppi and Spicer, 1966, 1967; Leppi *et al.*, 1967). In most cases, the high iron diamine and aldehyde fuchsin reactivities remained unaltered, indicating sites of sulfated mucins as judged by correlative ^{35}S-sulfate autoradiography. However, some of these mucins displayed resistance to the action of sialidase with or without prior exposure to mild alkali which has empirically resulted in an enhancement of the sialidase digestibility of certain mucins (Spicer and Duvenci, 1964). The susceptibility of mucins toward sialidase is probably influenced by the O- acetylation of the neuraminic acid involved and by the position of the attachment of the sialic acid to the adjacent monosaccharide (Gibbons, 1963). Some correlation was noted between the degree of resistance of certain ungulate mucins toward sialidase as judged by the residual alcianophilia following exposure to enzyme and the biochemically characterized forms of sialic acid known to be present in the same mucin (Leppi and Spicer, 1967).

That all carbohydrates of epithelial tissues may not exist as glycoproteins of the chemical classification is evident from the observations on the basophilia of certain cells in dog gastric mucosa which is labile toward the action of testicular hyaluronidase, an enzyme frequently employed for the histochemical differentiation of connective tissue polysaccharides (Spicer et al., 1967). Specifically, the autoradiographically proven (^{35}S-sulfate) sulfomucin-laden chief cells and cells of the cardiac and pyloric gland regions of dog stomach lose their basophilia following hyaluronidase digestion. These unexpected results indicate that there may be carbohydrate polymers with the β-$(1{\rightarrow}4)$ hexosaminidic linkage to uronic acid which is particularly susceptible to hyaluronidase. Such linkages are peculiar to the complex carbohydrates of mesodermal origin.

There has been limited applicability of enzymes in the electron histochemical localization of carbohydrates in epithelial secretions. The mouse rectosigmoid colon is a site which, being well-characterized by light microscopic histochemical means, contains two distinct acidic mucosubstances (Spicer, 1965). More superficially positioned goblet cells contain sulfomucin while deeper crypt cells contain sialidase-labile mucins as judged by loss of their alcianophilia after exposure to sialidase. Conversely, there is no loss of colloidal iron staining of these deep crypt cells in glutaraldehyde-fixed frozen thin sections following exposure to sialidase (Dr. M. Wetzel, personal communication). This resistance to such digestion in thin sections is difficult to explain in view of the results on paraffin sections. However, a histochemically proved site containing sialic acid, the sublingual gland of the mouse, does exhibit corresponding loss of colloidal iron staining in thin sections after sialidase digestion.

2. Specific Chemical Treatment

The alterations of dye binding of carbohydrate macromolecules by exposure of tissue sections to certain chemicals may help to establish the type of radical which may be stainable. In numerous studies of epithelial mucins, a battery of techniques have been applied to elucidate the chemical basis of staining with periodate oxidation and cationic dye methods. The frequently used techniques include (1) sulfation for the induction of ester sulfate residues on neutral (uncharged) and some acidic mucins to render them stainable (Spicer, 1960); (2) acetylation of vicinal hydroxyls to prevent their periodate oxidizability (McManus and Cason, 1950); (3) the attachment of phenylhydrazine on sites containing periodate-engendered dialdehydes which prevents their reaction with Schiff's reagent (Lillie, 1965, p. 276); (4) methylation to esterify carboxyl groups (Fraenkel-Conrat and Olcott, 1945) and to remove ester sulfate groups (Kantor and Schubert, 1957); and (5) saponification or demethylation to restore carboxyl-dependent staining by removal of methyl esters induced by methylation (Spicer and Lillie, 1959). The effects of these chemically based modifications, usually termed blocking and unblocking methods, together with results from certain enzymatic digestion and autoradiographic techniques, can be used advantageously to determine the specificity of histochemical staining.

In a critical evaluation of the effects of the methylation–demethylation sequence on the Alcian Blue staining of certain salivary glands, it was concluded that definitive identification of acid mucins was not possible unless the anionic radicals of these substances were chemically defined (Quintarelli *et al.*, 1964b). Depending on the temperature of the methylation solutions and duration of exposure, a variety of results were observed which also seemed to depend on the pH of dye solutions. Under usual conditions of histochemical application, the selectivity of methylation in this study was thought to be impaired because demethylation usually resulted in a further decrease in staining from that observed following methylation alone. This failure to recover alcianophilia following saponification was thought to be due to the hydrolysis of chemical groups other than ester sulfates. Sialic acid was considered a likely candidate since it is a ubiquitous component of epithelial mucins and may be quite susceptible to the action of 0.1 N HCl in absolute methanol for 4 hours at 60°C. This latter procedure is termed active methylation while acidified methanol for 4 hours at 37°C is referred to as a mild methylation. Mild methylation may result in the esterification of some carboxyls and leave ester sulfates unaffected. Strong methylation primarily effects the removal of ester sulfates but also may remove sialic acid. Other studies have reported some agreement between the effects of methylation–demethylation on staining and the chemical composition of carbohydrate in selected mucins (Spicer, 1965; Leppi and Spicer, 1966; Leppi and Kinnison, 1967; Leppi *et al.*, 1967; Leppi, 1968). The removal of the ^{35}S-sulfate labeling from these mucins by strong methylation corroborated the chemical basis for active methylation, i.e., removal of ester sulfates from complex carbohydrate.

Active methylation with other reagents may induce different alterations of reactive groups in tissue carbohydrates. Exposure of neutral formalin- or Carnoy-fixed hamster tissues to a 2% methanolic thionyl chloride solution probably esterifies sulfate groups rather than hydrolyzes them as occurs after methanolic HCl (Stoward, 1967; 1968). It is suspected that some hydrolytic desulfation does occur after methanolic thionyl chloride treatment. An important observation related to these experiments with methylating reagents was the increased affinity of mucosubstances toward Biebrich Scarlet at alkaline pH following exposure to methanolic thionyl chloride. This indicated an increase in the protein component of the mucins which might have been due to the conversion of protein amino groups to highly charged cationic groups. If these mucins were cationic as a result of this conversion, attempts to stain them by cationic reagents could possibly be blocked due to mutual repulsive forces since electrostatic forces are involved in the staining of most acid carbohydrates.

Protein interference in the staining of carbohydrates in certain epithelial mucins has been indicated due to the increased basophilia after pretreatment of tissue sections with crude proteolytic enzymes such as pepsin and papain (Quintarelli, 1963). Since this basophilia was shown to be sialidase labile, it was concluded that the carboxyl groups of sialic acid were masked somewhat by the presence of basic proteins. The staining of certain salivary mucosaccharides was completely abolished following this proteolysis, indicating that there was loss of stainable substrate. The blockage of the cationic staining of polysaccharides by certain proteins had been reported earlier (French and Benditt, 1953).

The adaptation of chemical modifications of staining to the electron microscope level of resolution has concentrated on the methylation of sections which were subsequently stained by colloidal metallic reagents. Revel (1964) reported that colloidal thorium staining of cat intestinal goblet mucus was lost following a 20-minute exposure to methanolic HCl at 60°C. Similarly, Wetzel *et al.* (1966) found that the colloidal iron reactivity of mouse colonic goblet cells containing histochemically demonstrable ester sulfate was abolished following a 6- to 18-hour exposure to acidified methanol at 60°C. Nearby sialic acid-containing mucins appeared to be unaffected by this methylation treatment which may be attributable to a deesterification of the methylated sialocarboxyls by the acidic iron solutions (Spicer, 1965).

D. Autoradiography

1. ^{35}S-Sulfate

The existence of ester sulfate as a component of the carbohydrates in epithelial mucins has been established in several studies on a variety of cells (Spicer, 1960, 1965; Spicer and Duvenci, 1964; Spicer *et al.*, 1961; Leppi *et al.*, 1967). These reports have all emphasized correlations between specific histochemical staining and the *in vivo* incorporation of $^{35}SO_4^{--}$ as observed in autoradiographs. The removal of labeling by methanolytic desulfation from several epithelial sites confirmed that the uptake of radioisotope was due to the incorporation of sulfates into complex carbohydrates. The intracellular site of the incorporation of ^{35}S-sulfate or sulfation of carbohydrates in mucus is the Golgi zone as established by the use of light and electron microscopic autoradiographic techniques (Lane *et al.*, 1964; Peterson and Leblond, 1964b; Neutra and Leblond, 1966b). Recent biochemical evidence for sulfated carbohydrates of epithelial origin has been correlated with histochemical data for their presence in several tissues (see Section II).

The stainability of sulfomucins seems to parallel that observed for sialomucins although the former group continues to stain when the pH of the dye solution is at or below 2.0. The ester sulfate group and the carboxylate of sialic acid can be visualized by most cationic stains although it has been noted that the high iron diamine and aldehyde fuchsin reagents show a special affinity for sulfated carbohydrates. These reactivities are often observed in epithelial sites which also incorporate considerable ^{35}S-sulfate (Leppi *et al.*, 1967).

2. *Labeled Carbohydrates and the Golgi Complex*

Up to now, the emphasis has been on the localization and characterization of epithelial mucins by a variety of techniques. This section will be devoted to a discussion of the dynamic intracellular events leading to the secretion of a mucus as followed by autoradiography. Beams and Kessel (1968) have thoroughly reviewed the structure and overall functions of the Golgi apparatus while Neutra and Leblond (1969) have compiled an excellent and comprehensible recollection of their involvement in elucidating the role of this cellular organelle in the synthesis of complex carbohydrates.

Much of the recent and probing investigations on the role of the Golgi complex in the synthesis of heterosaccharides have primarily involved the goblet cells in the intestine of the rat. This series of studies began by the subcutaneous injection of D-glucose-6-^{3}H into young rats which were sacrificed at various intervals ranging between 5 minutes and 3 hours after injections (Peterson and Leblond, 1964b). The tissues were removed at the appropriate time intervals, fixed, stained, and prepared for light microscopic autoradiography by the coating technique. Other rats received local injections of ^{3}H-labeled glucose in their small intestine and these tissues were removed 5 minutes after injections. Labeling was observed over the Golgi regions of intestinal goblet cells 5–15 minutes after injection. Local injections of ^{3}H-glucose resulted in a similar localization of silver grains over the Golgi zone as did systemic injections. At later times after injection, the labeling was observed over the intracellular secretory products of the goblet cells. From these results, it was concluded that the Golgi region of these cells is the site where glucose is utilized by the cell to form the carbohydrate portion of mucus. In order to rule out the possibility that the glucose-6-^{3}H was being incorporated as a fragmented sugar into other materials, such as proteins and nucleic acids, rats were injected with glucose labeled with ^{3}H in the 1 or 6 position and incorporation was followed at various intervals after injection (Peterson and Leblond, 1964a). Again, labeling with either isotope occurred over the Golgi zone at short time intervals, demonstrating that the 6-carbon chain must have been utilized as an intact unit by the carbohydrate portion of the glycoprotein in goblet mucus. This is necessary for the conversion of glucose to any one of the several monosaccharide building blocks of glycoproteins.

High resolution autoradiography was then selected as the tool to determine specifically the intracellular site of the synthesis of complex carbohydrates (Neutra and Leblond, 1966a). Slices of rat colon were removed, fixed, and prepared for autoradiography at 5, 20, and 40 minutes, 1, $1\frac{1}{2}$, and 4 hours after the administration of glucose-6-^{3}H. By 5 minutes following injection, substances in the flattened saccules of the Golgi complex in colonic goblet cells were labeled and by 20 minutes both the saccules and adjacent mucous granules were labeled. Lane et al. (1964) demonstrated that the Golgi saccules or even perhaps their membranes are the intracellular sites where sulfation of colonic goblet mucus occurs. These granules contained almost the total amount of detectable label by 40 minutes, and during the interval from 1 to 4 hours the label was traced from a supranuclear location to the apical plasma membrane. The final event was extrusion of the label from the colonic goblet cells. Taken together, these results strongly indicated the Golgi saccules are the sites where the carbohydrate of mucus is synthesized and added to protein to form the glycoprotein macromolecule. It was considered highly probably that there is a continuous renewal of Golgi stacks since it was estimated that a saccule is released by each stack every 2–4 minutes.

In a companion study (Neutra and Leblond, 1966b), another precursor of complex carbohydrates, galactose, was also followed by electron microscopic autoradiography in various secretory cells of the rat and results compared with those obtained for glucose. The conclusions were similar in that, when secretory cells were labeled by either isotope, label first ap-

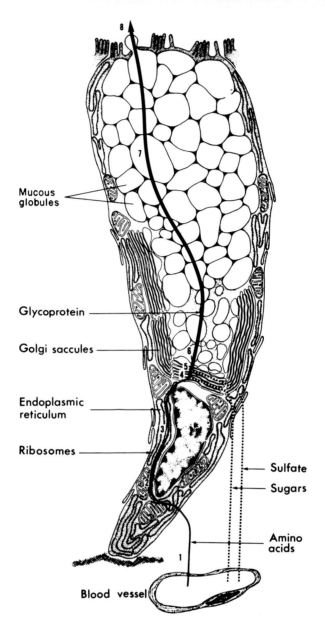

Mucous
globules

Glycoprotein

Golgi saccules

Endoplasmic
reticulum

Ribosomes

Sulfate

Sugars

Amino
acids

Blood vessel

Fig. 1. Schematic diagram of the mucus formation in a goblet cell. Precursors of the mucus enter the cell from a blood vessel (1). Amino acids are synthesized on ribosomes (2) into proteins, which move up through the endoplasmic reticulum (3) to enter the Golgi saccules. Meanwhile simple sugars are taken up into the saccules, there to combine with the incoming protein (4) to form glycoprotein, to which sulfate from the blood is also added (5). The saccules in which the glycoprotein is put together, are transformed into globules of mucus (6). The globules migrate to the top of the cell (7), ultimately leaving the cell and releasing the mucus to coat the surface of the intestine (8). (Courtesy of M. Neutra and C. P. Leblond, McGill University.)

peared over the Golgi region and later over the mucus. Amylase digestion eliminated the scattered cytoplasmic galactose label but did not affect glucose labeling. However, such digestion never affected labeling of the Golgi region by either isotope.

Thus, it was apparent from these correlated studies that the Golgi apparatus is the intracellular site of synthesis of the carbohydrate portion of mucus. After the carbohydrate is bonded to the protein, presumably in the Golgi, the intracellular route of the glycoproteins can be followed toward the apex of the cell and it can be observed to be eventually extruded from the cell in the form of mucous globules (Fig. 1.)

III. Histochemistry of Polysaccharides

The shapeless or amorphous matrix not occupied by cells or fibers of connective tissues is the domain of polysaccharides which are produced by connective tissue cells. This ground substance, a term synonymous with amorphous matrix which arose from histochemical studies of connective tissues, has a varied polysaccharide content depending on the functions served by a particular form of connective tissue. In the chemical sense, there is no generalized ground substance, but the high content of anionic carbohydrates seem to be common to most connective tissue matrices. Although the term *mucopolysaccharide* has common usage in both the chemical and histochemical literature, but particularly in the latter, the more recently acceptable terms appear to be simply connective tissue *polysaccharides* or *protein–polysaccharides* since most of these carbohydrates appear to be bound to protein rather than occurring in the free state (Schubert and Hamerman, 1968, p. 70). The following discussion of connective tissue histochemistry will be limited to some of the seven biochemically well-characterized, anionic polysaccharides whose structures have been elucidated largely through the investigations of Meyer and his colleagues. Several excellent reviews on the biochemistry of polysaccharides are available and these should be consulted for possible correlations with histochemical data in a connective tissue site (Hoffman and Meyer, 1962; Jeanloz, 1963; Schiller, 1966; Schubert and Hamerman, 1968).

Structural features that are common to all of the anionic polysaccharides so far characterized are (1) composed of unbranched chains of regularly repeating units consisting of two different saccharide units; (2) the disaccharide repeating unit is uauslly composed of a hexuronate linked to a hexosamine, but in one polysaccharide (keratan sulfate), a galactose residue substitutes for the uronic acid; (3) covalent bonding of the polysaccharide to a protein backbone; and (4) the presence of fixed negative charges in the form of carboxylate and ester sulfate groups which are regularly spaced on the uronic and hexosaminidic residues, respectively. The histochemistry of polysaccharides depends largely on these anionic groups for interactions with metachromatic and polyvalent cationic stains.

The precise, histochemical localization of the anionic polysaccharides in normal connective tissue ground substance is important from the standpoint of understanding their alteration during pathology of connective tissues. These disorders of polysaccharide formation may have a direct relationship bearing on the effectiveness by which the ground substance acts as the mainstream for passage of cell metabolites between the blood and cells.

A. FIXATION

To properly introduce this problem and some of its ramifications, the reader is referred to the critical discussion of Szirmai (1963) concerning the process of hopefully rendering polysaccharides sensitive to histochemical manipulation. The chemical events constituting fixation to permit the subsequent staining of highly charged macromolecules, such as protein–polysaccharides, most likely depends on the interaction of reagents, usually formaldehyde-based, with the protein moiety rather than with the carbohydrate portion. Thus, the actual fixation of polysaccharides may not occur under usual conditions of aqueous fixation, but rather the carbohydrate is precipitated as a conseuqence of being covalently bonded to protein. Despite this probable action of polysaccharide fixatives, many of the connective tissue carbohydrates are subject to partial and often total loss from tissue sections during fixation due to their highly hydrated state. This condition varies, of course, with the connective tissue being studied; the more highly hydrated the complex carbohydrate is, the greater the chances are for increased solubility. To circumvent or perhaps minimize this tendency to solubilize, there are a variety of fixative reagents that have been applied to the histochemical study of polysaccharides. Fixation with alcohol alone or in combination with certain acids such as acetic, as in Carnoy's fluid, has the potential of precipitating polysaccharides in an unaltered state. However, serious objections to these modes of fixation, such as tissue shrinkage and the chances for resolubilization during histological processing, detract from their effectiveness. The addition of cations in the form of metals or barium, sodium, or calcium to fixative solutions has provided investigators with relatively more tissue carbohydrates to study than with other methods (Szirmai, 1963).

The adaptation of a biochemical system for fractionating a wide variety of polyanions in biological materials for use in the histochemical visualization of anionic polysaccharides has proved also to be of significant value in their fixation (Scott, 1960). The addition of long-chain, positively charged, aliphatic quaternary ammonium salts such as cetylpyridinium chloride (CPC) to formalin solutions resulted in optimum fixation for anionic polysaccharides as judged by subsequent staining with various cationic dyes (Kelly *et al.*, 1963). Preservation of morphology following CPC–formalin paralleled that obtained following fixation with neutral formalin or neutral ethanol–formalin. In a comparative study to determine the effectiveness of aqueous formalin fixatives containing cationic substances in preserving the polysaccharides of human umbilical cord, Conklin (1963a) concluded that CPC–formalin retained the maximum stainable portion of this extracellular matrix. From a histochemical and biochemical analysis of the influence of various fixatives on the preservation of the acid polysaccharides in rabbit cornea, it was concluded that CPC–formalin at 28°C was the most effective fixative, while at room temperature it was the poorest, probably due to an increased hydration of corneal carbohydrates (Cejkova and Brettschneider, 1969). These reactions of cationic detergents with anionic polysaccharides are difficult to explain, especially when maximum retention of stainable complex carbohydrates is indicated following such fixation. Most of the problems encountered during fixation are secondary compared to the interaction of a cationic fixative with the reactant groups of the tissue, i.e., anions of carbohydrates, which are the basis for their staining. If one assumes a near total reaction of cations in the fixative with anions of the substrate, this results in very few sites left for attachment of dye cations. It is quite possible that the interactions of cations in fixatives or stains may be similar. Thus, Szirmai (1963) has obtained excellent results for the histochemical staining of polysaccharides in frozen sections exposed only to relatively high concentrations of cationic dyes capable of precipitating anionic carbohydrates. His procedure essentially avoided most of the routine tissue processing and thus probably avoided many of the pitfalls associated with fixation in polysaccharide histochemistry.

B. STAINING PROCEDURES

1. *Light Microscopy*

a. Vicinal Hydroxyl Methods. The use of periodic acid is helpful in the determination of polysaccharide structure, but it has limited applicability in the histochemistry of polysaccharides. The methodology of the periodic acid-Schiff reaction has been mentioned previously (see Section II,B, 1,a) and it was noted that the reaction was more effective in identifying complex carbohydrates of epithelial origin. When a connective tissue site is reactive toward the PAS sequence, this usually indicates the presence of uncharged (neutral) polysaccharides (Spicer *et al.*, 1967), or hexose or methyl pentose residues containing free 1,2-glycols (Leblond, *et al.*, 1957). Acid or charged polysaccharides are potentially PAS-reactive with an abundance of 1,2-glycols contained within their uronic acid moiety. However, PAS staining of these carbohydrates does not usually occur after the usual 10-minute exposure to periodate in the histochemical test. It is well known that the consumption of periodate by certain acid polysaccharides *in vitro* does occur, but it is a slow reaction on the order of days (Schubert and Hamerman, 1968, p. 67). Current evidence points to a mutal repulsion between anions of the polysaccharide chain and the periodate ion which inhibits access of periodate to 1,2-glycols in polymeric carbohydrates (Scott and Harbinson, 1968).

A probable exception to the generalized PAS unreactivity of most acid polysaccharides is the reactivity of keratan sulfate toward the PAS sequence much like that exhibited by the oligosaccharides of epithelial mucins. Recent studies on this atypical (no uronic acid) polysaccharide have revealed other forms of this polymer (Mathews and Cifonelli, 1965) with a few of these containing sialic acid as a terminal sugar (Bhavanandan and Meyer, 1968). The PAS reactivity of keratan sulfate could be due to sialic acid or neutral sugars, although Hirano *et al.* (1961) reported little consumption of periodate, i.e., 1 mole of periodate per chain length of 10 monosaccharide units.

Before the basic structure of keratan sulfate was known, it was noted that the PAS reactivity of costal cartilage matrix increased with age (Joel *et al.*, 1956) while the acid polysaccharide decreased during aging as determined by colloidal iron staining and by the decreased content of uronic acid (Stidworthy *et al.*, 1958). The increased PAS reaction was attributed to an increase of a neutral hexosamine-containing substance which contained galactose. Meyer *et al.* (1958) corroborated the fact that keratan sulfate of cartilage increases with age, and they also demonstrated that this polymer, composed basically of galactose and glucosamine, was increased in young adult cartilage matrix from individuals afflicted with Marfan's syndrome.

b. Single and Combination Methods. Saunders (1964) advocated the use of the fluorochrome, acridine orange, for identifying acid polysaccharides because it was demonstrated that this cationic dye can precipitate carbohydrate macromolecules much like cetylpyridinium chloride, a cationic detergent. In experiments on preparations of hyaluronic acid, chondroitin sulfate, and heparin, precipitates formed between acridine orange and these polysaccharides were redissolved in sodium chloride solutions with molarities varying from 0 to 1.8. This system is analogous to the fractionation technique for acid polysaccharides which relies on their precipitation by CPC and subsequent solution of precipitates by added inorganic salts (Scott, 1960). Under the experimental conditions of Saunder's studies, solution of the acridine orange– heparin precipitates occurred at the highest salt concentration while chondroitin sulfate was next followed at the lowest salt molarity by hyaluronic acid. This order was noted to be the same as that observed for solution of polysaccharide–CPC precipitates. Sections of umbilical cord, cock's comb, and rat tail tendon were fixed in Newcomer's solution to minimize the solubility of polyanions, treated with cetyltrimethylammonium chloride (acts like CPC), followed by ribonuclease digestion, and then stained by acridine orange. The same differentiation between the three polysaccharides was then possible when sections were differentiated in salt solutions of increasing molarity.

The matrix of amorphous ground substance of hyaline cartiliage has been subdivided into approximately five zones on the basis of a histochemical study employing a battery of methods on CPC–formalin-fixed cartilages (Conklin, 1963b). Through the use of certain empirical staining methods, e.g., Bismarck brown, it was determined that the affinity of the interterritorial matrix for this dye increased with age, suggesting that this reflects the well-known increase of keratan sulfate with age (Meyer et al., 1958).

Further studies of certain animal and human cartilages have emphasized comparisons between tissues of different embryological origin (Quintarelli and Dellovo, 1965) and the histochemically detectable changes which matrix undergoes during aging (Quintarelli and Dellovo, 1966). The application of various polyanionic staining techniques, including the Alcian Blue–periodic acid-Schiff sequence, Alcian Blue with different concentrations of electrolyte (critical electrolyte concentration method), and enzymatic and chemical modifications of staining led to definite conclusions regarding the distribution of chondroitin sulfate and keratan sulfate. In developing cartilages, the areas of appositional growth were found to synthesize mainly chondroitin sulfate while the territorial and interterritorial regions of matrix contain chondroitin mixed with keratan sulfate. With age, the interterritorial matrix loses much of the latter polysaccharide, but then is found in greater amounts immediately adjacent to chondrocytes. These studies have perhaps provided further insight into the exact location of keratan sulfate in old cartilage.

2. Electron Microscopy

a. Colloidal Reagents. The electron microscopic localization of extracellular acid polysaccharides has been reported in cartilages by colloidal
iron (Matukas *et al.*, 1967) and by colloidal thorium (Revel, 1964); in
loose connective tissue stroma of rodent intestine (Curran *et al.*, 1965;
Wetzel *et al.*, 1966) and of uterine cervix (Leppi *et al.*, 1968) by colloidal
iron; and in tissue cultures of fibroblasts by colloidal iron (Yardley and
Brown, 1965). There is generally denser staining of acid polysaccharides by
thorium than by the various iron reagents, a distinct advantage when one is
viewing otherwise unstained sections to determine the specificity of the
localization of stain deposits. Optimal conditions of exposure of sections
to the colloidal reagents seem to favor immersion of fixed, frozen, or nonfrozen sections in the staining solutions prior to embedding. Application of
colloidal stains to plastic sections or to nonembedded sections greater than
80 μ thick is not recommended, since penetration of stain micelles is poor.
Intracellular staining by thorium and iron has been localized to the Golgi
zone giving further credence to the notion that this organelle is involved
in the formation of polysaccharides (Revel, 1964; Wetzel *et al.*, 1966).

Artifactual accumulation of stain deposit has been a problem in the
identification of a hormonally controlled ground substance in the uterine
cervix of the mouse (Leppi *et al.*, 1968). Fixation of cervices with Karnovsky's (1965) glutaraldehyde–paraformaldehyde mixture at high osmolality (2010 milliosmols/kg) resulted in large accumulations of extracellular colloidal iron deposits which were clearly unrelated to adjacent
structures such as collagenous fibrils and fibroblasts. However, when an
aldehyde mixture with approximately one half the osmolality of the Karnovsky blend was utilized by diluting the original formula with buffer as
directed by Flickinger (1967), iron deposits were uniformly dispersed among
collagenous fibrils and bordering cell membranes with intracellular staining
confined to Golgi regions of activated fibroblasts. Of particular interest was
the intense iron staining between collagenous fibrils which occurred as
small, widely dispersed bundles in the walls of large cervices whose gross
structural features resembled those present at parturition. Conversely,
there was no intrafibrillar iron staining in cervices which were clearly
smaller and whole cervical canals were undilatable. These findings may
partly explain the drastic changes in connective tissue which the uterine
cervix undergoes during pregnancy, parturition, and postpartum.

b. Phosphotungstic Acid. Interaction between phosphotungstate radicals
and tissue polyanions at pH 1.2 may be possible for localizing polysaccharides, but somewhat doubtful for shorter sugar chains characteristic
of acid glycoproteins, as discussed elsewhere (see Section II,B,2,d). Strong

staining of various extracellular materials, including elastica and cartilage matrix, by phosphotungstic acid has been observed by Pease (1966b) in sections prepared for electron microscopy by "inert" dehydration (Pease, 1966a) with ethylene glycol and embedment in hydroxypropyl methacrylate to avoid the intermediate solvents of routine processing. The use of this embedding medium seems to be a general requirement of the PTA staining method since other media have given inconsistent results.

The basis for interpreting the specificity of PTA for polysaccharides is the affinity of the stain for materials which are PAS reactive in the light microscope. Polysaccharides equipped with anions are generally PAS unreactive as established by both histochemical and biochemical means (see Section III,B,1,a). Therefore, it is difficult to relate PTA reactivity to the presence of acid polysaccharides. If there are available groups in tissues prepared for staining by PTA, they may represent other histochemically unidentifiable radicals since the specificity of the reaction has not been attempted either by enzymatic or chemical modification. However, there is a pH dependency of the PTA reaction for sites containing polysaccharides since above pH 3.5 nucleoprotein staining increases and above pH 5.5, PTA acts as a general protein stain.

c. Ruthenium Red. This routine, botanical stain for the highly polymerized pectic materials of plant cell walls has been adapted to the electron microscopic localization of a variety of animal extracellular carbohydrates by combining ruthenium red (RR) and osmium tetroxide in a single reagent (Luft, 1964, 1965, 1966, 1968). It was noted early that cartilage matrix was stained red by RR in thick sections of Epon-embedded tissues (Luft, 1965, 1966). Adjacent thin sections of cartilage were not stained when viewed in the electron microscope. Coupling RR to osmium tetroxide resulted in brown staining of matrix in thick sections while thin sections revealed a cartilage matrix composed of dense, spherical particles 300 Å in diameter (Figs. 2 and 3). Subsequent heavy metal staining by uranyl and lead salts revealed a population of short, tapered threads (ca. 150 Å in diameter) extending between the 300 Å dense particles. The threads were less than 50 Å before heavy metal staining which suggested that any staining in addition to RR may add artifactually to thread size. Although Luft inferred that the dense, 300 Å particles in cartilage matrix, as visualized by RR, were polysaccharide in nature, Matukas *et al.* (1967) described particles of similar size (200–700 Å) in cartilage matrix which exhibited colloidal iron staining. This staining was labile toward testicular hyaluronidase indicating the presence of chondroitin sulfates.

In further testing of RR's specificity for acid polysaccharides, it was observed that this inorganic dye will precipitate solutions of heparin,

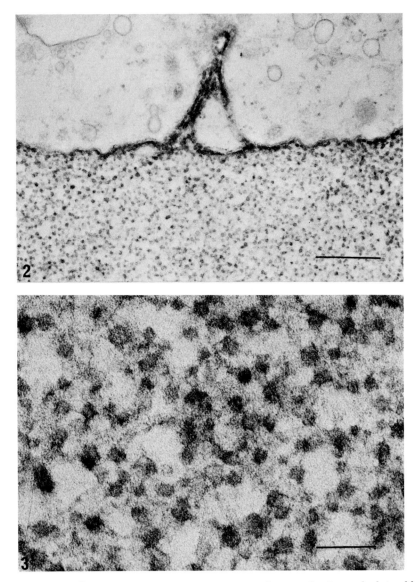

FIG. 2. A 800-Å thick section of frog cartilage exposed to a ruthenium red–glutaralde-hyde–OsO₄ mixture, but otherwise unstained. Lower half of the micrograph shows the matrix which is more densely stained than a portion of cartilage cell cytoplasm in the upper half of the section. Marker represents 0.5 μ. 34,000 ×.

FIG. 3. Higher magnification of section in Fig. 2 showing the densely stained granules of the cartilage matrix which presumably represent acid polysaccharides. Marker repre-sents 0.1 μ. 160,000 ×. (Figs. 2 and 3 courtesy of J. H. Luft, University of Washington.)

chondroitin sulfate, and pectin, all highly acidic carbohydrate polymers, while uncharged (neutral) substances such as plant gums are unaffected by RR.

Although cartilage has been the model tissue for investigating the specificity of RR for complex carbohydrates, other sites of reaction have been noted. These include (1) cell-coating materials such as the microvillar surface coat or "fuzz" of intestinal epithelia which is rich in carbohydrates; (2) intercellular materials of mouse diaphragm which are closely related to collagenous fibrils and those at relatively broad junctions between these fibrils and muscle cells; and (3) sheath materials surrounding collagenous fibrils and endothelial cells of capillaries, including their luminal surfaces.

The application of certain enzymatic and chemical modification procedures to RR-stained materials is necessary at this time to help establish the specificity of the reaction. This would not be difficult since fine structural detail is preserved rather well following RR–OsO$_4$ treatment and the relationships of staining to underlying structures could be made.

C. ALTERATIONS OF STAINING

1. *Enzymes*

The most commonly used polysaccharase for the histochemical differentiation of polysaccharides is testicular hyaluronidase. This enzyme was actually identified as the spreading factor in loose connective tissues much before its substrates, the polysaccharides, were known (Schubert and Hamerman, 1968, pp. 67–69). Chemically, hyaluronidases of testicular origin hydrolyze the hexosaminidic linkages of chondroitin 4- and 6-sulfates producing a variety of oligosaccharides in the reaction. This hyaluronidase does not affect keratan sulfate, heparin, heparan sulfate, or dermatan sulfate. The enzyme also acts on hyaluronic acid but less completely as compared to the chondroitins. Hyaluronidases of bacterial origin degrade only hyaluronic acid with the subsequent production of unsaturated saccharides. All of the polysaccharides which are susceptible to the action of testicular hyaluronidase contain potentially stainable acidic groups in the form of carboxyls and ester sulfates. In the usual histochemical test, the absence of cationic staining following exposure to hyaluronidase in fixed sections is related to the presence of stainable anionic groups on enzyme-susceptible polymers. Apparently, the degradation of long polysaccharide chains to shorter chains results in the decrease of sufficient groups of stainable anions. This relative decrease in charge density as produced originally by intact polysaccharide chains effectively prevents the accumulation of stain at reactive sites which may still be present, but are in a depolymerized state.

In the light microscopic histochemical examination of connective tissues, the absence of staining by cationic reagents such as Alcian Blue, colloidal iron, aldehyde fuchsin, and high iron diamine, among others, following hyaluronidase digestion, is attributed to the presence of one or more of the polysaccharides whose staining was readily apparent in enzyme buffer-control sections. The reader is referred to a critical discussion of the possible errors which may result in the use of enzymes for the localization of polysaccharides (Spicer *et al.*, 1967).

Testicular hyaluronidase is also used as a modifying reagent in electron microscopic studies which employ reagents capable of inducing electron-dense staining of complex carbohydrates. Revel (1964) has observed the complete loss of the colloidal thorium staining of cartilage matrix after

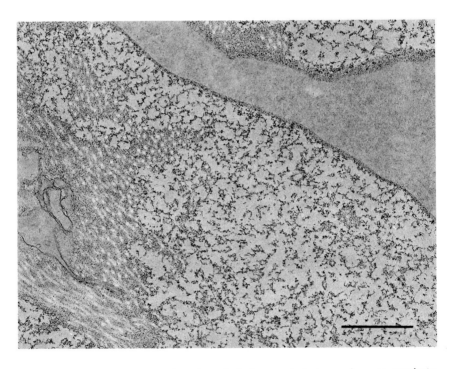

Fig. 4. Enzyme buffer control section of uterine cervical stroma from an ovariecto-mized mouse treated with estradiol and relaxin. The finely granular colloidal iron staining at pH 1.7 is limited to the extracellular region and does not deposit intracellularly as evidenced by a portion of an unstained fibroblast in the upper right corner of the micrograph. No poststaining. 19,000 ×.

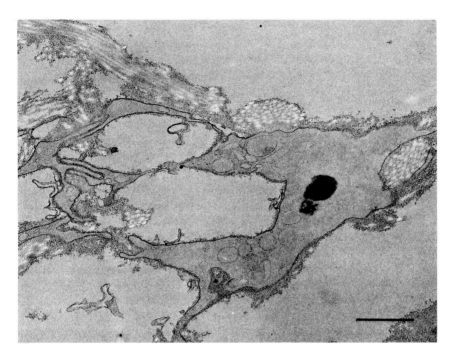

FIG. 5. Adjacent section of cervix treated with testicular hyaluronidase for 2 hours at 37° C. There is a marked reduction of the extracellular iron staining (cf. Fig. 4) but some staining remains, especially near collagenous fibrils which appear in negative image. No poststaining. 15,500 ×.

exposure of sections to hyaluronidase while Matukas et al. (1967) have noted a similar loss of colloidal iron staining of matrix particles following similar enzyme digestion. Both of these results imply the presence of sulfated carbohydrates since hyaluronic acid is not a normal constituent of cartilage matrix. The colloidal iron reactivity of materials in the loosened connective tissue stroma of uterine crevices from pregnant and hormonally treated mice was reduced following prior exposure to testicular hyaluronidase (Figs. 4 and 5) (Leppi et al., 1968).

Acid polysaccharides in close association with synovial collagenous fibrils have been demonstrable through use of a combination glutaraldehyde–ruthenium red solution as a fixative-staining reagent (Myers et al., 1969). The stainable polysaccharides appeared in several different forms, all of which were adjacent to the fibrils in human synovial lining tissue. Digestion with testicular hyaluronidase prior to staining resulted in varying degrees of lability toward the enzyme with staining of some forms of the polysaccharides completely abolished by enzyme while in others there was only partial removal. It is believed that staining was due to both chondroitin sulfate and hyaluronic acid since both of these polymers are chemically identifiable in synovial tissue.

2. Chemical Treatment

For connective tissues, this has been mainly limited to determining the effects of methylation on cationic staining as detailed elsewhere (Section II,C,2). The action of methylation in the hydrolytic removal of ester sulfates from polysaccharides has been more successfully demonstrated in sections stained for light microscopy (Quintarelli et al., 1964b; Spicer et al., 1967). Severe tissue damage has been reported in studies on the effects of hot, acidified methanol on colloidal thorium staining in thin sections of cartilage matrix (Revel, 1964). In this study, the staining was labile toward such treatment, but remaining morphology was difficult to interpret.

D. AUTORADIOGRAPHY

As pointed out earlier, the ester sulfate group of hexosamines in polysaccharides is the frequent target of histochemical staining procedures since it is the most acidic group available for complexing with stains. Of secondary importance is the carboxylate group of uronic acids which are not as amenable to histochemical manipulation as the sulfates. The injection of ^{35}S-sulfate and following its time-based course of incorporation into polymeric carbohydrate by light microscopic autoradiography permits comparison with sites stained by cationic dyes. Labeling of polysaccharides by radioactive sulfate in numerous connective tissue sites was slower than that observed for epithelial mucins (Spicer et al., 1967). In general, sacrifice of animals up to 24 hours after administration permitted adequate isotope incorporation into polysaccharides as visualized by autoradiographic labeling, whereas sulfate uptake into epithelial sugars occurred from 2 to 6 hours.

The selectivity of ^{35}S-sulfate incorporation into polysaccharides was proved by the biochemical recovery of such labeling as demonstrated for the chondroitin sulfates of cartilage (Dziewiatkowski, 1951). The effect of purified testicular hyaluronidase on sulfate uptake in complex polysaccharides is the removal of the autoradiographically demonstrable label (Curran, 1964). Exposure of autoradiographs, containing tissues from animals injected with isotope 2–12 hours prior to sacrifice, to hot, acidified methanol removes incorporated isotope from most polysaccharides (Spicer et al., 1961). Such treatment did not remove labeling of certain tissues from animals sacrificed beyond 24 hours after ^{35}S-sulfate administration (Spicer *et al.*, 1967). This labeling was present in tissues such as hair follicles which are rich in sulfur-containing proteins. Correlations between positive histochemical staining with certain cationic dyes, chemical modification of such staining, and ^{35}S-sulfate labeling of the same sites can provide believable data for the presence of sulfated polysaccharides.

The intracellular events leading to the release of sulfated polysaccharides into the extracellular milieu have received serious scrutiny. Utilizing sections of developing cartilage removed from fetal and newborn rats which were sacrificed at intervals from $1\frac{1}{2}$ minutes to 15 hours after intraperitoneal injections of ^{35}SO$_4^{--}$, it was demonstrated by electron microscopic autoradiography that radiosulfate was bound to Golgi vesicles of active chondrocytes 3 minutes after presentation of isotope *in vitro* (Godman and Lane, 1964). By 1 hour following injection of ^{35}S-sulfate, the labeling occurred at the margins of chondrocytes and in the surrounding matrix. Pretreatment with testicular hyaluronidase removed sulfate radioactivity from the matrix and chondrocytes which had been labeled *in vivo* at 60 minutes. These results indicated that the vesicular component of the Golgi complex is the site of sulfation of the chondromucoprotein with the protein moiety presumably synthesized in the endoplasmic reticulum while uniting of polysaccharide with protein occurred in the Golgi zone. Neutra and Leblond (1966b) reported localization of glucose-6-^{3}H and galactose-6-^{3}H radioactivity at early times following injection in the Golgi regions of chondroblasts as determined by light microscopic autoradiography. This labeling was also susceptible to digestion with testicular hyaluronidase as reported for ^{35}S-sulfate radioactivity in cartilage.

Biochemical studies on the subcellular sites for the synthesis of cartilage chondromucoprotein have suggested that the initial formation of this macromolecule begins with the protein core at the ribosome (Horwitz and Dorfman, 1968). Addition of the basic hexosamine and uronic acids occurred in both rough and smooth microsomal fractions while the sugars involved at linkage sites to the protein core are added primarily at the rough endoplasmic reticulum. Much of these data was derived from the assay of the *in vitro* enzymatic activities involved in the biosynthesis of chondroitin 4- and 6-sulfates. The patterns of activity were judged to be consistent with most theories dealing with the synthesis, transfer, and release of carbohydrate macromolecules.

In a combined biochemical and electron microscopic autoradiographic study of a nonsulfated polysaccharide, hyaluronic acid, the ultrastructural sites of its synthesis and storage were followed in cultures of human synovial cells (Barland *et al.*, 1968). In order to obtain an adequate uptake of glucosamine-6-^{3}H by synovial cells as a component of the disaccharide repeating unit of hyaluronic acid, it was necessary to employ a culture medium devoid of glucose but rich in pyruvate as the energy source. With this system, the autoradiographic localization of glucosamine-^{3}H was confined to the Golgi region at early times (5 minutes) after initial incubation. The recovery of the tritium label in the hyaluronic acid of the synovial cell cultures by biochemical procedures supported the autoradiographic findings which pointed to its intracellular localization. By as late as 30 minutes after initial incubation, the Golgi zone was still the predominantly labeled organelle.

REFERENCES

Barland, P., Smith, C., and Hamerman, D. (1968). Localization of hyaluronic acid in synovial cells by radioautography. *J. Cell Biol.* **37**, 13–26.

Beams, H. W., and Kessel, R. G. (1968). The Golgi apparatus: structure and function. *Int. Rev. Cytol.* **23**, 209–276.

Bhavanandan, V. P., and Meyer, K. (1968). Studies on keratosulfates. Methylation, desulfation, and acid hydrolysis studies on old human rib cartilage keratosulfate. *J. Biol. Chem.* **243**, 1052–1059.

Bignardi, C., Aureli, G., Balduini, C., and Castellani, A. A. (1964). Sulfosialopolysaccharide-peptide from dog submaxillary gland. *Biochem. Biophys. Res. Commun.* **17**, 301–312.

Bradbury, S., and Stoward, P. J. (1967). The specific cytochemical demonstration in the electron microscope of periodate-reactive mucosubstances and polysaccharides containing *Vic*-glycol groups. *Histochemie* **11**, 71–80.

Buddecke, E. (1966). Miscellaneous glycoproteins. *In* "Glycoproteins, Their Composition, Structure and Function" (A. Gottschalk, ed.), pp. 563–567, Elsevier, New York.

Cejkova, J., and Brettschneider, I. (1969). On the influence of fixations on the normal hydration of rabbit cornea and the total amount of acid mucopolysaccharides in the stroma. *Histochemie* **17**, 108–120.

Conklin, J. L. (1963a). Staining reactions of mucopolysaccharides after formalin-containing fixatives. *Stain Technol.* **38**, 56–59.

Conklin, J. L. (1963b). Staining properties of hyaline cartilage. *Amer. J. Anat.* **112**, 259–267.

Curran, R. C. (1961). The histological demonstration of connective-tissue mucopolysaccharides. *Biochem. Soc. Symp.* **20**, 24–38.

Curran, R. C. (1964). The histochemistry of mucopolysaccharides. *Int. Rev. Cytol.* **17**, 149–212.

Curran, R. C., Clark, A. E., and Lovell, D. (1965). Acid mucopolysaccharides in electron microscopy. The use of the colloidal iron method. *J. Anat.* **99**, 427–434.

Dziewiatkowski, D. D. (1951). Isolation of chondroitin sulfate-S^{35} from articular cartilage of rats. *J. Biol. Chem.* **189**, 187–190.

Flickinger, C. J. (1967). The postnatal development of the Sertoli cells of the mouse. *Z. Zellforsch. Mikrosk. Anat.* **78**, 92–113.

Fraenkel-Conrat, H., and Olcott, H. S. (1945). Esterification of proteins with alcohols of low molecular weight. *J. Biol. Chem.* **161**, 259–268.

French, J. E., and Benditt, E. P. (1953). The histochemistry of connective tissue: II. The effect of proteins on the selective staining of mucopolysaccharides by basic dyes. *J. Histochem. Cytochem.* **1**, 321–325.

Gad, A., and Sylvén, B. (1969). On the nature of the high iron diamine method for sulfomucins. *J. Histochem. Cytochem.* **17,** 156–160.

Gasic, G., and Berwick, L. (1962). Hale stain for sialic acid-containing mucins. Adaptation to electron microscopy. *J. Cell Biol.* **19,** 223–228.

Gasic, G. J., Berwick, L., and Sorrentino, M. (1968). Positive and negative colloidal iron as cell surface electron stains. *Lab. Invest.* **18,** 63–71.

Gerard, A., Lev, R., and Glass, G. B. J. (1967). Histochemical study of the mucosubstances in the canine stomach. *Amer. J. Dig. Dis.* **12,** 891–915.

Gibbons, R. A. (1963). The sensitivity of the neuraminosidic linkage in mucosubstances towards acid and towards neuraaminidase. *Biochem. J.* **89,** 380–391.

Godman, G. C., and Lane, N. (1964). On the site of sulfation in the chondrocyte. *J. Cell Biol.* **21,** 353–366.

Gottschalk, A. (1966). Definition of glycoproteins and their delineation from other carbohydrate-protein complexes. *In* "Glycoproteins, Their Composition, Structure and Function" (A. Gottschalk, ed.), pp. 20–28. Elsevier, New York.

Hardonk, M. J., and van Duijn, P. (1964). The mechanism of the Schiff reaction as studied with histochemical model systems. *J. Histochem. Cytochem.* **12,** 748–751.

Hirano, S., Hoffman, P., and Meyer, K. (1961). The structure of keratosulfate of bovine cornea. *J. Org. Chem.* **26,** 5064–5069.

Hoffman, P., and Meyer, K. (1962). Structural studies of mucopolysaccharides of connective tissue. *Fed. Proc. Fed. Amer. Soc. Exp. Biol.* **21,** 1064–1069.

Horwitz, A. L., and Dorfman, A. (1968). Subcellular sites for synthesis of chondromucoprotein of cartilage. *J. Cell Biol.* **38,** 358–368.

Inoue, S., and Yosizawa, Z. (1966). Purification and properties of sulfated sialopolysaccharides isolated from pig colonic mucosa. *Arch. Biochem. Biophys.* **117,** 257–265.

Jeanloz, R. W. (1960). The nomenclature of mucopolysaccharides. *Arthritis Rheum.* **3,** 233–237.

Jeanloz, R. W. (1963). Mucopolysaccharides (acidic glycosaminoglycans). *Comp. Biochem. Physiol.* **5,** 262–296.

Joel, W., Masters, Y. F., and Shetlar, M. R. (1956). Comparison of histochemical and biochemical methods for the polysaccharides with age. *J. Histochem. Cytochem.* **4,** 476–478.

Kantor, T. G., and Schubert, M. (1957). A method for the desulfation of chondroitin sulfate. *J. Amer. Chem. Soc.* **79,** 152–154.

Karnovsky, M. J. (1965). A formaldehyde–glutaraldehyde fixative of high osmolality for use in electron microscopy. *J. Cell Biol.* **27,** 137A–138A.

Kelly, J. W., Bloom, G. D., and Scott, J. E. (1963). Quaternary ammonium compounds in connective tissue histochemistry: I. Selective unblocking. *J. Histochem. Cytochem.* **11,** 791–798.

Lane, N., Caro, L., Otero-Vilardebó, L. R., and Godman, G. C. (1964). On the site of sulfation in colonic goblet cells. *J. Cell Biol.* **21,** 339–351.

Leblond, C. P., Glegg, R. E., and Eidinger, D. (1957). Presence of carbohydrates with free 1,2-glycol groups in sites stained by the periodic acid-Schiff technique. *J. Histochem. Cytochem.* **5,** 445–458.

Lehtonen, A., Kärkkäinen, J., and Haahti, E. (1966). Carbohydrate components in the epithelial mucin of hagfish, *Myxine glutinosa. Acta Chem. Scand.* **20,** 1456–1462.

Leppi, T. J. (1968). Morphochemical analysis of mucous cells in the skin and slime glands of hagfishes. *Histochemie* **15,** 68–78.

Leppi, T. J., and Kinnison, P. A. (1967). Histochemical evaluation of acidic carbohydrates in pig colonic mucosa. *J. Histochem. Cytochem.* **15,** 774.

Leppi, T. J., and Pratt, S. A. (1969). Variations in the appearance and iron staining of the microvillar surface coat. *J. Cell Biol.* **43**, 79A–80A.

Leppi, T. J., and Spicer, S. S. (1966). The histochemistry of mucins in certain primate salivary glands. *Amer. J. Anat.* **118**, 833–860.

Leppi, T. J., and Spicer, S. S. (1967). The histochemistry of carbohydrate-rich substances in certain ungulate salivary glands. *Anat. Rec.* **159**, 179–191.

Leppi, T. J., Spicer, S. S., Henson, J. G., and Fioravanti, J. (1967). Correlated histochemical staining and S^{35}-labeling of salivary gland mucosubstances. *J. Histochem. Cytochem.* **15**, 745–751.

Leppi, T. J., Kinnison, P. A., and Gaffney, S. P. (1968). Intercellular substances of the uterine cervix: electron microscopic histochemical studies of hormone-dependent changes in the mouse. *Proc. 26th Annu. Meeting Electron Microscopy Soc. Amer.*, pp. 60–61. Claitor, Baton Rouge, Louisiana.

Lev, R., and Gerard, A. (1967). The histochemical demonstration of protein in epithelial mucins. *J. Roy. Microsc. Soc.* **87**, 361–373.

Lillie, R. D. (1965). "Histopathologic Technic and Practical Histochemistry." pp. 194–204, 269–272, 276. McGraw-Hill, New York.

Luft, J. H. (1964). Electron microscopy of cell extraneous coats as revealed by ruthenium red staining. *J. Cell Biol.* **23**, 54A–55A.

Luft, J. H. (1965). The fine structure of hyaline cartilage matrix following ruthenium red fixative and staining. *J. Cell Biol.* **27**, 61A.

Luft, J. H. (1966). Fine structure of capillary and endocapillary layer as revealed by ruthenium red. *Fed. Proc. Fed. Amer. Soc. Exp. Biol.* **25**, 1773–1783.

Luft, J. H. (1968). Selective staining of acid mucopolysaccharides by ruthenium red. *Proc. 26th Annu. Meeting Electron Microscopy Soc. Amer.*, pp. 38–39. Claitor, Baton Rouge, Louisiana.

McManus, J. F. A., and Cason, J. E. (1950). Carbohydrate histochemistry studied by acetylation techniques. I. Periodic acid methods. *J. Exp. Med.* **91**, 651–654.

Mathews, M. B., and Cifonelli, J. A. (1965). Comparative biochemistry of keratosulfates. *J. Biol. Chem.* **240**, 4140–4145.

Matukas, V. J., Panner, B. J., and Orbison, J. L. (1967). Studies on ultrastructural identification and distribution of protein-polysaccharide in cartilage matrix. *J. Cell Biol.* **32**, 365–378.

Meyer, K., (1966). Problems of histochemical identification of carbohydrate-rich tissue components. *J. Histochem. Cytochem.* **14**, 605–606.

Meyer, K., Hoffman, P., and Linker, A. (1958). Mucopolysaccharides of costal cartilage. *Science* **128**, 896.

Mowry, R. (1958). Improved procedure for the staining of acidic polysaccharides by Müller's colloidal (hydrous) ferric oxide and its combination with the Feulgen and the periodic acid-Schiff reactions. *Lab. Invest.* **7**, 566–576.

Mowry, R. (1963). The special value of methods that color both acidic and vicinal hydroxyl groups in the histochemical study of mucins. *Ann. N. Y. Acad. Sci.* **106**, 402–423.

Myers, D. B., Highton, T. C., and Rayns, D. G. (1969). Acid mucopolysaccharides closely associated with collagen fibrils in normal human synovium. *J. Ultrastruct. Res.* **28**, 203–213.

Neuberger, A., and Marshall, R. D. (1966). Methods for the qualitative and quantitative analysis of the component sugars. *In* "Glycoproteins, Their Composition, Structure and Function" (A. Gottschalk, ed.), pp. 190–234, Elsevier, New York.

Neutra, M., and Leblond, C. P. (1966a). Synthesis of the carbohydrate of mucus in the Golgi complex as shown by electron microscope radioautography of goblet cells from rats injected with glucose-H³. *J. Cell Biol.* **30,** 119–136.

Neutra, M., and Leblond, C. P. (1966b). Radioautographic comparison of the uptake of galactose-H³ and glucose-H³ in the Golgi region of various cells secreting glycoproteins or mucopolysaccharides. *J. Cell Biol.* **30,** 137–150.

Neutra, M., and Leblond, C. P. (1969). The Golgi apparatus. *Sci. Amer.* **220,** (Feb.) 100–107.

Pease, D. C. (1966a). The preservation of unfixed cytological detail by dehydration with "inert" agents. *J. Ultrastruct. Res.* **14,** 356–378.

Pease, D. (1966b). Polysaccharides associated with the exterior surface of epithelial cells: kidney, intestine, brain. *J. Ultrastruct. Res.* **15,** 555–588.

Peterson, M. R., and Leblond, C. P. (1964a). Uptake by the Golgi region of glucose labeled with tritium in the 1 or 6 position, as an indicator of synthesis of complex carbohydrates. *Exp. Cell Res.* **34,** 420–423.

Peterson, M. R., and Leblond, C. P. (1964b). Synthesis of complex carbohydrates in the Golgi region, as shown by radioautography after injection of labeled glucose. *J. Cell Biol.* **21,** 143–148.

Pigman, W., and Gottschalk, A. (1966). Submaxillary gland glycoproteins. *In* "Glycoproteins, Their Composition, Structure and Function" (A. Gottschalk, ed.), pp. 434–445, Elsevier, New York.

Pigman, W., and Hashimoto, Y. (1964). Recent studies of mucins and blood-group substances. *Advan. Oral Biol.* **1,** 111–129.

Pratt, S. A., and Napolitano, L. (1969). Osmium binding to the surface coat of intestinal microvilli in the cat under various conditions. *Anat. Rec.* **165,** 197–209.

Quintarelli, G. (1961). Histochemistry of sialo-mucins in connective tissues. *Histochemie* **2,** 356–358.

Quintarelli, G. (1963). Histochemical identification of salivary mucins. *Ann. N. Y. Acad. Sci.* **106,** 339–363.

Quintarelli, G., and Dellovo, M. C. (1965). The chemical and histochemical properties of Alcian Blue. IV. Further studies on the methods for the identification of acid glycosaminoglycans. *Histochemie* **5,** 196–209.

Quintarelli, G., and Dellovo, M. C. (1966). Age changes in the localization and distribution of glycosaminoglycans in human hyaline cartilage. *Histochemie* **7,** 141–167.

Quintarelli, G., Scott, J. E., and Dellovo, M. C. (1964a). The chemical and histochemical properties of Alcian Blue. II. Dye binding of tissue polyanions. *Histochemie* **4,** 86–98.

Quintarelli, G., Scott, J. E., and Dellovo, M. C. (1964b). The chemical and histochemical properties of Alcian Blue. III. Chemical blocking and unblocking. *Histochemie* **4,** 99–112.

Rambourg, A. (1967). An improved silver methenamine technique for the detection of periodic acid-reactive complex carbohydrates with the electron microscope. *J. Histochem. Cytochem.* **15,** 409–412.

Rambourg, A., and Leblond, C. P. (1967). Electron microscope observations on the carbohydrate-rich cell coat present at the surface of cells in the rat. *J. Cell Biol.* **32,** 27–53.

Rambourg, A., Neutra, M., and Leblond, C. P. (1966). Presence of a 'cell coat' rich in carbohydrate at the surface of cells in the rat. *Anat. Rec.* **154,** 41–72.

Revel, J.-P. (1964). A stain for the ultrastructural localization of acid mucopolysaccharides. *J. Microsc. (Paris)* **3,** 535–544.

Saunders, A. M. (1964). Histochemical identification of acid mucopolysaccharides with acridine orange. *J. Histochem. Cytochem.* **12**, 164–170.

Saunders, A. M., and Rosan, R. C. (1966). Histochemical nomenclature of carbohydrate-rich components. *J. Histochem. Cytochem.* **14**, 869.

Schiller, S. (1963). Connective and supporting tissues: mucopolysaccharides of connective tissues. *Annu. Rev. Physiol.* **28**, 137–158.

Schubert, M., and Hamerman, D. (1968). "A Primer on Connective Tissue Biochemistry." Lea and Febiger, Philadelphia, Pennsylvania.

Scott, J. E. (1960). Aliphatic ammonium salts in the assay of acidic polysaccharides from tissues. *In* "Methods of Biochemical Analysis" (D. Glick, ed.), pp. 145–197. Interscience, New York.

Scott, J. E., and Dorling, J. (1965). Differential staining of acid glycosaminoglycans (mucopolysaccharides) by Alcian Blue in salt solutions. *Histochemie* **5**, 221–233.

Scott, J. E., and Harbinson, R. J. (1968). Periodate oxidation of acid polysaccharides. Inhibition by the electrostatic field of the substrate. *Histochemie* **14**, 215–220.

Scott, J. E., Quintarelli, G., and Dellovo, M. C. (1964). The chemical and histochemical properties of Alcian Blue. I. Mechanism of Alcian Blue staining. *Histochemie* **4**, 73–85.

Spicer, S. S. (1960). A correlative study of the histochemical properties of rodent acid mucopolysaccharides. *J. Histochem. Cytochem.* **8**, 18–34.

Spicer, S. S. (1961). The use of various cationic reagents in histochemical differentiation of mucopolysaccharides. *Amer. J. Clin. Pathol.* **36**, 393–407.

Spicer, S. S. (1962). Basic protein visualized histochemically in mucinous secretions. *Exp. Cell Res.* **28**, 480–488.

Spicer, S. S. (1965). Diamine methods for differentiating mucosubstances histochemically. *J. Histochem. Cytochem.* **13**, 211–234.

Spicer, S. S., and Duvenci, J. (1964). Histochemical characteristics of mucopolysaccharides in salivary and exorbital lacrimal glands. *Anat. Rec.* **149**, 333–357.

Spicer, S. S., and Henson, J. G. (1967). Methods for localizing mucosubstances in epithelial and connective tissues. *In* "Methods and Achievements in Experimental Pathology" (E. Bajusz and G. Jasmin eds.), Vol. 2, 78–112. Karger, New York.

Spicer, S. S., and Jarrels, M. H. (1961). Histochemical reaction of an aromatic diamine with acid groups and periodate engendered aldehydes in mucopolysaccharides. *J. Histochem. Cytochem.* **9**, 368–379.

Spicer, S. S., and Lillie, R. D. (1959). Saponification as a means of selectively reversing the methylation blockade of tissue basophilia. *J. Histochem. Cytochem.* **7**, 123–125.

Spicer, S. S., and Meyer, D. B. (1960). Histochemical differentiation of acid mucopolysaccharides by means of combined aldehyde fuchsin-alcian blue staining. *Amer. J. Clin. Pathol.* **33**, 453–460.

Spicer, S. S., and Warren, L. (1960). The histochemistry of sialic acid containing mucoproteins. *J. Histochem. Cytochem.* **8**, 135–137.

Spicer, S. S., Swarm, R. L., and Burtner, H. J. (1961). Comparison of basophilia with S^{35} label in normal and methylated mucopolysaccharides. *Lab. Invest.* **10**, 256–264.

Spicer, S. S., Leppi, T. J., and Stoward, P. J. (1965). Suggestions for a histochemical terminology of carbohydrate-rich tissue components. *J. Histochem. Cytochem.* **13** 599–603.

Spicer, S. S., Leppi, T. J., and Henson, J. G. (1967). Sulfate-containing mucosubstances of dog gastric mucosa. *Lab. Invest.* **16**, 795–802.

Stidworthy, G., Masters, Y. F., and Shetlar, M. R. (1958). The effect of aging on mucopolysaccharide composition of human costal cartilage as measured by hexosamine and uronic acid content. *J. Gerontol.* **13**, 10–13.

Stoward, P. J. (1966a). Studies in fluorescence histochemistry. I. The demonstration of sulphomucins. *J. Roy. Microsc. Soc.* **87**, 215–235.

Stoward, P. J. (1966b). Studies in fluorescence histochemistry. II. The demonstration of periodate-reactive mucosubstances with pseudo-Schiff reagents. *J. Roy. Microsc. Soc.* **87**, 237–246.

Stoward, P. J. (1966c). Studies in fluorescence histochemistry. III. The demonstration with salicylhydrazide of the aldehydes present in periodate-oxidized mucosubstances. *J. Roy. Microsc. Soc.* **87**, 247–257.

Stoward, P. J. (1967). The histochemical properties of some periodate-reactive mucosubstances of the pregnant Syrian hamster before and after methylation with methanolic thionyl chloride. *J. Roy. Microsc. Soc.* **87**, 77–103.

Stoward, P. J. (1968). The histochemical reactions of methanolic thionyl chloride with the anionic groups and basic protein component of sulphated mucosubstances. *J. Roy. Microsc. Soc.* **88**, 119–131.

Stoward, P. J., and Mester, L. (1964). Formazan reaction as a confirmatory test for aldehyde groups in histochemistry. *Nature (London)* **204**, 488–489.

Stoward, P. J., Baker, S. A., Kent, P. W., and Pearse, A. G. E. (1966). Some British comments on the histochemical nomenclature of mucosubstances. *J. Histochem. Cytochem.* **14**, 681.

Sumner, B. E. H. (1965a). Experiments to determine the composition of aldehyde fuchsin solutions. *J. Royal Microsc. Soc.* **84**, 181–187.

Sumner, B. E. H. (1965b). A histochemical study of aldehyde fuchsin staining. *J. Royal Microsc. Soc.* **84**, 329–338.

Szirmai, J. A. (1963). Quantitative approaches in the histochemistry of mucopolysaccharides. *J. Histochem. Cytochem.* **11**, 24–34.

Wetzel, M. G., Wetzel, B. K., and Spicer, S. S. (1966). Ultrastructural localization of acid mucosubstances in the mouse colon with iron-containing stains. *J. Cell Biol.* **30**, 299–315.

Yardley, J. H., and Brown, G. D. (1965). Fibroblasts in tissue culture. Use of colloidal iron for ultrastructural localization of acid mucopolysaccharides. *Lab. Invest.* **14**, 501–513.

Zobel, C. R., and Beer, M. (1965). The use of heavy metal salts as electron stains. *Int. Rev. Cytol.* **18**, 363–400.

CHAPTER 10

Calcification

George W. Bernard

The story of mammalian calcification has a very complicated, cloudy syntax. To begin with, normal mammalian calcification is seen in five different tissues: bone, calcified cartilage, dentin, enamel, and cementum. Each of these has an immature and a mature form. Four of them—enamel is the exception—are derived from mesenchyme and enamel is derived from ectoderm. Calcification in each tissue is preceded by the formation of an extracellular organic matrix, primarily a secretion by the lining cells. In two tissues, bone and cellular cementum, cells are embedded in the mineralized structure and are connected with peripheral cells by long cellular extensions, the canaliculi. In dentin, no cells, only cellular extensions, the odontoblastic processes, are embedded in the calcified substance. In acellular cementum and enamel, neither cells not their processes are found. In the enamel when it is completely formed, even the cells are shed from the surface, but the cementocytes remain to line the cementum. Calcified cartilage is an interim phase between the hyalin cartilagenous model and the calcification of certain bones (endochondral ossification). It is resorbed after bone has formed in contiguity with it. To complicate the structural variations even more, bone has an immature (woven) and a mature (lamellar) state and dentin has an immature (mantle) and mature (circumpulpal) phase. Bone also has two embryonic means by which it forms, intramembranous and endochondral.

There is yet another order of resolution concerned with the mechanism of calcification that complicates the picture even more.

Since 1953, when Neuman and Neuman espoused the epitaxial nucleation theory of calcification, the prevailing concept of mineralization involved the extracellular matrix as a nucleating site for hydroxyapatite, the calcium phosphate crystal of normal mammalian calcification. Because collagen makes up 65% of the dry weight of the organic matrix, it is not surprising

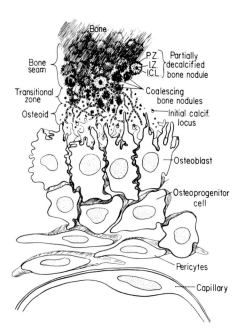

Fig. 1. Initial woven bone development is illustrated sequentially from the initial calcification locus (I.C.L.) to the bone nodule to the bone seam. Similar initial calcification is observed in calcifying cartilage and mantle dentin of the tooth. P.Z., peripheral zone of the bone nodule; I.Z., intermediate zone.

that a good deal of scientific effort was expended upon linking collagen with the nucleation site of calcium phosphate crystal formation (Fitton-Jackson, 1957; Glimcher, *et al.*, 1957; Robinson and Watson, 1955). Even so, other investigators held that the mucopolysaccharide component of the matrix was the site for nucleation (Sobel *et al.*, 1960), while still others implicated an extracellular lipid component (Irving, 1958). Clearly, the attention of researchers was focused on the matrix and not on the cell, despite the fact that in many phyla other than mammals, mineralization begins as an intracellular event (Pautard, 1966). With all of these histological varieties and mechanismic differences, are there some integrating factors that can help clarify the complexities and confusions? There are indeed, and these are termed "unifying factors" in mammalian calcification.

In 1966, using electron microscopic techniques, Bernard and Pease (1966) first reported that the initiation of calcification in fetal mouse membrane bone is a cellular phenomenon. The first crystals were demonstrated in cellular extensions or "buds" from osteoblasts (see Fig. 1). From these initial calcification loci (ICL), crystals, growing spheroidally, develop within a field of collagen into discrete units of woven bone termed the "bone nodules" (Bernard and Pease, 1967; Bernard, 1969; Bernard and Pease, 1969). This unit of immature bone, when decalcified, exhibits a defined organic structure; an inner core, which is the "initial calcification locus," an outer peripheral zone of collagen and an intermediate zone of apparently "decomplexed" collagen. At the peripheral layer of the bone nodule, the process of depolymerization of collagen appears to begin coincident with the appearance of discrete bone crystals. In the wake of this decomplexing process, collagen becomes fibrous and vesicular (Bernard and Pease, 1969).

During endochondral osteogenesis, immature, woven bone is indistinguishable from woven bone found in intramembranous osteogenesis. Calcification begins in a cellular initial calcification locus and develops the same nodular form, with the same organic substructure as in membrane bone (Bernard, 1969).

Recently, we have substantiated Anderson's (1969) finding that when cartilage is first calcified, it occurs in extracellular "vesicles" or cellular buds originating as part of chondrocytes (Bernard, 1970b). Crystal growth from this ICL determines the spheroidal shape of the calcified cartilaginous nodule much as is seen in the woven bone nodule. An interesting similarity is that the calcified cartilagenous nodule, which developes in poorly polymerized collagen, and the woven bone nodule, which grows in a matrix of well-polymerized collagenous fibrils, eventuate in very similar intermediate zones. This would imply that there is a simple organic fibrillar system in both to help orient the early development of immature calcification. Cartilage has a simple collagenous fibrillar system and in woven bone the route to simple fibrils appears to involve some change back to a less polymerized state of collagen within the bone nodule. In the tooth, the first calcification is that of dentin; in dentin the first calcification observed is in odontoblastic extensions, which are cellular initial loci of calcification, just as was seen in woven bone and calcified cartilage (Bernard, 1970a).

Unifying factor No. 1 in calcification is that the first calcifications seen embryologically, i.e., woven bone, calcified cartilage, and mantle dentin, are related to cellular processes (Fig. 2). These initial calcifying structures develop from precursor elements within the cells. Urist (1964) believes this to be a calcium proteinate while Posner et al. (1965), Termine and Posner (1966), and Eanes et al. (1965) present evidence for an amorphous calcium phosphate precursor to hydroxyapatite. Whatever the immediate precursor, it is evident that calcium and phosphate are both concentrated within the active calcifying cells (Kashiwa, 1966). There is indeed a growing body of information that links the mitochondrion with calcium concentra-

LINEAGE OF MAMMALIAN CALCIFICATION

Initial	Subsequential
Woven bone	Lamellar bone
Calcified cartilage	⟨ Lamellar bone ⟩ ∤ Woven bone??
Mantle dentin	⟨ Circumpulpal dentin ⟨ Enamel ∤ Cementum

Fig. 2. Division of the process of calcification by maturation. Initial is the first or non-precedent calcification in a tissue, which develops a nodular pattern. Subsequential calcification is more mature tissue growth from a calcified tissue previously formed. The two question marks after woven bone in the subsequential lineage indicates that woven bone is sometimes seen juxtaposed to calcified cartilage but may or may not be subsequentially calcified from the calcified cartilage.

tion within all cells and particularly within calcifying cells (Deluca and Sallis, 1965; Mathews *et al.*, 1968). Calcium and phosphate or calcium phosphate in some form then is packaged by the cell and exported into the organic matrix either as a membrane-bound cellular vesicle (Anderson, 1969) or as a "bud" from a cellular extension (Bernard and Pease, 1969; Bernard, 1969). In the extracellular matrix, calcium and phosphate ions are supersaturated in regard to hydroxyapatite and when the membranes of the buds break down, the ions bind onto the hydroxyapatite nucleation sites within the ICL. Calcium and phosphate ions deposit into the particular lattice structures—originated in the nucleation center—of hydroxyapatite and frank crystals appear. These crystals grow in a 360° pattern from the ICL, forming spheroids or nodules. The nodules grow together to form seams of calcified cartilage, mantle dentin, or woven bone and are the hallmark of initial embryonic calcification. The first step in the calcification process is cellularly derived and is involved with energy expenditure since the calcium must be actively transported into the cells, concentrated and packaged with phosphate, and then extruded into the matrix. After the nucleation sites in the initial calcification loci are exposed to calcium and phosphate ions in the extracellular space, crystals of hydroxyapatite can grow appositionally without energy loss. This is an excellent example of biological economy, energy being used to initiate a process which can continue developing by the nonenergy-expending physicochemical phenomenon of crystal growth.

After the first stages of crystal growth have transformed the initial calcification loci into the first or immature calcified tissues (woven bone, calcified cartilage, and mantle dentin), the more mature tissues quickly begin to develop. Unifying factor No. 2 is that mature tissues grow subsequential to the previously formed immature calcified tissues (Fig. 2). Organic matrix is secreted by the cells in a fashion more organized than before. Hydroxyapatite crystals probably grow by secondary crystallization; that is, by using already made crystals as nucleating sites for the new crystals forming in the new matrix. Energy is expended by the cells in producing organic matrix, but hydroxyapatite crystals still forms appositionally from calcium primarily by the fibrillar protein, collagen. Mature bone is lamellar bone forming concentric interlocking rings of calcified structure with entrapped osteocytes connected to each other and to osteoblasts by canaliculi. Circumpulpal dentin is the successor to mantle dentin and it too is primarily calcified collagen surrounding cellular processes of the odontoblasts which almost reach the dentinoenamel junction. Acellular cementum begins its growth at the dentinal border of the tooth root, with crystals of hydroxyapatite growing from the dentin into the collagenous matrix of the pre-cementum. Enamel forms when specialized enamel protein is laid down in juxtaposition to mantle dentin. This is either primarily fibrillar or macro-molecularly globular but secondarily fibrillar, the globules of protein lining up in a fibrillar pattern. Almost immediately upon secretion, enamel protein is calcified beginning with crystallization at the mantle dentinal–enamel protein interface much the same way that lamellar bone and cir-cumpulpal dentin calcify (Bernard, 1970a). In bone and dentin the crystals have virtually the same size and shape ranging between 25 and 75 Å in width and 200–500 Å in length (although some crystals are reported to be 3000–4000 Å long). The size and shape are primarily related to the orientation imposed upon the crystals by the collagenous framework. Enamel protein, being less well polymerized than collagen, provides a different orientation for hydroxyapatite growth and the crystals develop into long ribbons 400–1200 Å wide and 2000–1000 Å long (Frank and Sognnaes, 1960). It must be remembered, however, that the unit crystal of calcium hydroxyapatite is the same in all the tissues, the size and shape only vary as a consequence of the microenvironment created by the particular orienting protein.

The mature calcified tissue is a finite aggergation of the unique calcification units of that particular tissue and growth essentially ends when the tissue has reached its predetermined size and shape.

When the adult state has been reached, enamel loses its ability to metabolize and reorganize since its cells, the ameloblasts, are sloughed when the tooth erupts. Calcified cartilage is an interim tissue serving as a rigid embryomic framework until bone is formed, when the cartilage is resorbed. Bone, cellular cementum, and to a limited extent dentin, even in the adult state, is in a constant state of reorganization. Resorption and deposition of new crystals take place throughout life. Bone is the major storehouse for calcium in the body which is released when the blood levels fall below the norm of 10 mg/100 ml. Control of this release is by the parathyroid gland which secretes parathyroid hormone (PTH) when serum calcium levels fall. The exact mode of action of PTH is not known although histologically, osteoclasts, the resorptive cells of calcified tissues, increase in number and activity when PTH is administered experimentally. When the serum calcium level is higher than normal, calcium is redeposited in the bones. This is also affected by vitamin D which aids in the absorption of calcium across the surface absorptive cells of the small intestine and mimics the role of PTH in resorbing bone.

Bone will reorganize and will reshape its internal architecture depending upon the stresses to which it is exposed. The gross structural effects are products of resorption and redeposition in localized areas.

The role of collagen as nucleating sites for hydroxyapatite has been stressed. There is good reason to believe, however, that much of the ultrastructural evidence for this has been based upon interpretations of artifacticious material (Bernard, 1970b). Yet collagen does play a role as the microenvironment for hydroxyapatite crystalline growth. Pease and Boutelle (1969) have reported that complex polysaccharides play an important role in the polymerization of collagenous filaments. The shape and disposition of these polysaccharides fit perfectly the dimensional needs of hydroxyapatite crystals and probably represent the locale within the fibril into which the crystals grow. Unifying factor No. 3 is that both fibrous protein and mucopolysaccharides play a role as sites for hydroxyapatite crystal growth.

REFERENCES

Anderson, H. C. (1969). Vesicles associated with calcification in the matrix of epiphyseal cartilage. *J. Cell Biol.* **41,** 59–72.

Bernard, G. W. (1969). The ultrastructural interface of bone crystals and organic matrix in woven and lamellar endochondral bone. *J. Dent. Res. Suppl.* **48** [No. 5], 781–788.

Bernard, G. W. (1970a). Ultrastructural observations of initial calcification in dentin and enamel. *J. Ultrastruct. Res.* (in press).

Bernard, G. W. (1970b). *In* "Biology of Hard Tissue," (A. Budy, ed.), 5th Conf. Hard Tissues. N. Y. Acad. Sci. Interdisciplinary Commun. Program New York (in press).

Bernard, G. W., and Pease, D. C. (1966). The relationship of polysaccharides to the calcification of membrane bone. *J. Appl. Phys.* **37,** 3932.

Bernard, G. W., and Pease, D. C. (1967). The bone nodule, the developmental unit of bone. *J. Dent. Res. Suppl.*, March 1967.

Bernard, G. W., and Pease, D. C. (1969). An electron microscope study of initial intramembranous osteogenesis. *Amer. J. Anat.* **125,** 271–290.

Deluca, H. F., and Sallis, J. D. (1965). Parathyroid hormone: Its subcellular actions and its relationship to vitamin D. *In* "The Parathyroid Glands" (P. T. Gaillard, R. V. Talmage, and A. M. Budy, eds.), pp. 181–196, Univ. Chicago Press, Chicago, Illinois.

Eanes, E. D., Gillessen, I., and Posner, A. S. (1965). Intermediate states in the precipitation of hydroxyapatite. *Nature (London)* **208,** 365.

Fitton-Jackson, S. (1957). The time structure of developing bone in the embryonic foul. *Proc. Roy. Soc. London Ser. B* **146,** 270–280.

Frank, R. M., and Sognnaes, R. F. (1960). Electron microscopy of matrix formation and calcification in rat enamel. *Arch. Oral Biol.* **1,** 339–348.

Glimcher, M. J., Hodge, A. J., and Schmitt, F. O. (1957). Macromolecular aggregation states in relation to mineralization: The collagen hydroxyapatite system as studied *in vitro. Proc. Nat. Acad. Sci. U.S.* **43,** 860–867.

Irving, J. T. (1958). Sudanophil inclusions in ameloblasts, odontoblasts and cells of the oral epithelium. *Nature (London)* **181,** 569.

Kashiwa, H. K. (1966). Calcium in cells of fresh bone stained with glyoxal Bis (2-hydroxyanil). *Stain Technol.* **41,** 49.

Mathews, J. L., Martin, J. H., and Collins, E. J. (1968). Metabolism of radioactive calcium by cartilage. *Clin. Orthop.* **58,** 213–224.

Neuman, W. F., and Neuman, M. (1953). The nature of the mineral phase of bone. *Chem. Rev.* **53,** 1–45.

Pautard, F. G. E. (1966). A biomolecular survey of calcification. *In* "Calcified Tissues, 1965," (H. Fleisch, J. J. J. Blackwood, and M. Owed, eds.), pp. 108–122. Springer-Verlag, New York.

Pease, D. C., and Boutelle, M. (1969). Ultrastructural features of native collagen fibrils. *Proc. 27th Annu. Meeting Electron Microscopy Soc. Amer.*, pp. 214–215.

Posner, A. S., Harper, R. A., Muller, S. A., and Menczel, J. (1965). Age change in the crystal chemistry of bone apatite. *Ann. N. Y. Acad. Sci.* **131,** 737–742.

Sobel, A. T., Burger, M., and Nebel, S. (1960). Mechanisms of nucleii formation in mineralizing tissue. *Clin. Orthop.* **17,** 103–123.

Robinson, R. A., and Watson, M. L. (1955). Crystal-collagen relationships in bone as observed in the E.M. III. *Ann. N. Y. Acad. Sci.* **60,** 596.

Termine, J. D., and Posner, A. S. (1966). Infrared analysis of rat bone: age dependency of amorphous and crystalline mineral fractions. *Science* **153,** 1523–1525.

Urist, M. R. (1964). Recent advances in the physiology of calcification. *J. Bone Joint Surg.* **46,** 889–900.

Author Index

A

Abdel-Latif, A. A., 317, *321*
Abercrombie, M., 50, *79*, 226, *267*
Abood, L. G., 317, *321*
Abrams, R., 140, *146*
Adams, K., 61, *84*
Adamson, S. D., 172, *205*
Agarwal, P. S., 185, 186, *213*
Agate, F. J., 318, *328*
Agranoff, B. W., 311, 315, *321*, *322*
Alexander, P., 37, *42*
Alfert, M., 26, 34, *38*, *39*, *43*
Alho, A., 6, *23*
Alin-Slater, R. B., 297, *328*
Allen, E. R., 28, *39*
Allen, J. R., 318, *323*
Allerton, S. E., 230, *267*
Allfrey, V. G., 30, *41*, 157, 160, 162, 164, 165, 166, 167, *205*, *206*, *209*, *212*, *213*, *214*, *217*
Alpen, E., 60, *81*
Altman, K. I., 130, *145*
Amaldi, F., 118, *145*
Amano, M., 111, 130, *142*, *146*
Ambrose, E. J., 223, 226, 230, 231, 251, *267*, *275*
Amos, H., 251, *267*
Amsterdam, A., 197, *206*
Anderson, B., 260, *274*
Anderson, E. C., 3, *23*
Anderson, H. C., 375, 376, *378*
Anderson, N. G., 177, *206*
Ando, T., 159, *217*
Andrew, W., 88, 89, 95, 101, *104*
Anker, H. S., 295, *322*

Anker, P., 36, *44*
Ansell, C. B., 306, *322*
Anseth, A., 260, *267*
Appleton, T. C., 36, *38*
Arey, L. B., 92, *104*
Arold, R., 32, *38*
Arvidson, G. A. E., 317, *322*
Asao, T., 162, *206*
Atkins, N. G., 32, *38*
Attardi, B., 116, 117, 127, 128, *142*, 171, *206*
Attardi, G., 112, 116, 117, 118, 127, 128, *142*, *145*, 171, *206*
Atwood, K. C., 112, *149*
Aureli, G., 335, *366*
Awai, M., 202, *206*
Axelrod, A. E., 138, *151*
Azen, E. A., 175, *206*

B

Bacharach, A. D. E., 186, 189, 190, *210*
Bacon, R. L., 89, 95, *104*
Baglioni, C., 172, 174, *206*
Bahr, G. F., 34, *38*
Bailey, E., 309, *329*
Bailey, J. M., 297, *322*
Baird, G. R., 232, *271*
Baitsell, G. A., 249, *267*
Baker, S. A., 334, *371*
Balazs, E. A., 25, 259, 260, *267*
Baldini, A., 251, *272*
Balduini, C., 335, *366*
Bale, W. F., 20, *23*
Balint, J. A., 310, *322*

381

Balis, M. E., 183, *211*
Ballou, C. E., 311, *322*
Ballou, J. E., 282, 300, 320, *329*
Baltimore, D., 182, *206*
Bamforth, J., 71, *81*
Baranor, M. N., 316, *322*
Barbiroli, B., 139, 140, *142*
Bargmann, W., 292, *322*
Barka, T., 75, *79*
Barland, P., 365, *366*
Barlow, G. H., 228, 229, *272*
Barnard, E. A., 156, 157, *206*
Barnard, P. J., 231, 233, 248, *267*
Barnett, W. E., 127, 128, *142*, *144*
Barnett, S. R., 155, *208*
Barnum, C. P., 204, *206*
Barondes, S. H., 154, *206*
Barrett, J. C., 61, *84*
Barrows, C. H., 96, *106*
Bartley, W., 309, *329*
Barton, A. D., 35, *39*
Baseman, J. B., 174, *209*
Baserga, R., 180, 181, 182, *206*, 2, 3, *21*,
    60, 75, *79*, 140, *142*
Bass, A. D., 33, *40*
Bauer, H., 68, *81*
Baumber, J., 319, *322*
Bavetta, L. A., 224, 230, 232, 233, 243,
    245, 246, 248, 249, 250, 251, 252, 254,
    255, 256, 257, 259, 263, *267*, *274*
Beagrie, G. S., 71, *79*
Beals, T. F., 249, *273*
Beams, H. W., 350, *366*
Beattie, D. S., 170, *206*
Becker, J. E., 204, *215*
Becker, Y., *148*, 232, *271*
Beeken, W. L., 202, *206*
Beer, M., 343, *371*
Beierle, J. W., 224, 226, 230, 238, 250,
    254, *267*, *274*
Bell, B. M., 61, *83*
Bell, E., 136, *149, 150*
Bell, J., 28, *42*
Beller, J., 172, *217*
Bellini, O., 60, *81*
Bender, M. A., 158, 180, *215*, 110, 142, *149*
Bendich, A., 35, *40*
Benditt, E. P., 349, *366*
Benedetti, E. L., 230, *267*
Benfey, B. G., 313, *325*

Benjamins, J. A., 311, *322*
Berg, B. N., 301, *322*
Berg, N., 111, *142*
Bergerard, J., 33, *39*
Berlin, C. M., 203, *216*
Berman, M., 202, *212*
Bern, H. A., 34, *38, 39*
Bernard, G. W., 374, 375, 376, 377, 378,
    378
Bernfield, M. R., 241, 243, *267*
Bernhard, K., 281, 282, *322*
Bernhardt, D., 122, *142*
Bernstein, G., 202, *214*
Berry, J. F., 311, *326*
Bertalanffy, F. D., 14, *21*, 65, 68, *79, 80, 83*
Berwick, L., 344, *367*
Bessada, R., 130, 137, *144*
Betts, A., 60, *80*
Bhavanandan, V. P., 356, *366*
Bicknell, D. S., 68, *82*
Bignardi, C., 335, *366*
Billing, R. J., 139, 140, *142*
Billingham, R. E., 224, 240, *269*
Birge, W. J., 34, *44*
Birnboim, H. C., 116, 117, *151*
Birnstiel, M. L., 29, 30, *43*, 112, *143*, 162,
    206
Birren, J. E., 92, *104*
Bizzozero, G., 45, 49, *80*
Bjerknes, R., 71, *82*
Blair, S. M., 34, *39*
Blakley, R. L., 253, *267*
Blenkinsopp, W. K., 65, 68, 71, *80*
Bloch, D. P., 159, *206*
Bloch, K. E., 295, 296, 301, *322, 323, 329*
Block, P., 75, *80*
Bloom, G. D., 355, *367*
Bloom, S., 140, *143*
Blumenthal, H. T., 5, *21*, 97, 99, 100, *104*
Bly, C. G., 20, *23*
Boberg, J., 283, 320, *322*
Boiron, M., 121, *145*
Boivin, A., 26, *39*
Bok, D., 186, 188, 189, 190, *206, 210, 219*
Bolden, T. E., 94, *104*
Boling, M. E., *44*
Bond, V. P., 68, *82*, 109, 110, 111, 131, *144*
Bonner, J., 160, 161, 162, 166, 167, 168,
    169, *206, 208, 211, 213*
Boone, C. W., 232, *271*

Borck, E., 295, *322*
Borel, J., 202, *213*
Borges, W. G., 202, *209*
Borisy, G. G., 13, *21*
Borner, G., 61, *85*
Borokas, S., 228, 229, *272*
Borsook, J. L., 131, *143*
Borst, P., 125, *143*
Borun, T. W., 162, *207*, *215*
Bosmann, H. B., 180, *207*
Bourne, G. H., 101, *104*
Boutelle, M., 378, *379*
Bouvier, C. A., *207*
Bowie, M. A., 96, *105*
Box, H., 33, *42*
Boyce, R. P., 36, *39*
Boyen-Rikkers, I., 185, *209*
Brackett, F. S., 10, *23*
Bradbury, S., 342, *366*
Bradley, R. M., 311, 315, *321*, *322*
Brady, R. O., 303, 311, 315, *321*, *322*
Brassil, D., 260, *271*
Brettschneider, I., 355, *366*
Breuch, S. R., 92, *104*
Breuer, M. E., 27, *39*
Brewer, M., 318, *323*
Bringas, P., 224, 232, 233, 243, 250, 251, 254, 255, 256, 257, 263, *274*
Brizzee, K. R., 93, *104*
Brock, F. E., 200, *213*
Brockerhoff, H., 311, *322*
Brody, H., 89, 93, *104*
Bronner, F., *21*, *22*
Bro-Rasmussen, F., 131, *143*
Brown, D. D., 30, *39*, 112, 113, 121, 122, *143*
Brown, E. B., 202, *206*
Brown, D. H., 127, 128, *142*
Brown, G. B., 35, *40*, 358, *371*
Brown, J. M., 15, *21*
Brown, J. R., 305, *327*
Brown, R. E., 127, 129, *144*
Brownson, R. H., 88, 89, 93, *104*
Brück, K., 318, *322*
Brues, A. M., 35, *39*
Brunk, C. F., 36, *41*
Brunner, G., 309, *322*
Brutlag, D., 168, 169, *213*
Bucher, N. L. R., 77, *80*, 253, *267*
Buchner, T., 71, *84*

Buck, C. A., 128, *143*, *147*
Buddecke, E., 333, *366*
Bullet, F., 281, *322*
Bullough, W. S., 3, 5, 6, *21*, *22*, 74, 78, *80*
Burch, E. A., 71, *84*
Burger, M., 374, *379*
Burr, G. D., 280, *323*
Burr, M. M., 280, *323*
Burtner, H. J., 350, 364, *370*
Burton, R. M., 304, 320, *323*
Busch, H., 122, 123, *147*, *150*, 159, 161, 168, *207*, *211*, *217*
Buschke, W., 4, 10, *22*
Bustin, M., 161, *207*
Butler, J. A. V., 156, 161, *207*
Byers, T. J., 158, *207*
Bygrave, F. L., 308, 309, 317, *323*
Byrne, W. L., 203, *208*
Byvoet, P., 163, 165, *207*

C

Cahill, G. F., 318, 319, *328*
Cahn, R. D., 38, *39*
Carinie, A. B., 60, *80*, 180, *207*
Caldwell, I., 37, *42*
Callan, H. G., 30, *39*
Calvert, F., 108, *147*
Cameron, C. B., 199, *207*
Cameron, I. L., 5, *22*, 32, 39, 57, 60, 63, 64, 71, 72, 73, *80*, *84*, 132, 133, 134, *143*, 178, *210*, 319, *323*
Cameron, J., 233, 243, 253, 254, *274*
Campbell, R. M., 33, *39*
Canellakis, E. S., 156, *212*
Caro, L. G., 19, *22*, 292, *323*, 350, 351, *367*
Carrier, W. L., 36, *44*
Carter, H. E., 303, *323*
Carter, S. B., 227, *267*
Cason, J. E., 348, *368*
Caspersson, T. O., 108, *143*
Cassuto, Y., 318, *323*
Castellani, A. A., 335, *366*
Cave, M. D., 28, *39*, *42*
Cejkova, J., 355, *366*
Chaffee, R. R. J., 318, *323*

Chanana, A. D., 61, *85*
Charles, P., 36, *44*
Chatteryi, S., 185, 186, *213*
Chesterton, C. J., 297, *323*
Chevallier, F., 301, 302, *323*, *324*
Chiang, K. S., 126, *143*
Chigasaki, H., 60, *80*
Church, R. B., 140, *143*
Chvapil, M., 261, *268*
Cifonelli, J. A., 260, *272*, 356, *368*
Clamon, H. N., 179, *217*
Clark, A. E., 344, 358, *366*
Clark, F. I., 61, *85*
Clark, R., 185, *207*
Clarke, D. R., 61, *85*
Clark-Walker, B. F. C., 129, *144*
Clayton, R. B., 295, *323*
Cleaver, J. E., 14, *22*, 26, 37, 38, *39*, 54, 57, 60, *80*, 131, *144*
Clermont, Y., 68, *80*, *82*,, 180, *212*
Cohen, A. I., 186, *207*
Cohen, C., 264, 265, *268*
Cohen, J. H., 224, 242, 246, 247, 248, *269*, *276*
Cohen, S., 202, *207*, 223, *268*
Cohn, C., 204, 205, *207*
Cohn, N. S., 32, *39*
Cohn, W. E., 35, *39*
Colbeau, A., 288, 309, 317, *327*
Cole, J. W., 68, *80*, *81*
Cole, R. D., 159, 160, 161, 162, 163, 164, 166, 167, 168, *207*, *212*, *215*, *217*
Cole, R. S., 37, *41*
Coleman, R., 297, *323*
Collier, A., 170, *218*
Collier, R. J., 174, *207*
Collins, A., 203, *213*
Collins, E. J., 376, *379*
Comar, C. L., 9, 21, *22*
Comb, D. G., 164, *207*
Combes, B., 199, *207*
Comings, D. E., 162, 167, *207*
Comorosan, S., 127, 128, *144*
Conklin, J. L., 355, 357, *366*
Cook, G. M. W., 230, *268*
Cooper, E. H., 71, 75, *83*
Cooper, H. L., *149*
Copper, W. G., 109, 140, *150*
Corbin, K. B., 90, *104*
Cordova, C. C., 251, *272*

Corlette, S. L., 27, *44*
Cornatzer, W. E., 307, *327*
Cornforth, J., 295, *327*
Cornwell, D. G., 202, *209*
Couch, J. L., 36, *41*
Coutts, R. T., 190, 191, *207*
Cowdry, E. V., 101, *104*
Cowen, D. M., 71, 75, *83*
Cox, D. G., 14, *22*
Cox, M. C. L., 162, *217*
Craddock, C. G., *22*
Cravito, B., 171, *206*
Creamer, B., 71, *81*
Crick, F. H. C., 263, *273*
Crocker, T. T., 61, *83*, 109, *145*
Cronkite, E. P., 60, 61, 68, *81*, *82*, *85*, 111, 130, 131, *144*
Crouse, H. V., 28, *39*, *40*
Cruickshank, C. N. D., 75, *82*
Cuenid, M., 163, *214*
Cunningham, I., 233, 248, *271*
Curran, R. G., 334, 339, 344, 358, 364, *366*
Curtis, A. S. G., 226, 227, *268*
Cutright, D. E., 68, *81*

D

Dahmus, M. E., 160, 161, 167, *206*
Dallner, G., 171, 176, 177, *207*, *208*, 297, 306, 307, 309, 317, *323*
Dalton, A. J., 233, 237, *268*
Dan, K., 245, *268*, *272*
Darnell, J. E., 108, 112, 114, 115, 116, 117, 118, 120, 121, 122, 127, 128, *142*, *144*, *145*, *146*, *148*, *149*, *150*, *151*, 171, 172, 173, 174, *208*, *218*
Dashman, T., 203, *208*
Davenport, H. C., 196, *208*
David, I. B., 30, *39*
Davidova, S. Ya., 250, *268*
Davidson, E. A., 260, *268*, *272*
Davidson, E. H., 30, *40*, 130, *144*
Davidson, J. N., 26, 32, *40*, 108, 109, *150*
Davies, W. E., 303, 305, 320, *325*, *326*
Davis, B. D., 172, *217*, 228, 230, *268*
Davison, A., 301, *323*, *324*
Dawid, I. B., 125, *144*
Dawkins, M. J. R., 318, 321, *324*
Dawson, R. M. C., 311, 315, *324*

Dean, C. J., 37, *42*
DeBernard, B., 170, *208*
Decker, A. B., 281, *327*
DeDuve, C., 170, *214*
Defendi, V., 60, *81*, 238, *268*, 301, *326*
DeHaan, R. L., 225, *268*
DeLange, R. J., 161, *208*
de la Torre, L., 34, *44*
De llovo, M. C., 335, 348, 357, 364, *369*, *370*
De Luca, H. F., 311, *324*, 376, *379*
Dempster, G., 319, *328*
Den Tonkelaar, E. M., 32, *40*
de Reuck, A. V. S., 160, *208*
Desnuelle, P., 196, *208*
De Sombre, E. R., 138, *146*
Devi, S. K., 134, *149*
Devik, F., 71, *82*
Deynes, A., 319, *322*
Diermeir, H. F., 33, *40*
Dietschy, J. M., 295, 296, *324*
Dils, R. R., 317, *325*
Dische, Z., 245, *268*
di Stefano, H., 33, *40*
Dixon, G. H., 156, *211*
Dobbing, J., 301, *323*
Dodson, J. W., 246, *268*
Dohan, F. C., 61, *84*
Donaldson, J. T., 60, *81*
Dorfman, A., 194, *208*, 262, *275*, 365, *367*
Dorling, J., 336, 339, *370*
Dounce, A. L., 155, *208*
Downes, H. R., 294, *324*
Drabikowski, W., *328*
Dray, S., 251, *275*
Dreyfus, J. C., 20, *23*
Droz, B., 188, 189, 198, *208*, *218*, *219*
Druyan, R., 170, *208*
Drysdale, J. W., 202, *210*
Dubin, D. T., 127, 129, *144*
Dubryszycka, W., 202, *213*
Dulbecco, R., 224, *268*
Duncan, D., 91, *104*
Dunn, E. H., 90, *104*
Durell, J., 316, *324*
Durwald, H., 109, *148*
Duvenci, J., 340, 347, 350, *370*
Dziewiatkowski, D. D., 364, *366*

E

Eagle, H., 232, *268*, *271*
Eanes, E. D., 375, *379*
Eartly, H., 6, *22*
Ebert, J. D., 223, *268*
Edds, M. V., 249, *268*
Edelman, G. M., 156, *213*
Edwards, J. L., 60, *81*
Edwards, L. J., 156, 161, 162, *211*
Eggman, L. D., 313, *324*
Eichberg, J., 302, *324*
Eidinger, D., 356, *367*
Einem, G. E., 163, *210*
El-Aser, A. B. A., 157, *215*
Elden, H. R., 262, *269*
Elgjo, K., 76, *82*
Elkind, M. M., 141, *144*
Ellem, K. A. O., 116, *144*
Ellis, F., 11, *22*
Ellis, R. S, 92, *104*
Elson, D., 129, *144*
Ely, J. O., 33, *40*
Emmelot, P., 230, *267*
Enesco, M., 8, *22*, 47, 65, *81*
Eng, L., 301, 320, *328*
Enger, M. D., 141, *144*
Epifanova, O. I., 3, *22*, 60, 75, *81*
Epler, J. L., 127, 128, *142*, *144*
Epstein, J. H., 37, 38, *40*
Epstein, W. L., 37, 38, *40*
Erdos, T., 130, 137, *144*
Errera, M., 109, *148*
Evans, J., 224, 245, *270*, *276*
Evans, R. G., 37, *40*
Everett, N. B., 68, *81*
Eyer, J., 128, *150*

F

Fabrikant, J. I., 60, 71, *81*
Fallon, H. J., 203, *208*
Fambrough, D. M., 160, 161, 162, 167, *206*, *208*
Farquhar, M. G., 292, *324*
Faulkner, R., 164, *205*
Fausto, N., 140, *144*
Favarger, P., 199, *208*
Fawcett, D. W., 233, 237, 245, *269*, 297, *325*

Feigelson, P., 203, *208*
Feindegen, L. E., 177, *208*
Feinendegen, L. E., 14, 17, 21, *22*, 57, *81*, 109, 110, 111, 131, *144*
Felix, K., 156, 159, *208*
Ferris, W., 245, 264, *275*
Fessler, J. H., 261, *269*
Fieq, A., 27, *40*
Finch, C. A., 131, *144*
Finean, J. B., 297, *323*
Fioravanti, J., 333, 335, 340, 346, 348, 350, *368*
Fischberg, M., 112, *143*
Fitton-Jackson, S., 374, *379*
Flamm, W. G., 162, *206*
Fleischmajer, R., 224, 240, *269*
Fleischman, R. F., 232, *268*
Fleischmann, W., 4, 10, *22*
Fletcher, M. J., 18, *22*, 169, *208*, 309, *324*
Flickinger, C. J., 176, *208*, 336, 358, *366*
Fliedner, T. M., 60, 68, *81*, *82*
Flores, P., 250, 251, 256, 257, *274*
Folch-Pi, J., 301, *324*
Forbes, W. F., 185, *212*
Forget, B. G., 121, *144*
Forsell, K.-J., 6, *23*
Forssberg, A., 35, *43*
Fraenkel-Conrat, H., 348, *366*
Frame, J., 260, *274*
Francois, J., 185, *209*
Frank, R. M., 377, *379*
Frazer, S. C., 26, *40*
Freedman, M. L., 162, *209*
Freeman, T., 202, *207*
Freer, R. M., 155, *208*
Freese, H. L., 60, *81*
Freinkel, N., 313, *324*
French, J. E., 349, *366*
Frenster, J. H., 169, *209*
Fresco, J. R., 35, *40*, 108, 109, *144*
Friday, T. J., 71, *84*
Fridlender, B. R., 171, 173, *209*
Friedenwald, J. S., 4, 10, *22*
Frindel, E., 60, 61, *81*
Fry, R. J. M., 60, 61, 71, *81*, *83*, 97, 102, 103, *104*
Fujimara, F., 162, *208*
Fujiwara, Y., 141, *144*
Fukuski, T., 245, *272*

Fukuyama, K., 37, 38, *40*
Fulhorst, H. W., 134, *144*, *152*, 184, 185, *209*, *219*
Fuller, R. W., 204, 205, *209*
Furst, S. S., 35, *40*

G

Gabrusewycz-Garcia, N., 28, *40*
Gad, A., 340, *367*
Gaetani, M., 60, *81*
Gaffney, S. P., 358, 363, *368*
Gahan, P. B., 35, 36, 38, *43*
Galand, P., 60, *81*
Galanti, N., 228, 229, *269*
Galibert, F., 121, *145*
Gall, J. G., 29, 35, 38, *40*
Galliard, T., 311, *324*
Gallwitz, D., 137, *149*, 164, *216*
Galper, J. D., 127, 128, *145*
Ganong, W. F., 196, *209*
Garber, B., 225, 240, *269*, *275*
Garbus, J., 311, *324*
Garby, L. E., 202, *206*
Garcia, A. M., 32, 33, 38, *40*, *41*
Gardner, E., 88, 90, *104*, *105*
Garland, J. T., 316, *324*
Gasic, G., 228, 229, 238, 252, *268*, *269*, 344, *367*
Gasic, G. J., 344, *367*
Gasic, T., 252, *269*
Gaspar, A., 127, 128, *144*
Gaunt, W. A., 256, *269*
Gautheron, G., 301, *324*
Geiduschek, E. P., 108, *145*
Gelfant, S., 178, *209*
Gelehrter, T. D., 182, *217*
Georgiev, G. P., 156, 157, *209*
Gerard, A., 335, 336, *367*, *368*
Gerber, G., 130, *145*
Gerber, G., 130, *145*
Gershey, E. L., 165, *209*
Gesner, B. M., 252, *269*
Getz, G. S., 127, *145*, 170, *208*
Gibbons, R. A., 193, *209*, 346, 347, *367*
Gill, D. M., 174, *209*
Gillessen, I., 375, *379*
Ginsburg, V., 252, 253, *269*, *274*
Girard, M., 174, *218*

Gitlin, D., 202, *209*
Glass, G. B. J., 335, *367*
Gledhill, B. L., 34, 38, *41*
Gledhill, M. P., 34, 38, *41*
Glegg, R. E., 356, *367*
Glick, M. C., 172, *209*, 224, 232, 234, 250, *275*
Glimcher, M. J., 374, *379*
Go, V. L. W., 197, *209*
Godman, G. C., 350, 351, 365, *367*
Goel, S. C., 244, *269*
Goldfeder, A., 60, *81*
Goldstein, L., 109, *145*, 158, 159, 203, *207*, *209*
Goldsmith, B., 202, *218*
Goldsworthy, P. D., 202, *206*
Goodman, D. S., 302, 320, *324*
Gordon, J., 138, *146*
Gordon, M. P., *44*
Gorenstein, S. L., 68, *85*
Gorin, E., 320, *328*
Gorski, J., 138, *145*, *151*
Goss, R. J., 88, 101, *105*
Gottschalk, A., 190, *210*, 334, *367*, *369*
Gould, B. S., 261, *269*
Gould, R. G., 202, *213*
Grad, B., 6, *22*
Graffi, A., 125, *151*
Graham, A. F., 35, *41*
Granner, D., 182, *217*
Grasso, J. A., 131, *145*
Green, H., 140, *143*
Green, J. G., 177, *206*
Greenbaum, A. L., 14, *23*
Greenberg, M. L., 61, *85*
Greenlee, T. K., 245, *269*
Greulich, R. C., 53, 57, 60, 61, *80*, *81*, *83*, *85*, 97, 102, *105*, 178, *210*
Griem, M. L., 60, *81*
Griffith, M., 317, *326*
Grillo, H. C., 246, *269*
Grinstein, M., 20, *22*
Grisham, J. W., 75, *82*
Grobstein, C., 224, 226, 232, 240, 241, 242, 245, 246, 248, 249, 252, 262, *269*, *270*
Groehler, K., 197, *218*
Gröschel, U., 193, *210*
Gros, F., 134, *149*
Gross, J., 224, 246, *270*
Gross, M. J., 126, 127, *145*

Gross, P. R., 224, *270*
Grossman, D., 157, *210*
Grossman, L. I., 125, *150*
Grossman, M. I., 196, 197, *210*
Grynfeltt, J., 293, *324*
Guha, A., 251, *272*
Gupta, A. K., 185, 186, *213*
Gurdon, J. B., 182, *210*
Gurley, L. R., 161, 163, 166, *210*, *212*
Gurney, E. G., 126, 127, *145*
Gurr, M. I., 309, *324*
Gustafson, T., 226, 245, *270*
Guttes, E. W., 127, *145*
Guttes, S., 127, *145*

H

Haahti, E., 335, *367*
Hackney, E. J., 205, *208*
Haguenau, F., 233, 237, *268*
Hajra, A. K., 305, *324*
Halberg, F., 204, *206*, *210*
Hale, A. J., 32, *41*
Hall, D. A., 261, *270*
Hall, M. O., 186, 188, 189, 190, *210*
Halvorson, H. O., 127, *150*
Hamerman, D., 353, 356, 361, 365, *366*, *370*
Hamilton, T. H., 138, 139, 140, *145*, *150*, *151*, 168, *217*
Hammarsten, E., 35, *41*
Hammond, J. D. S., 202, *210*
Hanawalt, P. C., 36, *41*, *43*, *145*
Hander, P., 190, 191, *218*
Handler, S. D., 204, 205, *212*
Hanna, C., 68, 71, *82*, 134, 135, 136, *145*, 185, *210*
Harbinson, R. J., 332, 356, *370*
Hardeland, R., 204, *210*
Hardin, J. A., 163, *210*
Hardin, J. M., 163, 166, *210*
Harding, C. V., 75, *82*
Harding, J. J., 185, *210*
Hardonk, M. J., 338, *367*
Hargie, M. P., 228, 229, *272*
Hargreaves, T., 199, *210*
Harkness, R. D., 14, *23*
Harper, R. A., 375, *379*
Harris, M., 10, *22*

Harrison, D. D., 183, *218*
Harrison, R. G., 225, *270*
Hartman, J. L., 245, *269*
Haselkorn, R., 108, *145*
Hashimoto, Y., 334, *369*
Haupt, H., 193, *216*
Haus, E., 204, *210*
Hauschka, S. D., 224, 246, *271*
Hauser, G., 302, 315, *324, 326*
Hawthorne, J. N., 297, 306, 309, 311, *322, 324, 327*
Hay, E. D., 241, 244, 245, 249, *270, 273*
Hayashi, K., 315, *324*
Haymaker, W. E., 68, *82*
Healy, G. M., 35, *41*
Heard, D. H., 230, *268, 270*
Heaysman, J. E. M., 226, *267*
Hecht, L. T., 35, *41*
Heinmets, F., 228, 263, *270*
Hell, A., 109, *148*
Hell, E., 14, *22*, 75, *82*
Heller, C. G., 68, *82*
Henriksen, O., 131, *143*
Henry, J. L., 14, *22*, 68, *82*
Henson, J. G., 333, 334, 335, 339, 341, 346, 347, 348, 350, 356, 362, 364, 365, *367, 370*
Heppleston, A. G., 71, *84*
Herbert, E., 172, *205*
Heremans, J. F., 199, 201, 202, 203, *216*
Heringa, G. C., 259, *270*
Herron, W. L., 190, *210*
Herscovies, A., 192, 195, *218*
Herskovitz, I., 27, *41*
Heston, W. E., 203, *215*
Heubner, D., 312, *325*
Hevesy, G., 35, *41*
Hey, A. E., 156, 161, 162, *211*
Hiatt, H. H., 137, 138, *145, 149*
Hicks, S. J., 202, *210*
Highton, T. C., 363, *368*
Higoshi, K., 122, *150*
Hill, H. Z., 138, *151*
Himms-Hagen, J., 321, *325*
Hirano, S., 356, *367*
Hirsch, C. A., 137, *145*
Hirschowitz, B. I., 197, *211*
Hnilica, L. S., 155, 156, 159, 161, 162, *211, 213*

Hoagland, M. B., 130, 137, 138, *151*
Hodge, A. J., 265, *273*, 374, *379*
Hodge, L. D., 142, *145*, 180, *211*
Hodgson, G., 75, *82*
Hodnett, J. L., 122, 123, *147*
Hölzl, J., 311, 312, *329*
Hörhammer, L., 311, 312, *329*
Hoffert, D., 294, *326*
Hoffman, J., 64, *84*, 97, 98, *105*
Hoffman, P., 260, *274*, 353, 356, 357, *367, 368*
Hofmann, A. F., 197, *209*
Hokin, L. E., 312, 313, 314, 315, *324, 325*
Hokin, M. R., 312, 313, 315, *325*
Holbrook, D. J., 166, *210*
Holland, J. J., 142, *146*, 175, 176, *212*
Hollweg, S., 61, *83*
Holman, R. T., 281, *325, 329*
Holt, C. E., 126, 127, *145*
Holtfreter, J., 249, 255, *270*
Holtzer, H., 223, 240, *270*
Holtzman, E., 112, 118, 119, *148*
Honig, G. R., 162, *209*
Hopkins, J. W., 118, *147*
Horton, D. L., 97, 98, *106*
Horvath, S. M., 318, *323*
Horwitz, A. L., 365, *367*
Horwitz, B. A., 318, *328*
Hotta, Y., 178, *211*
Howard, A., 2, 3, *22*, 27, *43*
Howard, G. A., 172, *205*
Howard, E. F., 28, *41*
Howard, R. E., 304, *323*
Howard-Flanders, P., 36, 37, *39, 41*
Howell, R. R., 137, *146*
Howk, R., 169, *211*
Howton, D. R., 281, *326, 328*
Huang, A. S., 182, *206*
Huang, R. C., 160, 161, 166, 167, *206, 211*
Huberman, J. A., 112, *145*
Hübscher, G., 317, *325*
Hughes, W. L., 35, *41*, 68, *82*, 111, 131, *144*, 202, *209, 216*
Hull, D., 321, *324*
Humphrey, R. M., 142, *150*, 180, *217*
Humphreys, T., 226, 228, 229, 249, *270*
Hunt, E. A., 319, *325*
Hunt, J. A., 131, 132, *146*, 173, *211*

Hunt, N., 140, *146*
Hunt, T., 132, *145*
Hunt, T. E., 319, *325*
Hunter, T., 132, *145*
Hurlbert, R. B., 156, 161, 162, *211*, *213*
Hurwitz, J., 156, *214*
Hurych, J., 261, *268*
Hwang, M. L. H., 116, 117, *142*

I

Imondi, A. R., 183, *211*
Ingles, C. J., 159, *211*
Inoue, S., 335, *367*
Inukai, T., 89, 92, *105*
Iorio, R., 32, *41*
Irvin, J. L., *210*
Irving, J. T., 374, *379*
Ito, S., 233, 234, *270*, *273*
Iversen, O. H., 71, 76, *82*
Izawa, M., 30, *41*

J

Jacklin, A. J., 68, *82*
Jackson, C. W., 71, *84*
Jacob, M., 116, 117, *150*
Jacobs-Lorena, M., 172, 174, *206*
Jacoby, F., 75, *82*
Jaéjle, M. F., 202, *213*
James, D. W., 227, *270*
James, J., 33, *41*
James, M. C. M., 233, 248, *271*
Jamieson, J. D., 198, *211*
Jamroz, C., 133, *146*
Janeway, C. A., 202, *209*
Jardetzky, C. D., 204, *206*
Jarnum, S., 202, *211*
Jarrels, M. H., 339, 346, *370*
Javorska, H., 28, *42*
Jeanloz, R. W., 334, 353, *367*
Jeanteur, P., 118, *145*
Jellum, E., 167, *211*
Jensen, E. V., 138, *146*
Jesseph, J. E., 68, *82*
Joel, C. D., 318, *325*
Joel, D. D., 61, *85*
Joel, W., 356, *367*
Johns, E. W., 161, *207*
Johnson, F. R., 75, *83*

Johnson, G. E., 319, *328*
Johnson, H. A., 68, *82*
Johnson, P., 303, *323*
Johnson, W. W., 35, 38, *40*
Johnston, M. C., 225, *270*
Johnston, T. C., 142, *146*
Jones, A. L., 297, *325*
Jones, B. M., 233, 248, *271*
Joseph, D., 204, 205, *207*
Julku, E. J., 136, *148*
Jungblut, P. W., 138, *146*
Jurand, A., 244, *269*

K

Kärkkäinen, J., 335, *367*
Kahl, F. R., 248, *270*
Kahn, R., 34, *38*
Kai, M., 315, *324*
Kajiwara, K., 141, *146*, 163, *216*
Kalckar, H. M., 263, *270*
Kalf, G. F., 127, 129, *148*
Kaliszewski, B. F., 91, *105*
Kallman, F., 241, 242, 245, 246, 247, *270*
Kamen, M. D., 20, *22*
Kammen, H. O., 156, *212*
Kanner, L. C., 36, *41*
Kano, E., 141, *144*
Kanoh, T., 315, *324*
Kantor, T. G., 348, *367*
Karnovsky, M. J., 336, 358, *367*
Karnovsky, M. L., 302, *324*
Kashiwa, H. K., 375, *379*
Kastberg, M. L., 132, 133, 134, *143*
Katz, J. H., 202, *212*
Katzberg, A. A., 68, *82*, 97, 98, *105*
Kauffman, S. L., 60, *82*
Kavanau, J. L., 77, 78, *85*
Kawashima, T., 138, *146*
Kearns, K. E., 251, *267*
Keese, M., 60, *81*
Keir, H. M., 156, *212*
Kelley, D. E., 113, 121, 122, *148*
Kelly, J. W., 355, *367*
Kemp, R. B., 233, 248, *271*
Kennedy, E. P., 281, 289, 306, 308, 310, 311, 316, *325*, *327*, *329*
Kenney, F. T., 203, *212*
Kent, P. W., 334, *371*
Kern, H. L., 260, *271*

Kessel, R. G., 350, *366*
Keyl, H.-G., 28, *40, 41*
Kiehn, E. D., 175, 176, *212*
Kim, J. H., 141, *146*
Kim, S., 164, *212*
Kim, Y. S., 203, *216*
King, R. J. B., 138, *146*
Kinkade, J. M., 161, *212*
Kinnison, P. A., 335, 348, 358, 363, *367, 368*
Kinosita, R., 12, *23*
Kischer, C. W., 161, *212*
Kishimoto, Y., 303, 305, 320, *325, 326*
Klein, G., 35, *43*
Kleinschmidt, A. K., 125, *150*
Kleinsmith, L. J., 164, 165, 166, *206, 212*
Klenk, E., 281, *326*
Klevecz, R. R., 141, *146*, 180, 181, *212*
Klingman, J. D., 315, *326*
Kloch, A. L., 60, *81*
Kloep, L., P., 319, *327*
Knight, E., 121, 127, 128, 129, *146, 148*
Knight, J., 160, *208*
Knoop, A., 292, *322*
Knoop, F., 278, *326*
Knopf, P., 172, *218*
Knowlton, N. P., 11, *22*, 68, *82*
Knox, W. E., 203, *209*
Knudtson, K. P., 68, *82*
Koburg, E., 71, *82, 84*
Koch, W. E., 232, 254, *271*
Kohn, H. I., 60, 61, 71, *81, 83*, 97, 101, 102, 103, *105*
Kohn, R. R., 88, *105*
Kollar, E. J., 232, *271*
Koningsberg, I. R., 224, 246, *271*
Kornberg, A., 306, *326*
Kornfeld, R., 253, *271*
Kornfeld, S., 253, *271*
Kosterlitz, H. W., 33, *39*
Kotaki, A., 314, *329*
Kovach, J. S., 130, 131, *147*
Kraemer, P. M., 232, *271*
Krakow, J. S., 156, *212*
Kritchevsky, D., 301, *326*
Kroon, A., 125, *143*
Kroon, D. B., 259, *270*
Kruh, J., 20, *23*
Küntzel, H., 127, 129, *146*
Kumatori, T., 11, *23*

Kurnick, N. B., 27, *41*
Kuroda, Y., 229, *271*
Kyriakides, E. C., 310, *322*

L

Lagasse, A., 30, *44*
Laing, R., 118, *151*
Lahtiharju, A., 6, *23*
Lajtha, L. G., 9, 11, *23*, 130, *146*
Lala, P. K., 60, *82*, 130, *146*
Lamerton, L. F., 60, *80*, 180, *207*
Landman, O. L., 126, *149*
Lane, N., 350, 351, 365, *367*
Lang, K., 157, *210*
Lang, W., 61, *84*
Langan, T. A., 156, 164, 167, 169, *212*
Langham, W. H., 163, *210*
Lapiere, C. M., 224, 246, *270*
Larrabee, M. G., 315, 316, *326*
Larsen, C. L., 121, *144*
Lash, J. W., 240, 252, *271*
Lasher, R., 38, *39*
Laskowski, M., 156, *212*
Lasnitzki, I., 35, *41*
Lassen, N. A., 202, *211*
Latham, H., 117, *146*, 174, *218*
Latte, M. B., 60, *81*
Lau, C., 65, 68, *80*
Laurence, E. B., 5, *22*
Laurent, T. C., 260, *267*
Lavin, F., 204, 205, *207*
Lawrence, J. S., 9, *22*
Laycock, D. G., 131, 132, *146*, 173, *211*
Lazarow, A., 245, *271*
LeBaron, F. N., 315, *326*
LeBaron, R. D., 232, 233, 243, 254, 255, 257, 263, *274*
Leblond, C. P., 6, 7, 8, 19, *22, 23*, 36, 38, *42*, 47, 49, 50, 52, 53, 56, 65, 68, *80, 81, 82, 83, 84, 85*, 111, 130, *142, 146*, 177, 180, 192, 194, 195, 198, *212, 214*, *218*, 233, 244, 252, *273*, 292, *327*, 342, 350, 351, 356, 365, *367, 369*
LeBouton, A. V., 137, 138, *146*, 199, 200, 201, 202, 204, 205, *212*
Ledeen, R., 302, 303, *326*
Leeman, L., 30, *41, 42*
Lehmiller, D. J., 6, 9, *22*, 75, *83*
Lehtonen, A., 335, *367*

Leicht, W. Z., 315, 316, *326*
Leighton, F., 170, *214*
Lelong, J. C., 121, *145*
Lemahieu, M. A., 139, *148*
Lengyel, P., 108, *146*, 171, *212*
Lennartz, K. J., 60, 61, *83*
Leong, G. F., 75, *84*
Lepper, M. H., 202, *218*
Leppi, T. J., 333, 334, 335, 336, 337, 339,
    340, 341, 346, 347, 348, 350, 356, 358,
    362, 363, 364, 365, *367, 368, 370*
Lerman, S., 136, *152*, 185, *207, 212*
Lesher, S., 60, 61, 71, *81, 83*, 97, 102, 103,
    105
Leslie, I., 26, 32, *40*
Lett, J. T., 37, *42*
Leuchtenberg, C., 34, *42*
Leuchtenberger, R., 26, 34, *42*
Lev, R., 335, 336, *367, 368*
Levak-Svajzer, B., 240, *271*
Levi, P. E., 71, 75, *83*
Levine, E. M., 232, *271*
Lewallen, C. G., 202, *212*
Lewin, K., 197, 212
Lewis, N., 309, *326*
Li, C. H., 193, *210*
Liau, M. C., 156, 161, 162, 173, *211, 213*
Libby, P. R., 166, *213*
Lieberman, I., 140, *146, 151*
Lilien, J. E., 226, 229, 230, *271*
Lillie, R. D., 337, 348, *368, 370*
Lima-de-Faria, A., 26, 28, 29, *42*
Lindahl, T., 156, *213*
Lindsay, D. T., 163, *210*
Lindsley, D. L., 112, *149*
Lingrel, J. B., 131, *143, 146*
Linker, A., 257, 260, *272*, 356, 357, *368*
Linnane, A. W., 129, *144*
Lipkin, M., 61, *83*, 183, *211*
Lippman, M., 249, 250, 253, 263, *271*
Lison, L., 26, *43*
Lissau, Ä., 311, 312, *329*
Littau, V. C., 160, 162, *205*
Lloyd, L., 30, *39*
LaChang, T. C., 312, *326*
Lockard, R. E., 131, *146*
Locke, M., 233, *271*
Lodge, J. R., 34, *44*
Loeb, J. N., 137, *146*
Loening, U., 118, *151*

Loewenstein, W. R., 223, 251, *271*
Logan, R., 108, *150*
London, I. M., 134, *149*
Loomas, M. E., 311, *324*
Loran, M. R., 61, *83*
Lord, B. I., 68, *83*
Lorenson, M. G., 140, *147*
Lorenzsonn, V., 197, *218*
Lovell, D., 344, 358, *366*
Low, F. N., 245, *271*
Lowe, C. U., 33, *42*
Lucas, A. M., 133, *146*
Luck, J., 161, *215*
Luck, J. L., 129, *151*
Luft, J. H., 359, *368*
Lushbaugh, C. C., 68, *85*
Lyama, V. T., 232, *268*
Lynen, F., 281, *326*

M

McCarthy, B. J., 140, *143*
McConkey, E. H., 118, *147*
McCreight, C. E., 97, 98, *105*
MacDonald, R. A., 68, *83*
McEwen, B. S., 157, *213*
McFarlane, A. S., 202, *207, 213*
MacGillivray, A. J., 166, *213*
Macgregor, H. C., 29, 30, *42, 43*
McIndoe, W. M., 108, 109, *150*
McKalen, A., 68, *80, 81*
Mackenzie, C. G., 297, *326*
Mackenzie, J. B., 297, *326*
MacLean, I. S., 294, *326*
McLeenan, J. E., 246, *269*
McManus, J. F. A., 348, *368*
McMinn, R. M. H., 9, *23*, 68, 75, *83*
McMurray, W. C., 311, *326*
McNary, J. E., 319, *327*
MacPherson, S., 36, *42*
Madden, R. E., 202, *213*
Madden, S. C., 201, *213*
Maden, B. E. H., 174, *213*
Mahler, H. R., 169, *218*
Majerus, P. W., 309, *326*
Makinodan, T., 61, *84*
Malaise, E. P., 60, *81*
Maley, F., 140, *147*, 178, *213*

Maley, G. F., 140, *147*, 178, *213*
Malik, S. R. K., 185, 186, *213*
Maloney, M. A., 60, *82*, 130, *146*
Malt, R. A., 116, 134, *150*, *151*
Mandel, P., 116, 117, *150*, 253, *271*
Mandelstam, J., 232, *272*
Manson, L. A., 60, *81*, 230, *272*
Marcaud, L., 117, 118, 134, *149*
Marcker, K. A., 127, 128, *150*
Marcus, P. I., 141, 142, *149*, 232, *272*
Margoliash, E., 228, 229, *272*
Margolis, F., 203, *208*
Marinetti, G. V., 317, *326*
Marks, J. N., 196, 197, *210*
Marks, P. A., 130, 131, *147*
Marmur, J., 125, *150*
Marshak, A., 108, 109, *144*, *147*
Marshall, R. D., 346, *368*
Martin, D. Jr., 182, *217*
Martin, F. B., 305, *327*
Martin, J. H., 376, *379*
Marushige, K., 160, 161, 167, 168, 169, *206*, *213*
Marver, H. S., 170, 203, *213*, *218*
Marwah, A. S., 89, 96, 97, 99, *105*
Mason, C., 318, *323*
Masoro, E. J., 278, 279, 280, 282, 302, 321, *326*, *327*
Masters, Y. F., 356, *367*, *370*
Mathews, J. L., 376, *379*
Mathews, M. B., 260, 262, 263, *272*, 356, *368*
Matsuyuki, Y., 9, *22*
Matsuzawa, T., 61, *83*
Mattern, C. F. T., 11, *23*
Mattingly, A., *44*
Matukas, V. J., 358, 359, 363, *368*
Maurer, W., 60, 61, *83*, *84*
Maurice, P. A., *207*
Mauritzen, C. M., 161, *217*
Mayall, B. H., 33, 34, *42*
Mayhew, E., 250, *275*
Mazia, D., 156, *213*
Mead, J. F., 281, *326*, *327*, *328*
Means, A. P., 139, 140, *145*
Menczel, J., 375, *379*
Mendelsohn, M. L., 61, *84*
Messier, A., 68, *80*
Messier, B., 36, 38, *42*, 68, *84*

Mester, L., 338, *371*
Meyer, D. B., 340, *370*
Meyer, J., 14, *22*, 68, *82*, 89, 96, 97, 99, *105*
Meyer, K., 260, *268*, *272*, *274*, 334, 353, 356, 357, *366*, *367*, *368*
Meyer, R. R., 126, 127, *147*
Meyerzum Gottesberge, A., 71, *84*
Michelazzi, L., 251, *272*
Michell, R. H., 297, *327*
Micou, J., 109, *145*
Midgely, A. R., 249, *273*
Mikulicich, A. G., 134, *147*
Miles, A. E. W., 256, *269*
Miller, J. E., 307, *327*
Miller, L. L., 20, *23*
Miller, O. L., Jr., 29, 30, *42*, 127, *150*
Millette, R. L., 131, *143*
Mirsky, A. E., 26, 30, *41*, *42*, *44*, 157, 160, 162, 164, 165, 166, *205*, *206*, *212*, *213*, *214*, *217*
Mitmaker, B., 292, *327*
Monesi, V., 61, *84*
Monroy, A., 130, *147*
Montjar, M., 138, *151*
Moore, C. V., 20, *22*
Moore, H. A 61 *84*
Moore, M. O., 251, *267*
Moore, R., 182, *213*
Moore, W. J., 169, *218*
Moretti, J., 202, *213*
Morgan, R., 301, *323*, *324*
Moriyama, Y., 122, 123, *147*
Morrill, G. A., 179, *215*
Morrison, E. S., 310, *322*
Morrison, G. R., 200, *213*
Morton, L. T., 278, *327*
Moscona, A. A., 130, *147*, 226, 228, 229, 233, 238, 249, *269*, *271*, *272*
Moscona, M. H., 233, 240, *272*
Moses, M. J., 29, *42*
Moustacchi, E., 170, *213*
Mowry, R., 344, *368*
Moyer, E. K., 91, *105*
Mueller, G. C., 139, 141, *146*, *148*, *149*, *150*, 163, 181, 182, *213*, *216*
Mukeryee, H., 245, *272*
Muller, S. A., 375, *379*
Munkres, K. D., 171, *218*
Munro, A., 132, *145*

Munro, H. N., 202, *210*
Muramatsu, M., 122, 123, *147*
Murphree, S., 141, *150*
Murray, K., 159, 160, 161, 168, *213*, *215*
Musilova, H. A., 116, *151*
Myers, D. B., 363, *368*
Myers, O. E., 190, *210*

N

Nachbaur, J., 288, 309, 317, *327*
Nachmansohn, D., 316, *327*
Nachtwey, D. S., 57, *84*
Nadler, N. J., 111, 130, *142*, 180, 198, *212*, *213*, 292, *327*
Nagata, Y., 316, *326*
Nagy, K. P., 68, *80*
Nakamura, T., 122, 123, *147*
Nakasato, D., 202, *209*
Nanni, G., 251, *272*
Napolitano, L., 318, 319, *327*, 336, 337, *369*
Nash, D., 28, *42*
Nass, M. M. K., 124, 125, 126, 127, 128, *143*, *147*
Naylor, J. M., 27, 28, *44*
Nebel, S., 374, *379*
Neelin, J. M., 161, *218*
Nemeth, A. M., 203, *214*
Neuberger, A., 346, *368*
Neubert, D., 125, 126, *147*
Neufield, E., 253, *271*
Neuman, M., 373, *379*
Neuman, W. F., *379*
Neupert, W., 309, *322*
Neutra, M., 177, 192, 194, 195, *214*, 252, *273*, 342, 350, 351, 365, *369*
Nichol, C. A., 204, *216*
Nicolette, J. A., 139, *148*
Nilsson, B., 28, *42*
Niu, L. C., 251, *272*
Niu, M. C., 251, *272*
Norman, A., 37, *40*
Novogrodsky, A., 156, *214*
Novelli, A., 251, *272*
Novelli, G. D., 108, *148*
Nunn, L. C. A., 281, *327*

O

Oakberg, E. F., 53, 68, 71, *84*
Oberdisse, E., 126, *147*

O'Brien, J. E., 68, 71, *82*
O'Brien, P., 253, *271*
O'Brien, T. W., 127, 129, *148*
Ocumpaugh, D. E., 188, *210*, *214*
Odell, T. T., Jr., 71, *84*
Oehlert, W., 71, 75, *80*, *84*
Ohad, I., 197, *206*
Ojha, G., 71, *85*
Okada, S., 4, *23*
Okazaki, K., 245, *272*
Olcott, H. S., 348, *366*
Oliver, R., 11, 15, *21*, *22*
Olson, B. J., 10, *23*
Omura, T., 309, *327*
Oncley, J. L., 202, *209*
Oppenheimer, J. H., 202, *214*
Orbison, J. L., 358, 359, 363, *368*
Ord, M. G., 162, 164, 165, 167, *214*, *217*
Orlova, L. V., 163, *214*
Orr, S., 175, *206*
Osawa, S., 171, *214*
Osgood, E. E., 179, *214*
Otero-Vilardebo, L. R., 350, 351, *367*
Ottesen, J., 35, *41*
Ove, P., 140, *146*
Owen, M., 36, *42*

P

Paik, W. K., 164, *212*
Painter, R. B., 37, 38, *42*, *43*, 109, 110, *144*
Painter, T. S., 27, 29, *42*
Palade, G. E., 19, *22*, 171, 176, 177, 198, *207*, *208*, *211*, *215*, *216*, 292, 306, 307, 309, 317, *323*, *327*
Panner, B. J., 358, 359, 363, *368*
Pannese, E. J., 257, *273*
Papaconstantinou, J., 136, *148*, *150*
Pappenheimer, A. M., Jr., 174, *209*
Parker, R. C., 35, *41*
Parnas, H., 116, 117, *142*
Parshley, M. S., 250, *273*
Parsons, J. A., 127, *148*
Pascaud, M., 309, *327*
Pasteels, J., 26, *43*
Patkin, J. K., 282, 321, *327*
Patt, H. M., 3, *23*, 53, 60, *82*, *84*, 130, *146*
Pauling, E. C., 36, *41*
Paulus, H., 311, *327*
Pauly, J. E., 204, 205, *216*

Pautard, F. G. E., 374, *379*
Pavan, C., 27, 28, *39, 40, 43*
Payling Wright, G., 301, *323, 324*
Peachey, L. D., 230, 233, *273*
Pearse, A. G. E., 196, 197, *215*, 334, *371*
Pearson, R. W., 248, *270*
Pease, D. C., 233, 237, 245, 252, *273* 345, 359, *369*, 374, 375, 376, 378, *378, 379*
Pelc, S. R., 2, 3, *22*, 27, 31, 34, 35, 36, 38, *38, 41, 43, 44*
Pene, J. J., 121, *148*
Pengelley, E. T., 318, *323*
Penman, M., 112, 116, 117, 118, 119, 120, 121, 127, 128, *148, 151*
Penman, S., 112, 116, 117, 118, 119, 120, 121, 122, 123, *148, 151*, 162, *214*
Peraino, C., 203, *214*
Perez, A. G., 141, *146*
Periera, J. P. M., 57, *83*
Perkowska, E., 29, 30, *43*
Perrotta, C. A., 139, *148*
Perry, R. P., 109, 113, 121, 122, *148*, 173, *213*
Pesch, L. A., 199, *214*
Peterman, M. L., 129, *148*
Peters, T., Jr., 202, *214*
Peters, T. J., 260, *274*
Petersen, D. F., 3, *23*
Peterson, M. R., 19, *23*, 192, *214*, 350, 351, *369*
Pethica, B. A., 226, *273*
Petit, L., 301, *324*
Petruska, J. A., 265, *273*
Pettijohn, D. E., 36, *41, 43*
Pettit, B. J., 33, *43*
Pfeifer, U., 61, *85*
Pfeiffer, S. E., 141, *148*
Phillips, D. M. P., 161, *207*
Phillips, T. L., 75, *84*
Pierce, G. B., 244, 245, 249, *272, 273*
Piez, K. A., 232, 260, 261, 266, *268, 273*
Pigman, W., 334, *369*
Piha, R. S., 163, *214*
Piko, L., *148*
Pilgrim, C., 61, *83, 84*
Pinzino, C. J., 164, *207*
Pitot, H. C., 203, 204, *214, 215*
Platt, D. B., 158, *207*
Plaut, W., 28, *41, 43*
Pogo, A. O., 164, 165, 166, *214*

Pogo, B. G. T., 164, 165, 166, *206, 214*
Pollister, A. W., 26, *43*
Pool, B., 170, *214*
Popják, G., 295, 307, *327*
Post, J., 61, *84*, 97, 98, *105*
Potter, V. R., 35, *41*, 204, *215*
Pover, W. F. R., 317, *325*
Posner, A. S., 375, *379*
Power, D. R., 230, *267*
Pratt, S. A., 336, 337, *368, 369*
Prescott, D. M., 108, 109, 110, 133, 142, *143, 148, 149, 150*, 158, 159, 163, 178, 179, 180, 181, 182, *209, 215*
Prestayko, A. W., 122, 123, *147*
Preston, B. N., 129, *149*
Price, G., *44*
Price, V. E., 203, *215*
Price, W. E., 306, *326*
Priest, R. E., 68, *82*
Prottey, C., 309, *324*
Puck, T. T., 11, *23, 24*
Puga, A., 28, *42*
Pullman, M. E., 315, *327*

Q

Quastler, H., 3, *23*, 53, 61, 71, *84*
Quincey, R. V., 154, *215*
Quintarelli, G., 333, 334, 335, 348, 349, 357, 364, *369, 370*

R

Rabaey, M., 185, *209*
Rabinowitz, M., 126, 127, *145*, 162, 170, *208, 209*
Radin, N. S., 303, 305, 320, *324, 325, 326, 327*
Radley, J. M., 182, *213*
Rall, J. E., 202, *212*
Ralph, R. K., 122, *151*
Ram, J. S., 249, *273*
Rambourg, A., 233, 244, 252, *273*, 342, 343, *369*
Rand, R. N., 33, *42*
Randolph, M. L., *44*
Raper, H. S., 294, *327*
Rapp, F., 123, *147*

Rappaport, A. M., 199, *215*
Rasch, E. M., 33, *43*
Rasch, R. W., 33, *43*
Rasmussen, P., 161, *215*
Rasmussen, R. E., 37, 38, *43*
Ratcliffe, T., 231, 233, 248, *267*
Rayns, D. G., 363, *368*
Rechcigl, M., Jr., 201, 203, *213*, *215*
Redman, C. M., 171, *215*
Reeder, R., 136, *149*
Reeve, E. B., 202, *217*
Reid, B. R., 162, *215*
Reid, E., 157, *215*
Reinsch, I., 126, *147*
Reiskin, A. B., 61, *84*
Reiss, O. K., 297, *326*
Reith, E. J., 257, *273*
Rennels, E. G., 71, *85*
Rensing, L., 204, *210*
Revel, J. P., 233, 234, 241, 244, 245, 249, *270*, *273*, 344, 349, 358, 362, 364, *369*
Revel, M., 138, *149*
Révész, L., 35, *43*
Rexroth, A. K., 169, 170, *217*
Reynolds, W. E., 202, *206*
Rice, L. I., 297, *328*
Rich, A., 172, *218*, 263, *273*
Richards, B. M., 32, *38*
Richardson, C. C., 156, *215*
Richart, R. M., 68, *84*
Richert, D. A., 203, *217*
Richter, W. R., 228, 229, *272*
Ridgler, R., Jr., 34, 38, *41*
Riecken, E. O., 196, 197, *215*
Riegel, B. W., 190, *210*
Riley, E. F., 134, *149*
Ringertz, N. R., 34, 38, *41*
Ris, H., 26, *42*, 44, 127, *147*
Ritosso, F. M., 112, *149*
Rittenberg, D., 10, *23*, 295, 300, 301, *322*, *327*
Robbins, E. R., 141, 142, *145*, *149*, 162, 179, 180, 181, 182, *207*, *211*, *215*
Roberts, J. C., 317, 318, *328*
Robertson, A. L., Jr., 300, *327*
Robertson, J. D., 237, *273*
Robertson, J. S., 60, *81*
Robinson, R. A., 374, *379*
Rodionov, V. M., 163, *214*
Rodman, T. C., 28, *44*

Roeder, R. G., 156, 157, *216*
Roels, H., 26, 30, 33, *44*
Rogers, P. J., 129, *149*
Roll, P. N., 35, *40*
Ron, A., 159, *209*
Roodyn, D. B., 124, 127, 129, *149*, 170, *216*
Rosan, R. C., 334, *370*
Rosen, F., 204, *216*
Rosenberg, M. D., 225, 226, 238, *273*
Rosenthal, O., 96, *105*
Ross, M. H., 33, *40*
Ross, R., 245, *269*
Rossi, E., 190, *216*
Rossiter, R. J., 311, *326*, *329*
Rovery, M., 196, *208*
Rozijin, T. H., 162, *218*
Rubin, A. D., 140, *149*
Rubin, H., 238, 239, 249, *273*
Rubin, M. I., 190, *210*
Rubini, J. R., 68, *82*
Ruddle, F. H., 180, 181, *212*
Rudkin, G. T., 27, *44*
Rueckert, R. R., 141, *149*
Ruiz, E. E., 315, *326*
Rupp, W. D., 37, *41*
Russell, P. J., 35, *40*
Rustad, L. C., 178, *216*
Rustad, R. C., 178, *216*
Rutter, W. J., 156, 157, *216*
Ruttenberg, G. J. C. M., 125, *143*
Ryter, A., 126, *149*
Ruyter, J. H. C., 259, *270*

S

Sado, T., 61, *84*
Saffran, M., 313, *325*
Sagan, L., 129, *149*
Salb, J., 142, *149*
Salisbury, G. W., 34, *44*
Sallis, J. D., 376, *379*
Samuels, H. H., 182, *217*
Sanadi, D. R., 18, *22*, 169, *208*, 309, *324*
Sandritter, W., 32, *38*
Sandru, D., 127, 128, *144*
Saponara, A. G., 141, *144*
Sarkaria, D. S., 33, *42*
Saroja, I. S., 161, *217*

Sarzala, M. G., *328*
Sasaki, T., 61, *84*
Saunders, A. M., 334, 356, *370*
Savkar, N., 164, *207*
Scanu, A., 202, *216*
Scaro, J. L., 131, *143*
Schaeffer, J. R., 180, *217*
Schally, A. V., 313, *325*
Schapira, F., 20, *23*
Schapiro, G., 20, *23*
Scharff, M. D., 141, 142, *145*, 162, 180, *207*, *211*
Schatz, G., 315, *327*
Schenck, T. R., 228, 229, *272*
Scherrer, K., 114, 115, 117, 118, 134, *148*, *149*
Scheving, L. E., 204, 205, *216*
Schiefer, H. G., 317, *328*
Schiller, S., 353, *370*
Schimke, R. T., 203, *216*
Schlessinger, D., 171, 172, *216*
Schmidtberger, R., 193, *216*
Schmieder, M., 126, *147*
Schmitt, F. O., 374, *379*
Schnaitman, C. A., 175, *216*
Schönbaum, E., 319, *328*
Schoenheimer, R. J., 279, 281, 282, 294, 300, 320, 321, *322*, *327*, *328*
Schotz, M. C., 297, *328*
Schour, I., 14, *22*, 68, *82*
Schramm, M., 197, *206*
Schubert, M., 266, *274*, 348, 353, 356, 361, *367*, *370*
Schultz, J., 108, *143*
Schultze, H. E., 193, 199, 201, 202, 203, *216*
Schutt, M., 125, *151*
Schutz, G., 137, *149*
Schwartz, V. G., 232, *272*
Schwartze, M., 202, *211*
Schweizer, E., 127, *150*
Scopes, J. W., 318, *324*
Scott, J. E., 332, 335, 336, 339, 348, 355, 356, 357, 364, *367*, *369*, *370*
Scott, R. B., 134, 136, *150*
Seaman, G. V. F., 230, *268*, *280*
Segal, H. L., 203, *216*
Seiter, I., 75, *80*
Sekeris, C. E., 137, *149*, 164, *216*

Sekeris, K. E., 164, *216*
Sellers, E. A., 319, *328*
Seno, N., 260, *274*
Serafini-Francassini, A., 260, *274*
Setlow, R. B., 36, *44*
Sewall, E. L., 60, *80*
Shaeffer, J. R., 142, *150*
Shafrir, E., 320, *328*
Shapiro, B., 288, *328*
Shapiro, L., 125, *150*
Shapot, U. S., 250, *268*
Shea, S. N., 61, *84*
Shelanski, M., 181, 182, *215*, *216*
Shemen, D., 101, *23*
Shen, L., 252, *274*
Sheperd, G. R., 161, *212*
Sheridan, J. W., 116, *144*
Sherlock, P., 61, *83*
Sherman, F. G., 61, 71, *84*
Sherwood, N., 93, *104*
Shetlar, M. R., 356, *367*, *370*
Shiffer, L. M., 61, *85*
Shimizu, S., 315, *324*
Shock, N. W., 87, 88, 89, 94, 96, 101, 104, *105*, *106*
Shoemaker, W. J., 204, 205, *207*
Shorter, R. G., 68, 71, *81*, *84*
Showacre, J. L., 109, *150*
Shreeve, W. W., 109, 110, *144*
Shyamala, G., 138, *145*, *151*
Siebert, G., 157, *215*, *216*
Siekevitz, P., 171, 176, 177, 198, *207*, *208*, *215*, *216*, 306, 307, 309, 317, *323*, *327*
Silverman, W. A., 318, *328*
Silvestrini, R., 60, *81*
Siminovitch, L., 35, *41*
Simnet, J. D., 71, *84*
Simpson, M. V., 126, *147*
Sims, R. T., 158, *216*
Sinclair, J. C., 318, *328*
Sinclair, J. H., 127, *150*
Siperstein, M. D., 295, 296, *324*
Sirlin, J. L., 112, *143*
Sisken, J. E., 12, *23*
Sjostrand, F. S., 233, *274*
Skougaard, M. R., 71, *79*
Slaton, W. H., Jr., 281, *327*, *328*
Slavkin, H. C., 224, 226, 229, 232, 233, 237, 243, 245, 246, 248, 249, 250, 251, 252, 254, 255, 256, 257, 259, 263, *274*

Smail, G. A., 190, 191, *207*
Smedley-MacLean, I., 281, *327*
Smellie, R. M. S., 32, *40*, 108, 109, 139, 140, *142, 150*
Smith, A. E., 127, 128, *150*
Smith, C., 365, *366*
Smith, C. G., 92, *105*
Smith, D. W., 36, *41*, 127, *150*
Smith, E. L., 161, 190, 191, *208, 218*
Smith, I., 112, 118, 119, *148*
Smith, J. L., 202, *214*
Smith, J. W., 260, *274*
Smith, M., 159, *211*
Smith, M. E., 301, 303, 304, 305, 315, 317, 320, *328*
Smith, R. E., 317, 318, 319, *323, 328*
Smith, S. J., 122, *150*
Smith, T., 317, *326*
Smithies, O., 175, *206*
Smits, G., 251, *270*
Snoddy, H. D., 204, *209*
Sobel, A. T., 374, *379*
Soeiro, R., 116, 117, 120, 121, *150, 151,* 173, *218*
Söll, D., 171, *212*
Sognnaes, R. F., 377, *379*
Soll, D., 108, *146*
Solursh, M., 38, *39*
Sonnenbichler, J., 168, *216*
Sorrentino, M., 344, *367*
Spalding, J., 163, *216*
Speidel, E., 245, *291*
Spencer, H., 68, 71, *84*
Spencer, W. A., 319, *328*
Sperry, W. M., 301, *329*
Spicer, S. S., 333, 334, 335, 336, 337, 338, 339, 340, 341, 344, 346, 347, 348, 349, 350, 356, 358, 362, 364, 365, *368, 370,* 371
Spiegelman, S., 112, *149*
Spink, J. M., 89, 91, *106*
Spiro, M. J., 193, 194, *216*
Spiro, R. G., 190, 191, 192, 193, *216, 217*
Spitzer, H. L., 310, *322*
Srere, P. A., 295, *328*
Srinivasan, B. D., 75, *82*
Sri Ram, J., 245, *272*
Starbuck, W. C., 161, *217*
Starr, J. L., 108, *150*
Stayanoff, V. A., 301, *329*

Stedman, Edgar, 159, *217*
Stedman, Ellen, 159, *217*
Steel, G. G., 60, 61, *80, 84*, 180, *207*
Steele, W. J., 112, *150*
Steffensen, D. M., 28, *44*
Steffen, J., 11, *23*
Steggles, A. W., 138, *146*
Stein, O., 283, 284, 285, 286, 287, 288, 289, 290, 292, 293, 310, 320, *328*
Stein, Y., 283, 284, 285, 286, 287, 288, 289, 291, 292, 293, 310, 320, *328*
Steinberg, G., 281, *326, 328*
Steinberg, M. S., 226, 229, 230, 249, *274*
Steiner, G., 318, 319, *328*
Steinhauser, H., 281, *322*
Steinschneider, H., 129, *150*
Stella, E. J., 203, *209*
Stellwagen, R. H., 159, 160, 162, 163, 164, 166, 167, 168, *215, 217*
Stemler, R. S., 202, *206*
Stern, H., 179, *211*
Stevely, W. S., 164, *217*
Stevenin, J., 116, 117, *150*
Stevens, B. J., 127, *150*
Stevens, C. E., 49, 68, *83, 84*
Stevens-Hooper, C. E., 14, *23*, 51, 52, *85*
Steward, D. L., 142, *150*, 180, *217*
Stewart, J. A., 136, *150*
Stich, H. F., 27, 28, *44*
Stidworthy, G., 356, *370*
Stocken, L. A., 162, 164, 165, 167, *214, 217*
Stocker, E., 61, 75, *85*
Stoffel, W., 317, *328*
Stogsdill, R., 202, *206*
Stoll, E., 190, *216*
Stone, G. E., 127, *150*
Storer, J. B., 68, *85*
Storey, W. F., 68, *85*
Stoward, P. J., 334, 338, 341, 342, 349, *366, 370,* 371
Strange, J. L., 169, 170, *217*
Strauss, B. S., 37, *44*
Strehler, B. L., 5, *23*, 88, *105*
Strickland, K. P., 311, *326, 329*
Strong, F. M., 311, *324*
Stroun, M., 36, *44*
Stryckmans, P. A., 61, *85*
Stubblefield, E., 141, *146, 150*
Stumpf, P. K., 281, *329*

Stumpf, W. E., 138, *146*
Subrahmanyam, D., 311, *329*
Subramanian, A. R., 172, *217*
Sueoka, N., 126, *143*
Sugiyama, T., 127, 128, 129, *146*
Sulkin, N. M., 97, 98, *105*
Sumerskill, W. H. J., 197, *209*
Sumner, B. E. H., 340, *371*
Surks, M. I., 202, *214*
Sutton-Gilbert, H., 141, *144*
Suyama, Y., 128, *150*
Suzuki, K., 159, *217*
Suzuki, T., 138, *146*
Swaffield, M., 253, *267*
Swann, M. M., 178, 179, *217*
Swarm, R. L., 350, 364, *370*
Sweeley, C. C., 312, *326*
Sweeney, E. W., 203, *216*
Sweeney, P., 249, *268*
Swick, R. A., *217*
Swick, R. W., 169, 170, *217*
Swift, H., 26, 32, *38, 43, 44*, 131, *145*
Sylvén, B., 340, *367*
Szirmai, J. A., 354, 355, *371*

T

Taguay, R., 60, *80*
Takeda, Y., 202, *217*
Takeuchi, J., 250, *274*
Takuma, S., 257, *274*
Tal, M., 156, *214*
Talmage, D. W., 179, *217*
Tanzer, M. L., 224, 246, *270*
Tarbit, M. H., 36, *38*
Tarentino, A. L., 203, *217*
Tarver, H., 199, *217*
Tata, J. R., 139, 140, *145*
Tauro, P., 127, *150*
Taylor, A. C., 240, *276*
Taylor, A. N., 29, *42*
Taylor, C. B., 309, *329*
Taylor, E. W., 13, *21*
Taylor, C. W., 161, *211, 217*
Taylor, E., 181, *216*
Taylor, J. N., 109, *150*
Taylor, M., 75, *83*
Tchen, T. T., 296, *329*
Teir, H., 6, *23*

Teng, C. S., 138, 139, 140, *145, 150, 151*,
    168, *217*
Tepperman, J., 33, *40*
Terasima, T., 141, *151*
Termine, J. D., 375, *379*
Tershikh, V. V., 3, *22*
Thaler, M. M., 162, *217*
Thompson, E. B., 182, *218*
Thompson, R. C., 282, 300, 320, *329*
Thompson, W., 311, *329*
Thomson, R. Y., 32, *40*
Thorp, D. E., *275*
Thrasher, J. D., 57, 61, *85*, 97, 102, 103,
    105, 111, *142*, 178, 180, *210, 217*
Throp, F. K., 251, 262, *275*
Thuringer, J. M., 97, 98, *105*
Tidwell, T., 164, *217*
Tiedemann, H., 223, 240, *274, 275*
Timiras, P. S., 93, *104*
Tishoff, G. H., 155, *208*
Titchener, E. B., 129, *149*
Tobey, R. A., 3, *23*, 141, *144*
Todaro, G. J., 140, *143*
Toft, D., 138, *145, 151*
Toivonen, S., 223, *275*
Tolmach, L. J., 141, *148, 151*
Tomkins, G. M., 182, *217*
Tompkins, G. T., 137, *146*
Tongiani, R., 30, *44*
Tonino, G. J. M., 162, *218*
Topper, Y. J., 199, *214*
Toto, P. D., 71, *85*
Tracy, M. M., 35, *39*
Trakatellis, A. C., 138, *151*
Traub, A., 156, *214*
Traugh, J. A., 174, *207*
Trevithick, J. R., 159, *211*
Trier, J. S., 197, *218*
Trott, J. R., 68, *85*
Truex, R. C., 89, 94, *105*
Tsai, T. H., 204, 205, *216*
Tschudy, D. P., 170, 203, *213, 218*
T'so, P., 160, *206*
Tsukada, K., *151*
Tuan, D. Y. H., 160, 161, 167, *206*
Tubiana, M., 60, 61, *81*
Tuchmann-Duplessis, H., 33, *39*
Turner, M. K., 157, *215*
Tyler, A., *148*
Tyler (Caffrey), R. W., 68, *81*

U

Uren, J., 182, *213*
Urist, M. R., 249, 254, *275*, 375, *379*

V

Valleron, A. J., 60, 61, *81*
Van Duijn, P., 32, *39*, *40*, 338, *367*
van Heyningen, H. E., 198, *218*
Van Lancker, J. L., 140, *144*
Vasama, Raimo, 5, *23*
Vasama, Ritva, 5, *23*
Vassort, F., 60, 61, *81*
Vaughan, M. H., 172, 174, *213*, *218*
Vaughn, M., 120, *150*
Vendrely, C., 26, 33, 34, *39*, *42*, *44*, 47, *85*
Vendrely, R., 26, 33, 34, *39*, *42*, *44*, 47, *85*
Venkataraman, P. R., 33, *42*
Verel, D., 202, *210*
Vesco, C., 116, 117, 127, 128, *148*, *151*, 172, 174, *206*
Vidali, G., 161, 165, *209*, *218*
Vignais, P. M., 288, 309, 317, *327*
Villee, C. A., 162, *217*
Vincent, P. C., 61, *85*
Vinograd, J., *148*
Viola-Magni, M. P., 30, 31, 38, *43*, *44*
Vitols, E., 253, *267*
Volwiler, W., 202, *206*
von Hungen, K., 169, *218*
von Volksman, R., 53, *85*
Vulpe, M., 65, 68, *83*

W

Wachstein, M., 200, 201, *218*
Waelsch, H., 163, *214*, 301, *329*
Wagner, E., 118, *151*
Wagner, H., 311, 312, *329*
Wagoner, G., 96, *105*
Wajda, M., 301, *324*
Wakil, S. J., 282, *329*
Walker, B. E., 68, 71, *83*, *85*
Walker, P. M. B., 12, 13, *23*
Walker, R., 97, 99, *106*
Wall, P. D., 92, *104*
Wallace, H., 112, *143*
Wang, D. Y., 14, *23*
Wang, K. M., 155, 156, 174, *218*

Wang, T. Y., 155, 156, 167, 169, 174, *211*, *218*
Ward, P. D., 230, 231, *275*
Warner, J. R., 112, 116, 117, 121, *151*, 172, 173, 174, *218*
Warren, L., 172, 175, 176, *209*, *218*, 224, 228, 230, 232, 235, 250, *268*, *275*, 346, *370*
Warshawsky, H., 198, *218*
Wasserman, F., 262, *275*
Watanabe, I., 4, *23*
Watanabe, M., 204, *215*
Watkins, J. C., 316, *329*
Watson, J. D., 122, *151*
Watson, M. L., 20, *23*, 374, *379*
Weber, C. S., 112, 113, 121, 122, *143*
Weber, E. J., 303, *323*
Weber, F., 199, *218*
Webster, H. L., 183, *218*
Wegener, K., 61, *83*
Weinberg, R. A., 118, 122, 123, *151*
Weinmann, J. P., 14, *22*, 68, *82*, 89, 96, 97, 99, *105*
Weiss, L., 224, 226, 228, 230, 231, 233, 248, 250, 267, *275*
Weiss, P., 77, 78, *85*, 225, 238, 240, 245, 249, 255, 264, *275*, *276*
Weiss, S. B., 306, 310, 316, *325*, *329*
Weissmann, B., 251, 260, *272*
Weissman, S., 202, *218*
Weissman, S. M., 121, *144*
Wessel, N. W., *270*
Wessels, N. K., 224, 245, *276*
Westerfield, W. W., 203, *217*
Weston, J. A., 225, *276*
Wettstein, F. O., 171, 173, *209*
Wetzel, B. K., 336, 337, 344, 349, 358, *371*
Wetzel, M. G., 336, 337, 344, 349, 358, *371*
Whipple, G., 201, *213*
White, A., 190, 191, *218*
Whiteley, H. J., 97, 98, *106*
Whur, P., 192, 195, *218*
Widholm, J., 167, *206*
Widnell, C. C., 139, 140, *145*
Widner, W. R., 11, *22*, 68, *82*, *85*
Wied, G. L., 34, *38*
Wilgram, G. F., 289, 308, *329*
Wilhelm, D. L., 75, *85*
Wilkie, D., 124, 127, 129, *149*, 170, *216*

Wilkins, B. M., 37, *41*
Willems, M., 112, 116, 118, 119, 120, 121, *151*
Williams, G. E. G., 75, *85*
Williamson, D. H., 170, *213*
Williamson, J. R., 298, 299, 300, *329*
Wilson, R., 61, *83*
Wilson, S. H., 130, 137, 138, *151*, 154, *215*
Wimber, D. E., 15, 16, *24*, 63, *85*
Wimber, D. R., 61, 71, *86*
Winkelstein, A., 9, *22*
Winston, R. A., 180, *207*
Winzler, R., 202, *218*
Wirsen, G., 283, 285, *329*
Wirtz, K. W. A., 310, *329*
Wiss, O., 199, *218*
Witten, P. W., 281, *329*
Wolfort, F. G., *269*
Wolfsberg, M. F., 61, *85*
Wolpert, L., 226, 245, 246, *270*
Wood, D. D., 129, *151*
Woodin, A. M., 260, *276*
Woodland, H. R., 182, *210*
Woods, P. S., 109, *151*
Woodward, D. O., 171, *218*
Woodward, J. W., 131, *145*
Wright, E. A., 89, 91, *106*
Wünnenberg, B., 318, *322*
Wunderlich, V., 125, *151*
Wurtman, R. J., 204, 205, *207*

Y

Yagi, K., 314, *329*
Yamada, E., 233, *276*
Yamada, M., 11, *24*
Yamada, T., 223, *276*
Yamashina, I., 193, *219*
Yamazoe, S., 315, *324*
Yardley, J. H., 358, *371*
Yates, H. B., 12, 13, *23*
Yiengst, M. J., 89, 94, 96, *105*, *106*
Yosizawa, Z., 335, *367*
Youcis, P., 60, *81*
Young, B. A., 292, *327*
Young, R. W., 60, *85*, 134, *144*, *147*, *152*, 184, 185, 186, 187, 188, 189, 190, *209*, *210*, *214*, *219*

Z

Zajdela, F., 134, *149*
Zamelis, A., 318, *328*
Zigman, S., 136, *152*, 185, *207*, *212*
Zilversmit, D. B., 310, *329*
Zimmermann, B. U., 313, *325*
Zobel, C. R., 343, *371*
Zolokar, M., 109, *152*

SUBJECT INDEX

A

Acetate,
  cholesterol synthesis and, 294–295
  phosphatidylethanolamine and, 317
Acetylation,
  histones, 165–166, 167
  mucin staining and, 338, 343, 348
Acetylcholine,
  gangliosides and, 304
  phosphatidylinositol synthesis and, 312,
    313, 314, 316
Acetyl coenzyme A, histones and, 165
N-Acetylgalactosamine,
  glycoproteins and, 193
  mucopolysaccharides and, 191
N - Acetylgalactosamine - 4(6) - sulfate,
  mucopolysaccharides and, 191
N-Acetylglucosamine,
  glycoproteins and, 193
  mucopolysaccharides and, 191
N-Acetylglucosamine-6-sulfate, mucopolysaccharides and, 191
N-Acetylhexosamine, glycoproteins and,
  334
Acheta, oocytes, 28–29
α_1-Acid glycoprotein, synthesis and turnover, 202
Acridine orange, acid polysaccharides and,
  356–357
Actinomycin D,
  cell cycle and, 141, 181
  protein synthesis,
    enzymes, 140
    erythrocytes, 134
    lens, 136
  ribonucleic acids and,
    liver, 137
    nucleoplasmic, 116–117
    transfer, 122
  transcription and, 121
Adenohypophysis, phosphatidylinositol
  and, 313

Adenosine deaminase, cell differentiation
  and, 183
Adenosine triphosphate, colchicine and, 14
S-Adenosylmethionine, histone methylation and, 164
Adenylate deaminase, cell differentiation
  and, 183
Adipose tissue,
  brown,
    cell cycle phase duration, 59
    cold and, 318–319, 321
    distribution of, 318
    lipid of, 318–319, 321
    structure, 318
  fatty acid synthesis in, 282
Adrenal cortex,
  cell cycle phase duration in, 58
  cell turnover time in, 70
  deoxyribonucleic acid, constancy of,
    33–34
  mitotic rate, age and, 100
Adrenalectomy, enzyme induction and,
  204–205
Adrenaline, phosphatidylinositol and, 313
Adrenal medulla,
  deoxyribonucleic acid, constancy of,
    30–32
  phosphatidylinositol and, 313
Age,
  cell cycle and, 5
  cell turnover time and, 71
Aging,
  cartilage and, 356, 357
  changes in, 87–88
  intestinal mucosal cells and, 97, 101,
    102–103
  mitotic rates and, 97, 98–100
  nervous system and, 88–94
  other tissues and, 94–96
  variability and, 101
Alanine transaminase, induction of, 204
Alanine transferase, turnover rate, 170
Albumin, synthesis and turnover, 201–202

Albuminoid(s),
  lens, formation of, 185
Alcian Blue,
  cartilage and, 357
  mucins and, 335–336, 338, 339–341, 346–
    347, 348
Alcohol, polysaccharide fixation and, 354
Alcohol dehydrogenase, liver acinus and,
  200
Aldolase, half-life of, 20
Alkaline phosphatase, cell differentiation
  and, 183
Amberlite GC-50, histone separation on,
  161
Ameloblasts, cell cycle phase duration in,
  59
Amethopterin, synchronized cells and, 141
Amino acid(s),
  histone, 161
  incorporation,
    lens and, 184–185
    rods and cones and, 187–188
  labeled,
    liver acinus and, 201
    membranes and, 175–176
  protamines, 159
Aminoacyl transferase II, ribosomes and,
  174
δ-Aminolevulinate synthetase, turnover
  rate, 170, 203
Aminopterin, mitochondrial protein synthesis and, 128
Ammonium sulfide, mucin electron microscopy and, 342
Amnion cells,
  human, ribonucleic acid synthesis in, 109
Amoeba proteus,
  cytonucleoproteins of, 158
  Golgi complex, biogenesis of, 176
  mitosis, critical mass and, 179
Amphibia,
  deoxyribonucleic acid, constancy of, 29–
    30
Amylase, mucin staining and, 338, 342,
  346, 353
Anesthetics, cell cycle studies and, 4
Antibody,
  formation, cell cycle phase duration and,
    58

Arachidonate,
  biosynthesis of, 281
  lecithin and, 307
  occurrence of, 280
Arbacia punctulata,
  embryo, histones of, 162
Arginase, turnover of, 203
Arginine,
  histones and, 160, 161, 165–166
  protamines and, 159
Ascites cells, trypsin and, 231
Atropine, intestinal secretion and, 197
Autoradiography,
  mucins and, 349–353
  polysaccharides, 364–366
Autoregulators,
  tissue, cell cycle and, 6
Azure A, mucins and, 338, 339

B

Basal lamina, epithelial-mesenchymal interactions and, 244–245
Basic dyes, mucin staining and, 339–341
Beef,
  lymphocytes, cell cycle phase duration
    in, 60
Biebrich Scarlet, mucin staining and, 349
Birds, erythroid cell differentiation in,
  132–134
Bismarck brown, cartilage and, 357
Bladder,
  cell proliferation, stimulation of, 75
  cell turnover time, 67
Blood-group compounds, glycoprotein, 192
Bone,
  calcification in, 374–375, 376
  calcium storage in, 378
  cell cycle phase duration in, 59, 60
Bone marrow,
  cell turnover time, 65, 68
  proliferation of, 9, 49
  x-irradiation of, 11
Brain,
  cholesterol,
    localization, 301–302
    synthesis, 295, 301
    turnover, 301
  histone, half-life, 163
  lipids, turnover of, 320

5-Bromodeoxyuridine, cell cycle and, 141
Bronchus, cell turnover time, 67, 69
Brown fat, *see under* Adipose tissue
Brunner's gland,
    Golgi complex, labeling of, 194

C

Calcification, different types of, 373
Carbohydrate,
    cell surface and, 229, 252
    general considerations, 331–334
    labeled, Golgi complex and, 350–353
Carboxyl groups, cell surface, 230–231
Cardiolipin, content of membranes, 278
Carnoy fixative,
    mucin and, 336
    polysaccharide fixation and, 354
Cartilage,
    calcification of, 375, 376
    cell cycle phase duration in, 59
    cells, age and, 96
    ground substance, nature of, 357
    labeled sulfate and, 365
    polysaccharides of, 356
    ruthenium red and, 359–360
Cat,
    nervous system, age and, 89, 91
    tissues, cell turnover time in, 66–67
Catalase,
    synthesis, rate of, 203
    turnover rate, 170
Cataract, lens proteins and, 185–186
Cation(s), polysaccharide fixation and, 354
Cationic dyes, polysaccharide fixation and, 355
Cell(s),
    counting of, 10
    eucaryotic, genome size, 266
    G_0 phase, ribonucleic acid synthesis in, 140
    interphase, activity of, 154, 178
    proliferating, ribonucleic acid synthesis in, 140–142
    soluble phase, turnover of, 177–178
    tissue culture, membrane proteins, 175
Cell adhesion, differentiation and, 226
Cell cycle, 2–3
    duration of phases, 56–64
    factors affecting, 3–7

histone synthesis and, 163
proteins, 178–180
    synthesis and, 180–182
ribonucleic acid synthesis and, 139–142
Cell membranes, *see also* Membranes, Plasma membranes
    architecture of, 233–237
    unit membrane concepts, limitations, 237–239
Cell outer surface,
    characterization of, 230–231
    ribonucleic acid in, 250–251
    specific ligands of, 228–230
    turnover of, 232–233
Cell population,
    cell cycle, 2–3
        factors affecting, 3–7
    classification based on proliferative behavior, 64–74
    nature of, 7–8
    neoplastic, 73–74
    renewing, 73
    separation of, 183
    slowly renewing, 73
    static, 73
    types of, 8–9
    very slowly renewing, 73
Cell proliferation,
    embryonic and postnatal periods, 46–48
    methods for study, 48–64
    regulation of, 74–79
Cell renewal, methods for study, 9–16, 48–64
Cementum, formation of, 377
Cephalin, *see* Phosphatidylethanolamine
Cerebral cortex, *see also* Brain, Nervous system
    phosphatidylinositol and, 313
Cerebroside,
    nature and distribution, 303
    turnover of, 304–305, 320
Cerebroside sulfate, distribution of, 303
Cervical mucin, carbohydrate composition, 193
Cetylpyridinium,
    mucins and, 335–336
    polysaccharide fixation and, 355, 357
Chalones, mitosis and, 6, 78
Chick,
    embryo, ribosomal proteins, 171–172

Chinese hamster cells,
  histones, turnover of, 163
Chironomus,
  cytonucleoproteins of, 158
  polytene chromosomes of, 28
Chloramphenicol, mitochondrial protein
  synthesis and, 129
Cholesterol,
  acetylcholine binding and, 304
  biosynthesis, 294–296
  content of membranes, 278
  structure, 293
  subcellular distribution, 297–300
  turnover of, 300–302, 304, 320
Chondrocytes,
  calcification and, 375
  Golgi complex, labeling of, 194
Chondroitin, composition and location,
  191
Chondroitin sulfate(s),
  acridine orange and, 357
  composition and location, 191
  cornea and, 260
  differentiation and, 250
  hyaluronidase and, 361
  protein and, 263
  ruthenium red and, 361
Chromatin, ribonucleic acid synthesis and,
  112–113
Chromomeres, nature of, 168
Chromomycin succinate, cell cycle and,
  141
Chromosomes,
  lympbrush, deoxyribonucleic acid of, 30
  polytene, deoxyribonucleic acid con-
    stancy in, 27–28
  proteins of, 156, 167–168
Citric acid cycle,
  enzymes, nucleus and, 157
Clupeine,
  nature of, 159
  ribonucleic acid synthesis and, 159
Colchicine,
  cell cycle studies and, 13–14, 16, 51–53
  cell turnover time and, 65–67
  microtubule protein and, 181
Cold, brown adipose tissue and, 318, 319,
  321
Collagen,
  calcification and, 373–374, 375, 377, 378

cornea and, 259–260
differentiation and, 224, 246–248
epithelial differentiation and, 241–244
fibers, factors influencing formation,
  261–262
hydroxyapatite crystallization on, 238
mucopolysaccharides and, 262–264
polymerization of, 242, 245
self-assembly of, 264–266
Collagenase, epidermis and, 248
Colloidal iron,
  mucin staining and, 338, 341, 344, 347,
    349
  polysaccharides and, 356, 358, 359, 363
Colloidal metals,
  mucin electron microscopy and, 343–
    345, 349
  polysaccharide staining and, 358
Colon, *see also* Intestine
  cell cycle phase duration in, 58, 60
  cell turnover time, 67, 69
Cones,
  outer segments, renewal of, 187–190
Connective tissue, glycoproteins of, 192
Contact guidance, differentiation and,
  225–226
Contact inhibition, differentiation and,
  226–227
Coriphosphine, mucin staining and, 341
Cornea,
  cell cycle and, 4
  cell proliferation, stimulation of, 75
  cell turnover time, 65, 66, 69
  collagen and noncollagenous protein
    complexes, 259–260
Cortisol,
  enzyme induction by, 204
  liver histone acetylation and, 166
Critical electrolyte concentration, Alcian
  Blue staining and, 335–336, 339–340
Critical mass, mitosis and, 178, 179
Crystallin(s),
  cataracts and, 185–186
  formation of, 185
Cycloheximide,
  nucleolar ribonucleic acid synthesis and,
    120–121
  ribosomal proteins and, 174
  zymogen granules and, 198
Cysteine, histones and, 167

Cytidine diphosphate diglyceride, phosphatidylinositol synthesis and, 311
Cytidine triphosphate, lecithin synthesis and, 306
Cytochrome *a*,
  localization of, 175
  site of synthesis, 170, 171
Cytochrome *b*,
  localization of, 175
  site of synthesis, 170, 171
  turnover rate, 170
Cytochrome b_5,
  localization of, 175
  turnover rate, 170
Cytochrome *c*,
  site of synthesis, 170
  turnover of, 169–170
Cytochrome oxidase, cell differentiation and, 183
Cytonucleoprotein(s), 169
  behavior of, 158
Cytoplasm,
  histone synthesis in, 162
  ribosomal proteins in, 174

D

Dentin,
  calcification of, 375, 376
  formation of, 255–256
Deoxycholate, nuclear proteins and, 155
Deoxycytidylate deaminase,
  cell cycle and, 181
  synthesis of, 140
Deoxyribonuclease(s), nuclear, 156
Deoxyribonucleic acid,
  constancy, 25–26
    deviations, 27–34
    hypothesis, 26
  content of nucleus, 12–13, 47
  mitochondrial, 125–127
    half-life of, 126–127
  repair of, 36–37
  stability-renewal of, 20–21, 25–26, 35–37
  synthesis,
    cell cycle and, 2
    colchicine and, 14
    diurnal rhythm and, 204
    enzymes and, 181
    erythroid cell differentiation and, 130–132, 132–134

histone phosphorylation and, 164–165
histone synthesis and, 163
lens differentiation and, 134–137
polysaccharide synthesis and, 253
ribonucleic acid synthesis and, 141
x-rays and, 11
Deoxyribonucleic acid ligases, nuclear, 156
Deoxyribonucleic acid polymerase,
  cell cycle and, 181
  chromosomal, 169
  mitochondrial, 126
  nuclear, 156
  synthesis of, 140
Dermatan sulfate, differentiation and, 250
Diastase, mucin staining and, 342, 346
Diazomethane, cell surface and, 230
Diazonium compound(s), mucin staining and, 338
Differentiation,
  cellular, extracellular matrix and, 248–266
  control of, 182–184
  glycosaminoglycans and, 249–253
  regulation, epigenetic controls, 223–227
Digitonin, cholesterol and, 295
Dihydrouridylate, chromosomal ribonucleic acid, 167
N,N-Dimethylphenylenediamine, isomers, mucins and, 338, 340
Dimethylsulfoxide, ribosomal ribonucleic acid and, 121
Diphtheria toxin, aminoacyl transferase and, 174
Disulfide bonds,
  cataract and, 185
  histones and, 167
Diurnal rhythms,
  cell cycle and, 5, 50, 52–53, 74
  liver metabolism and, 204–205
Dog,
  tissues,
    cell cycle phase duration in, 60
    cell turnover time in, 67
Duodenum, *see also* Intestine
  cell cycle phase duration in, 58, 59
  cell turnover time, 66, 69
Drosophila, ribosomal ribonucleic acid synthesis in, 112
Dytiscus, oocytes, 28–29

E

Ear,
  epidermis,
    cell cycle phase duration in, 57, 58
    cell turnover time, 66, 69
Egg white, glycoproteins of, 192
Ehrlich ascites cells,
  cell cycle phase duration in, 59, 61
  histones, methylation of, 164
Elastin, formation of, 245
Electrolytes, subcellular renewal, 21
Electron microscopy,
  mucin histochemistry and, 341–346
  polysaccharide staining and, 358–361
Electron transport chain, localization of, 175
Electrophoresis,
  cell outer surface and, 230
  membrane proteins, 175
Embryogenesis,
  morphogenetic aspects, epithelial-mesen-
    chymal interactions, 240–244
Embryonic period, cell proliferation and
  growth, 46–48
Embryonic tissues,
  cell cycle phase duration in, 57, 58
  mitochondrial deoxyribonucleic acid, 125
Enamel, formation of, 377
Endoplasmic reticulum,
  carbohydrates and, 345
  cholesterol and, 297
  chondromucoprotein synthesis and, 365
  development, phospholipid and, 307–308
  lipid uptake and, 289, 292, 293
  phosphatidylinositol and, 312, 314
  proteins, 175
    derivation of, 176–177
  ribosomes and, 171
  rough, role of, 19
Energy reservoir, mitosis and, 178, 179
Enzymes,
  alteration of staining,
    mucins, 346–347
    polysaccharides, 361–364
  digestive, synthesis of, 196
  inducible, turnover of, 170, 203–204
  membranes and, 175
  nuclear, 156–157
  specificity, isotopes and, 17

Epidermis,
  cell cycle phase duration in, 59
  cell proliferation, 49, 53
    stimulation of, 75
  cell turnover time, 65, 66, 69
  differentiation, collagen and, 246
  mitotic inhibitor in, 78–79
  mitotic rate, age and, 98
  tritiated thymidine and, 15
Epididymis,
  cell turnover time, 70
  Golgi complex,
    differentiation and, 176
    labeling of, 194
Epinephrine, mitosis and, 5, 74
Epithelia,
  cells, age and, 96
  collagen production and, 241–244
  keratinizing, deoxyribonucleic acid con-
    stancy in, 34
  mitotic rate, age and, 98, 99
  ribonucleic acid turnover in, 130
Epithelial-mesenchymal interactions, 239–
  240
  basal lamina and, 244–245
  extracellular microfibrils and, 245–246
  morphogenetic aspects,
    collagen and, 246–248
    embryogenesis and, 240–244
Epithelial tumor, cell cycle phase duration
  in, 59
Erythroblasts, heterogeneous ribonucleic
  acid and, 117
Erythrocytes,
  chicken, histone synthesis in, 162
  life span of, 10
  lipid, turnover, 320
  loss, age and, 89, 94
  maturation,
    nucleic acid and hemoglobin synthesis
      and, 130–132, 132–134
    time, 70
  membrane,
    lipid composition, 278
    proteins of, 175
  sialomucopeptide of, 231
Erythropoietin, cell proliferation and, 9
Escherichia coli,
  genome, size of, 266

ribonucleic acid polymerase, clupeine and, 159

Esophagus,
cell turnover time, 65, 66, 69
epithelium, cell cycle phase duration in, 58

Esterase, cell differentiation and, 183

Estradiol, uterine histone acetylation and, 166

Estrogen, uterine ribonucleic acid synthesis and, 138–139, 140

Ethylenediaminetetraacetate, cell surface and, 230, 231, 232–233, 248

Ethylene glycol, "inert" dehydration and, 359

Euchromatin,
histone, acetylation of, 166, 167

Euplotes,
cell cycle, histone synthesis and, 163

Evolution, histones and, 166–167

F

Fat(s), turnover time, 282, 320

Fatty acid(s),
biological half-lives, 282–283
biosynthesis of, 280–282
chemistry and occurrence, 279–280
monolayers, cell attachment to, 238–239
oxidation of, 278–279
phosphatidylethanolamine, 316
ultrastructural localization, 284–293

Feeding,
regimen, liver metabolism and, 205

Ferritin, messenger ribonucleic acid and, 202

Feulgen stain,
cell cycle studies and, 12, 16
deoxyribonucleic acid physical state and, 32–33, 34

Fibrinogen, synthesis and turnover, 202

Fibroblast(s),
cell surface material, 230
Chinese hamster, ribonucleic acid synthesis in, 109
contact inhibition and, 227
cultures, cell orientation and, 225
mitochondrial deoxyribonucleic acid of, 127

stationary, ribonucleic acid synthesis in, 140

Fibrosarcoma, cell cycle phase duration in, 59, 60

Fixation,
mucin histochemistry and, 336–337
polysaccharides, 354–355

Fluorescence, mucin stains and, 341

Follicle-stimulating hormone, carbohydrate composition, 193

Fontinine, nature of, 159

Formaldehyde,
mucin fixation and, 336, 342, 344
polysaccharide fixation and, 354, 355

Fucose, glycoproteins and, 191, 193

G

Galactosamine, glycoproteins and, 191

Galactose,
anionic polysaccharide and, 353
complex carbohydrates and, 351, 353
labeled, glycoproteins and mucopolysaccharides, 192, 194–195
glycoproteins and, 191, 193
mucopolysaccharides and, 191

Galactose-6-sulfate, mucopolysaccharides and, 191

Gall bladder,
cell proliferation, stimulation of, 75

Galline, nature of, 159

Gangliosides, nature and distribution, 303, 304

Genes,
activation, 165–166
rate of transcription, 154

Globulin(s), nuclear, 155

Glucosamine,
glycoproteins and, 191
labeled, hyaluronate synthesis and, 365–366

Glucosamine-6-sulfate, mucopolysaccharides and, 191

Glucose,
labeled, glycoproteins and mucopolysaccharides, 192, 194–196
mucus secretion and, 350–351
occurrence in mammalian cells, 251–252

Glucose-6-phosphatase, Golgi complex and, 176

Glucose-6-phosphate, enzyme induction and, 204
Glucose-6-phosphate dehydrogenase, cell cycle and, 181
  cell differentiation and, 183
Glucuronate, mucopolysaccharides and, 191
Glucuronate-2-sulfate, mucopolysaccharides and, 191
Glutamate-pyruvate transaminase, half-life of, 203
Glutaraldehyde,
  mucin fixation and, 336, 337, 342, 343, 347
  polysaccharide fixation and, 358, 363
Glycerol,
  turnover of, 320
  uptake into lipids, 289
Glycerol-3-phosphate, acylation of, 306
L-α-Glycerophosphate dehydrogenase, half-life, 203
Glycogen,
  liver, diurnal rhythm, 204
  mucin staining and, 342, 346
Glycolipids,
  glucose and, 251
  synthesis, cell cycle and, 180–181
Glycolysis,
  enzymes,
    localization of, 175
    nucleus and, 157
Glycoprotein(s),
  basal lamina and, 244
  collagen fibrillogenesis and, 242
  composition of, 191, 193
  structural features, 334
  synthesis, cell cycle and, 180
  synthesis and transport, 190–196
Glycosaminoglycans, cell differentiation and, 249–253
Glyptotendipes, polytene chromosomes of, 28
Goblet cells, heterosaccharide synthesis in, 350–351
Golgi complex,
  carbohydrates, 344, 345
    sulfation of, 350
  hyaluronate synthesis and, 366
  labeled carbohydrates and, 350–353
  labeled sulfate and, 365
  lipid uptake and, 289, 292, 293

  membranes, biogenesis of, 176–177
  phosphatidylinositol and, 312, 314
  polysaccharides and, 358
  role of, 19
  sulfate incorporation in, 192, 194, 195
  zymogen granules and, 196–198
Gonads, mitosis in, 49
Guinea pig,
  tissues, mitotic rates of, 97, 99–100

H

Hair follicle, cell cycle phase duration in, 58
Haliclona occulata,
  cells, aggregation of, 228–229
Hamster,
  tissues, cell cycle phase duration in, 60
Haptoglobulin,
  carbohydrate composition, 193
  synthesis and turnover, 202
Heart,
  cell cycle phase duration in, 59
  cells, age and, 95–96
  fatty acid uptake by, 283
HeLa cells,
  histone synthesis in, 162, 163
  mitochondrial ribonucleic acid of, 127–128, 129
  ribonucleic acid synthesis, 109, 110
    ribosomal, 112
  ribosomes of, 171, 172
  sialate, replacement of, 232
Hemoglobin,
  renewal studies, 20
  synthesis, erythroid cell differentiation and, 130–132, 132–134
Heparin,
  acridine orange and, 357
  differentiation and, 250
  ruthenium red and, 359
Heparitin sulfate,
  composition and location, 191
  differentiation and, 250
Hepatectomy,
  partial, histone acetylation and, 166
Hepatocytes,
  differentiating,
    Golgi complex of, 176
    ribosomes of, 171

Hexosamine,
  anionic polysaccharides and, 353–354
  content of cornea, 260
Hexuronate, anionic polysaccharides and, 353–354
High iron diamine, mucin staining and, 340–341, 346, 350
Histidine, protamines and, 159
Histone(s),
  acetylation, cell division and, 140
  acidic nuclear proteins and, 168–169
  classification of, 160–162
  function of, 159–160
  methylation, acetylation and phosphorylation of, 163–166
  ribonucleic acid synthesis and, 165–168
  synthesis,
    site, 162
    time and turnover, 163, 165
  uterine chromatin, estrogen and, 138
Homeostasis, isotope effects and, 17
Hormones,
  cell cycle and, 6
  cell proliferation and, 79
  glycoprotein, 192
Human,
  nervous system, age and, 89–94
  tissue,
    cell cycle phase duration in, 60
    cell turnover time in, 66–68
    mitotic rates of, 97–99
Hyaluronate,
  acridine orange and, 357
  composition and location, 191
  differentiation and, 250
  extracellular matrix and, 264
  synthesis of, 365–366
Hyaluronidase,
  cartilage staining and, 359
  mucin staining and, 347
  polysaccharide staining and, 361–364 365
Hydroxyapatite, calcification and, 373–374, 375–376, 377, 378
Hydroxypropyl methacrylate, embedding in, 359

I

Iduronate, mucopolysaccharides and, 191
Ileum, see also Intestine
  cell cycle phase duration in, 58, 59
  cell turnover time, 67

Inducer(s),
  differentiation and, 223
  mechanism of, 240
Induction, substratum and, 254–259
Insects, deoxyribonucleic acid constancy in, 27–29
Intestine, see also Duodenum etc.
  cell populations, separation of, 183
  epithelium, surface coat, 233–235, 336–337
  Golgi complex, labeling of, 194
  heterosaccharide synthesis in, 350–352
  histone, half-life, 163
  mitosis in, 49
  mucosal cells, changes with age, 97, 101, 102–103
  secretory products, 196, 197
  sterol synthesis in, 295–296
Invertase, cell differentiation and, 183
Iridine, nature of, 159
Isotopes, cell cycle studies and, 16–20

J

Jejunum, see also Intestine
  cell cycle phase duration in, 58–60
  cell turnover time, 67

K

Karyotype, continuous proliferation and, 182
Keratan sulfate,
  cartilage and, 356, 357
  composition and location, 191
  content of cornea, 260
  differentiation and, 250
  periodate-Schiff reaction and, 356
  structure of, 353
Kidney,
  cell proliferation, stimulation of, 75, 79
  cell turnover time in, 70
  Golgi complex, labeling of, 194
  mitotic rate, age and, 98
  ribonucleic acid turnover in, 130
Kinetic effects, isotopes and, 17
Kynurenine hydroxylase, localization of, 175

L

Lacrimal gland,
  mitotic rate, age and, 99

Lactate dehydrogenase, cell cycle and, 181
Lacustrine, nature of, 159
L-cells,
    mitochondrial deoxyribonucleic acid of, 127
    ribonucleic acid synthesis in, 113
    surface membranes, turnover of, 232
Lead salts, cartilage staining and, 359
Lecithin, *see* Phosphatidylcholine
Lens,
    cell proliferation, stimulation of, 75
    differentiation, nucleic acid and protein synthesis and, 134–137
    immature and adult, protein synthesis in, 184–186
Leucine aminopeptidase, cell differentiation and, 183
Leukemia L5178Y, cell cycle phase duration in, 59
Leukocytes,
    deoxyribonucleic acid, constancy of, 32–33
Light,
    liver metabolism and, 204, 205
    retinal protein synthesis and, 188
Light microscopy,
    mucins, 337–341
    polysaccharide staining and, 355–357
Lignocerate, occurrence of, 303
Linoleate,
    fatty acid deficiency and, 280–281
    occurrence of, 280
Linolenate,
    fatty acid deficiency and, 280
    occurrence of, 280
Lipid,
    calcification and, 374
    droplets, fatty acid uptake by, 284, 292
    membrane composition, 278
    synthesis, cell cycle and, 180–181
α_1-Lipoprotein, synthesis and turnover, 202
S_{f3-9}(B) Lipoprotein, synthesis and turnover, 202
Liporibonucleoprotein, cell surface and, 250
Liver,
    acinus,
        diurnal rhythms, 204–205

    protein metabolism, 200–201
    structure, 199–200
    synthesis and turnover of plasma proteins and inducible enzymes, 201–204
    cell cycle, 2–3
        phase duration, 60, 61
    cell proliferation, stimulation of, 75, 76–77
    cell turnover time, 67, 70
    cholesterol synthesis in, 295–296
    deoxyribonucleic acid, constancy of, 33
    fatty acid synthesis in, 281–282
    Golgi complex, labeling of, 194
    histone,
        acetylation of, 165
        half-life, 163
        methylation of, 164
        phosphorylation of, 164
    metabolism of, 198–199
    mitochondrial
        deoxyribonucleic acid, 125
        ribonucleic acid, 128
    mitotic rate, age and, 98
    palmitate incorporation by, 289–293
    protein, turnover of, 20
    regenerating, ribonucleic acid synthesis in, 140
    ribonucleic acid,
        synthesis, 137–138
        turnover, 130
Lung,
    cell turnover time, 67, 69
    morphogeneisis, collagen and, 247
Lymphatic tissue, mitosis in, 49
Lymphocytes,
    cell cycle phase duration in, 60
    histones of, 162, 166
    phytohemagglutinin stimulated, ribonucleic acid synthesis in, 140
    proliferation of, 9
Lymphoma cells,
    protein synthesis, cell cycle and, 180
Lysine,
    histones, 160, 161–162
        acetylation of, 165
        methylation of, 164
    protamines and, 159
Lysosomes, intestinal, 197

M

Macromolecules,
  synthesis, cell cycle and, 179
  turnover of, 19–21
Magnesium ions, ribosomal subunits and, 172
Malate dehydrogenase, half-life, 203
Mammals,
  deoxyribonucleic acid, constancy of, 30–34
  erythroid cell differentiation in, 130–132
Mammary gland, triglyceride synthesis in, 292–293, 320
Mammary tumor, cell cycle phase duration in, 59
Mannose, glycoproteins and, 191, 193, 195
Matrix,
  extracellular, differentiation and, 248–266
  odontogenesis and, 256–259
Mealybug(s), histones of, 162
Megakaryocytes, maturation time, 70
Melanocytes, orientation of, 225
Membranes, see also Cell membrane, Plasma membrane
  lipid composition of, 278
  mitochondrial, 175
    turnover of, 170
  proteins, synthesis and turnover, 175–177
  ribonucleic acid and, 223–224
Mesenchyme, odontogenesis and, 254–259
Mesodermal cells,
  heart-forming, orientation of, 225
Methylation,
  histones, 164, 167
  mucin staining and, 348–349
  polysaccharide staining and, 364
  ribosomal ribonucleic acid, 174
ε-N-Methyllysine, histones and, 161, 164
Mevalonate, cholesterol synthesis and, 297, 301–302
Microcinematography, cell cycle studies and, 12
Microciona prolifera,
  cells, aggregation of, 228–229
Microfibrils,
  extracellular, epidermal-mesenchymal interactions and, 245–246

Microfilaments, plasma membrane and, 233–237
Microsomes, lipid composition, 278
Microtubules,
  colchicine and, 13
  protein, synthesis of, 181–182
Minerals, subcellular renewal, 21
Mitochondria,
  brown adipose tissue, 318
  calcification and, 375–376
  fatty acids,
    synthesis, 281
    uptake, 284, 288–289, 292, 293
  membrane, lipid composition, 278
  nucleic acids of, 124–129
  phospholipids,
    half-lives, 304, 315, 320
    origin of, 308–309, 314–315, 317
  proteins, turnover of, 169–171
  turnover of, 18–19
Mitosis,
  anesthetics and, 4
  cell cycle and, 2
  cell proliferation and renewal and, 48–50
  cell surface glycosaminoglycans and, 253
  connective tissue extracts and, 249–250
  control of, 182
  differential, 179, 180
  "trigger" and, 178–180
Mitotic apparatus, proteins of, 156
Mitotic figures, counting of, 10–11
Mitotic index, estimation of, 49–50
Mitotic rates, age and, 97, 98–100
Monoamine oxidase, localization of, 175
Morphogenesis,
  collagen and, 246–248
  problems of, 221–223
Mouse,
  intestinal mucosa, aging and, 97, 102–103
  nervous system, age and, 89, 91, 93
  ribonucleic acid synthesis in, 111
  tissues,
    cell cycle phase duration in, 58–59
    cell turnover time in, 66–70
    mitotic rates of, 97, 98
    water drinking habits of, 64
Mucigen granules, transport of, 195
Mucin(s),
  histochemistry, 334–336
    alterations of staining, 346–349

autoradiography, 349–353
  fixation, 336–337
  staining procedures, 337–346
Mucopolysaccharide,
  calcification and, 374, 378
  cell surface and, 237
  collagen and, 262–264
  collagen fibrillogenesis and, 242
  synthesis, photoreceptor cells, 188–189
  synthesis and transport, 190–196
  types and composition, 191
Mucous secretions, glycoprotein, 192
Muscle,
  aldolase, half-life, 20
  cells, age and, 96
  differentiation, collagen and, 246
  red fibers, fatty acid and, 283
  ribonucleic acid turnover in, 130
Myelin,
  lipid composition, 278
  phospholipids, half-lives of, 304, 315, 320
Myofibrils, oleate uptake by, 284

N

Nerve,
  axons, orientation of, 225
Nervonate, occurrence of, 303
Nervous system, *see also* Brain, Cerebral
  cortex
  cells and fibers, changes with age, 88–94
Neural crest cells, movements of, 225
Neuraminate, glycoproteins and, 191
Neuraminidase, cell outer surface and,
  230–231, 232
Neurospora,
  mitochondrial ribonucleic acid of, 128,
  129
  respiratory mutants, 170–171
  ribonucleic acid synthesis in, 109
Newcomer's solution, polysaccharide fixation and, 357
Newt,
  embryos, histones of, 162
Nicotinamide adenine dinucleotide,
  colchicine and, 14
  reduced, liver acinus and, 200
Nicotinamide adenine dinucleotide-cyto-
  chrome *c* reductase,
  cell differentiation and, 183
  localization of, 175, 176

Novikoff hepatoma, histone synthesis in,
  162
Novikoff hepatoma ascites cells, low molecular weight ribonucleic acid of, 123
Nucleolus,
  deoxyribonucleic acid constancy and,
    29–30
  histone synthesis in, 162
  proteins of, 156
  ribonucleic acid synthesis in, 118–122
  ribosomal proteins and, 173, 174
Nucleoside phosphorylase(s), cell differentiation and, 183
Nucleotide kinase(s), nuclear, 157
Nucleotide phosphatase(s), nuclear, 157
Nucleotidyl transferase,
  terminal, nucleus and, 156
Nucleus,
  cholesterol in, 297
  deoxyribonucleic acid content, 12–13
  histone synthesis in, 162
  proteins,
    acidic, 168–169
    classification, 155–156
    cytonucleoproteins, 158–159
    enzymes, 156–157
    histones, 159–168
    protamines, 159
  ribonucleic acid synthesis, 108–109
  sites of, 112–113
Nutrition, cell cycle and, 5

O

Odontoblasts, calcification and, 375
Oleate,
  incorporation of, 284, 288
  lecithin and, 307
  occurrence of, 280
Oocytes, deoxyribonucleic acid bodies in,
  28–29
Oral cavity, cell turnover time, 65, 66
Organelles, turnover of, 18–19
Ornithine transferase, turnover rate, 170
Orosomucoid, carbohydrate composition,
  193
Osmium tetroxide,
  mucin fixation and, 336, 337, 344
  mucin staining and, 342
  polysaccharide staining and, 359

Osteoblasts, calcification and, 374–375
Ovary, cell turnover time, 67
Oxygen,
  consumption, cell cycle and, 179–180

P

Palladium, contact inhibition and, 227
Palmitate,
  lecithin and, 307
  occurrence of, 279
  turnover of, 320
  uptake into liver lipids, 289–293
Palmitoleate, occurrence of, 279–280
Pancreas,
  cell cycle phase duration, 59
  cell turnover time in, 70
  development, collagenase and, 247
  Golgi complex, labeling of, 194
  membranes, protein of, 177
  phosphatidylinositol and, 312, 313
  ribonucleic acid synthesis in, 111
  ribosomes of, 171
  secretory products, 196
    synthesis and transport, 198
  zymogen granules, transport time, 177
Paneth cells,
  enzymes of, 196, 197
  zymogen granules, transport time, 177
Papain, mucin staining and, 349
Paraformaldehyde, polysaccharide fixation
  and, 358
Pararosaniline, mucin staining and, 337,
  338
Parathyroid gland,
  mitotic rate, age and, 100
Parathyroid hormone, bone and, 378
Parotid gland,
  phosphatidylinositol and, 313
  zymogen granules, transport time, 177
Pea,
  histones, 160, 161, 162
    synthesis of, 162
Pectin, ruthenium red and, 361
Pepsin, mucin staining and, 349
Periodate,
  mucins and, 334, 335, 337, 338
  polysaccharide staining and, 355–356,
    357

Periodate-pentafluorophenylhydrazine,
  mucin electron microscopy and, 342
Periodate-silver methenamine, mucin electron microscopy and, 342–343
Phagocytosis, photoreceptor outer segments and, 190
Pharynx,
  epithelium, cell cycle phase duration in,
    58
Phenylhydrazine, mucin staining and, 338,
  343, 348
Phosphate groups, cell surface, 231
Phosphatidylcholine,
  acetylcholine binding and, 304
  biosynthesis of, 306
  brain, half-life, 304
  content of membranes, 278, 306
  oleate incorporation into, 288, 309
  turnover of, 308–309, 320
  ultrastructural localization, 310
Phosphatidylethanolamine,
  biosynthesis of, 316–317
  brain, half-life, 304
  content of membranes, 278, 316
  oleate incorporation into, 288, 317
  turnover of, 308, 317
Phosphatidylinositol,
  biosynthesis of, 310–312
  content of membranes, 278
  distribution of, 312
  functional activity, 312–314
  half-life in brain tissues, 304
  turnover of, 314–316, 320
Phosphatidylserine,
  brain, half-life, 304
  content of membranes, 278
Phosphodiesterase(s), nuclear, 157
3-Phosphoglycerate dehydrogenase, half-
  life, 203
Phospholipid(s),
  content of membranes, 278
  function of, 306
  structure of, 306
Phosphorylation, histones, 164–165, 167
Phosphotransferase(s), nuclear, 157
Phosphotungstate,
  mucin electron microscopy and, 345–346
  polysaccharide staining and, 358–359
Physarum polycephalum, deoxyribonucleic
  acid of, 126, 127

Phytohemagglutinin, histone acetylation and, 166
Pigment cells, orientation of, 225
Pigment epithelium, photoreceptor outer segments and, 190
Pilocarpine, gastric secretion and, 197
Plasma,
    cholesterol, turnover of, 302
    glycoproteins of, 192
    proteins, synthesis and turnover, 201–203
Plasma membrane, *see also* Cell membrane, Membranes
    cholesterol and, 297
Platelets, phosphatidylcholine synthesis and, 309
Polyacrylamide gels, ribosomal protein and, 174
Polynucleotide kinase, nuclear, 156
Polysaccharide(s),
    anionic, structural features, 353–354
    biosynthesis of, 253
    cell recognition sites and, 252
    histochemistry, 353–354
        alterations of staining, 361–364
        autoradiography, 364–366
        fixation, 354–355
        staining procedures, 355–361
    hydroxyapatite crystals and, 378
Polysomes,
    heterogeneous ribonucleic acid and, 117
    proteins of, 172
Postnatal period, cell proliferation and growth, 47–48
Potassium ferrocyanide, colloidal iron staining and, 344
Prealbumin, synthesis and turnover, 202
Proline, incorporation by salivary gland, 247
Pronase,
    cell surface and, 229, 231
    polysaccharide synthesis and, 252
Prophase, colchicine and, 14, 51
Protamine(s), nature and types of, 159
Protein(s),
    carbohydrate staining and, 349
    cell cycle and, 178–184
    cytoplasmic systems, turnover of, 169–178
    enamel formation and, 377

estrogen acceptor, 138–139
extracellular matrix, 263–264
    self-assembly, 264–266
lens, synthesis of, 184–186
liver acinus,
    diurnal rhythm and, 204–205
    metabolism, 199–201, 204–205
    synthesis and turnover, 201–204
membrane, synthesis and turnover, 175–177
mitochondrial, turnover of, 169–171
noncollagenous, cornea and, 260
nuclear,
    acidic, 168–169
    classification, 155–156
    cytonucleoproteins, 158–159
    enzymes, 156–157
    histones, 159–168
    protamines, 159
polysaccharide fixation and, 354
ribosomal, turnover of, 171–174
structure, self-assembly and, 264
synthesis,
    lens differentiation and, 134–137
    mitosis and, 142
    phospholipid synthesis and, 307, 309
turnover of, 20
weakly basic, nuclear, 161
zymogenic cells, synthesis and transport, 196–198
Purine phosphoribosyl transferase, cell differentiation and, 183
Puromycin,
    cell cycle and, 181
    nucleolar ribonucleic acid synthesis and, 120–121
    thyroglobulin synthesis and, 195

R

Rabbit,
    tissues, cell turnover time in, 66
Rat,
    dystrophic, rod outer segments of, 190
    embryo, number of cells in, 47
    nervous system, age and, 89–94
    tissues,
        cell cycle phase duration, 59–60
        cell turnover time, 66–69
        histone half-life, 163
        mitotic rates, 97–99

Repressors, translation and, 182
Reticulin, formation of, 245
Retina,
 cells, aggregation of, 229–230
 rods and cones, structure of, 186, 187
Rhodopsin, synthesis and turnover, 189–190
Ribonuclease(s),
 nuclear, 157
 polysaccharide staining and, 357
Ribonucleic acid,
 cell differentiation and, 183–184
 cell surface and, 250–251
 chromosomal, histones and, 167–168
 heterogeneous, synthesis of, 116–118
 liver acinus and, 200, 201
 liver, half-lives, 154
 membranes and, 223–224
 messenger,
  amount of, 113–114
  cell cycle and, 180, 182
  mitochondrial, 127–128
  plasma proteins and, 202
  ribosomes and, 172
  synthesis of, 112–113
  turnover time, 130
 mitochondrial, 127–129
 nucleolar, synthesis of, 109–110
 nucleoplasmic, half-life of, 117
 ribosomal,
  amount of, 113–114
  mitochondrial, 129
  origin of, 112
  synthesis of, 118, 122
  turnover time, 130
 small molecular weight, synthesis of, 122–123
 5S, synthesis of, 121–122
 7S, synthesis of, 121
 synthesis,
  acidic nuclear proteins and, 169
  cell cycle and, 139–142
  diurnal rhythm, 204
  erythroid cell differentiation and, 130–132, 132–134
  histones and, 160, 165–168
  kinetics in tissue culture cells, 109–110
  kinetics in vivo, 110–111

lens differentiation and, 134–137
liver and, 137–138
nucleus and, 108–109
short and long term labeling, 113–116
special cell systems, 129–139
uterus and, 138–139
transfer,
 amount of, 114
 N-formylmethionyl, 128–129
 mitochondrial, 128–129
 synthesis of, 112, 122
 turnover time, 130
Ribonucleic acid polymerase(s), nuclear, 157
Ribonucleoprotein,
 ribosomal, maturation of, 173
Ribosome(s),
 cycle of, 171–173
 embryonic development and, 29
 histone synthesis and, 162
 membrane bound, cell type and, 171–172
 proteins, 156
  turnover of, 171–174
 subunits, components of, 172
Rods,
 outer segment, renewal of, 187–190
Ruthenium red, polysaccharide staining and, 359–361, 363

S

Salicylhydrazide, mucin staining and, 338
Salivary gland,
 cell cycle phase duration in, 59
 cell turnover time in, 70
 Golgi complex, labeling of, 194
 products, 196, 197
 proline incorporation by, 247
Salmine, nature of, 159
Salt gland, phosphatidylinositol and, 313
Saponification, mucin staining and, 348
Sarcoplasmic reticulum, oleate uptake by, 284
Scanning electron microscopy, fibroblasts, 227
Schiff's reagent,
 mucins and, 337–338, 340, 341, 346, 350
 polysaccharides and, 356, 357
Scombrine, nature of, 159

Sea urchin,
  egg, histone disulfide bonds, 167
  embryos, histones of, 162
Secretory granules, renewal of, 19
Seminal vesicles, nuclear labeling in, 35–36
Sephadex, cell ligands and, 229
Serine,
  histone, 164
  phosphatidylethanolamine and, 316–317
Serine dehydrase,
  half-life, 203
  induction of, 204
Sialate,
  cell surface, 230–231
    replacement of, 232
  gangliosides and, 303
  glycoproteins and, 193, 334, 335, 340–
    341, 346, 350
  keratan sulfate and, 356
  nature of, 191
Sialidase, mucin staining and, 340, 346–
  347, 349
Sialomucopeptide,
  cell surface and, 231
  intestinal epithelium, 233–234
Skin,
  lipids, turnover of, 320
Sperm,
  deoxyribonucleic acid, constancy of, 34
  maturation time, 70
  proteins of, 159
Spermatogonia,
  cell cycle phase duration in, 58
  cell turnover time in, 68
Sphingolipid(s),
  content of membranes, 278
  distribution in tissues, 303
  nature of, 302
  turnover of, 303–304
Spindle tumor, cell cycle phase duration
  in, 59
Spleen,
  cell cycle phase duration in, 59
  cell proliferation, stimulation of, 75
  cell turnover time in, 68, 70
  histone, half-life, 163
  macrophages, age and, 89
  ribonucleic acid turnover in, 130

Staining procedures,
  mucin,
    alterations of, 346–349
    electron microscopy, 341–346
    light microscopy, 337–341
  polysaccharides,
    alterations of, 361–364
    electron microscopy, 358–361
    light microscopy, 355–357
Starvation, liver metabolism and, 205
Stearate,
  occurrence of, 279
  sphingolipids and, 303, 304
Stomach,
  cell cycle phase duration in, 58
  cell turnover time, 66, 69
  Golgi complex, labeling of, 194
  ribonucleic acid synthesis in, 111
  secretory product, 196
  synthesis and transport, 197
Stress,
  cell cycle and, 5
  deoxyribonucleic acid and, 30–32
Sturine, nature of, 159
Subcellular renewal,
  general considerations, 16–18
  macromolecules, 19–21
  minerals, electrolytes and water, 21
  organelles and, 18–19
Substratum, cell orientation and, 225–226
Sulfate,
  labeled, mucopolysaccharides and, 192,
    194, 195
  mucins and, 335, 340–341, 348, 349–350
  polysaccharide labeling by, 364–365
Sulfation, mucin staining and, 348
Sulfurous acid, mucin staining and, 338
Superior cervical ganglion, phosphatidylinositol and, 313, 314, 315–316
Synovial cells, hyaluronate synthesis by,
  365–366

                          T

Temperature, cell cycle and, 4–5
Testis, ribonucleic acid turnover in, 130
Testosterone, mitotic activity and, 6
Tetrahymena,
  cell cycle, histone synthesis and, 163
  ribonucleic acid synthesis in, 109

Tetrahymena pyriformis,
  mitochondria,
    deoxyribonucleic acid of, 127
    ribonucleic acid of, 128
Thionyl chloride, mucin staining and, 338, 349
Thorium,
  mucin electron microscopy and, 344–345, 349
  polysaccharide staining and, 358, 362, 364
Threonine, histone, 164
Thrombin, platelet lipid and, 309
Thymidine,
  tritiated,
    administration of, 63–64
    adrenal medulla and, 31
    amphibian oocytes and, 29–30
    cell cycle studies and, 14–16, 53–64
    cell turnover time and, 65–70
    deoxyribonucleic acid repair and, 37
    polytene chromosomes and, 27, 28
    seminal vesicles and, 35–36
Thymidine kinase,
  cell cycle and, 178, 180, 181
  cell differentiation and, 183
  synthesis of, 140
Thymidylate, turnover time, 177
Thymidylate kinase, cell cycle and, 181
Thymidylate phosphatase, cell differentiation and, 183
Thymidylate synthetase, cell cycle and, 181
Thymus,
  cell turnover time in, 68, 70
  histones, 160, 161
    half-life, 163
    methylation of, 164
    synthesis of, 162
Thyroglobulin,
  carbohydrate composition, 193
  labeling of, 195–196
Thyroid gland,
  deoxyribonucleic acid, constancy of, 33–34
  mitotic rate, age and, 99
  phosphatidylinositol and, 313
Thyrotropin, phosphatidylinositol and, 313
Thyroxin, mitotic activity and, 6
Tipula, oocytes of, 28–29

Tissues,
  decaying, 9
  embryonic and hyperplastic, 8
  neoplastic, 9
  slow or nonrenewing, 8–9
  steady state, 8
  transiently responsive, 9
Tissue culture cells,
  ribonucleic acid synthesis, kinetics, 109–110
Tobacco,
  cells, histone synthesis in, 162
Toluidine blue, mucins and, 339
Tomatine, cholesterol and, 295
Tongue,
  cell turnover time, 66, 69
  epithelium,
    cell cycle phase duration in, 58, 59
    stimulation of mitosis, 75
Tooth primordia,
  differentiation, heterotypic tissues and, 254–259
  extracellular matrix, ribonucleic acid in, 250–251
Toxic effects, cell cycle and, 6–7
Trachea,
  cell proliferation, stimulation of, 75
  cell turnover time, 67, 69
  Golgi complex, labeling of, 194
Transferrin,
  carbohydrate composition, 193
  synthesis and turnover, 202
Transmutation, isotopic effects and, 17–18
Triglycerides,
  biosynthesis of, 284–285, 288, 292
  composition of, 279–280
  turnover of, 320
Triturus, ribonucleic acid synthesis in, 109
Trophoblasts, cell cycle phase duration in, 58
Tropocollagen,
  fibrils and fibers, 260–264
  synthesis, epithelium and, 241
Truttine, nature of, 159
Trypsin,
  ascites cells and, 231
  surface cell and, 229, 230, 231, 232–233, 248, 252
  histones and, 161

Tryptophan pyrrolase,
  half-life, 203
  induction of, 204, 205
Tumors,
  cell cycle phase duration in, 59, 60
  mitochondrial deoxyribonucleic acid of,
    125
Tympanic membrane,
  cell proliferation, stimulation of, 75
Tyrosine transaminase,
  half-life, 203
  induction of, 204, 205

U

Ultraviolet radiation, deoxyribonucleic
  acid repair and, 37
Uranyl salts, cartilage staining and, 359
Urea,
  contact inhibition and, 227
  lens proteins and, 185
  ribosomal ribonucleic acid and, 121
Ureter, cell turnover time, 67
Ureteric buds,
  development, collagen and, 247
Uridine nucleotides, polysaccharide synthesis and, 253
Uterus,
  cell proliferation, stimulation of, 75
  cell turnover time, 67
  cervix, polysaccharides of, 358
  epithelium, cell cycle phase duration in,
    58
  ribonucleic acid synthesis, estrogen and,
    138–139, 140

V

Vagina,
  cell turnover time, 67
  epithelium, cell cycle phase duration in,
    58
Vicia faba, ribonucleic acid synthesis in,
  109

Vicinal hydroxyl method,
  mucin staining and, 337–339
  polysaccharide staining and, 355–356
Vitamin D, bone and, 378

W

Walker carcinosarcoma,
  histones, half-life, 163
Water, subcellular renewal, 21
Wilm's tumor, extracellular components,
  230
Wound repair, cell proliferation and, 9,
  74–79

X

Xenopus,
  anucleolate, ribonucleic acid synthesis
    in, 109, 112–113, 122
Xenopus laevis,
  ovary, thymidine uptake by, 29–30
Xeroderma pigmentosum, deoxyribonucleic acid repair in, 37
X-rays, cell cycle and, 11–12, 16, 53

Y

Yeast,
  histones of, 162
  mitochondria
    deoxyribonucleic acid of, 127
    ribonucleic acid of, 129
  respiratory mutants, 170
Yoshida sarcoma, cell cycle phase duration
  in, 59, 60

Z

Zymogen granules,
  phosphatidylinositol and, 312
  transport times, 177
Zymogenic cells, protein synthesis and
  transport in, 196–198